CONTEMPORARY ISSUES IN
WOMEN'S
CANCERS

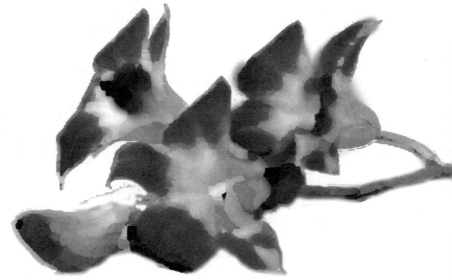

SUZANNE LOCKWOOD, PHD, RN, OCN®, CHPN

Editor

Associate Professor, Nursing
Director, Center for Oncology Education and Research
Texas Christian University

 SOCIETY OF GYNECOLOGIC
NURSE ONCOLOGISTS

JONES AND BARTLETT PUBLISHERS
Sudbury, Massachusetts
BOSTON   TORONTO   LONDON   SINGAPORE

World Headquarters

Jones and Bartlett Publishers
40 Tall Pine Drive
Sudbury, MA 01776
978-443-5000
info@jbpub.com
www.jbpub.com

Jones and Bartlett Publishers Canada
6339 Ormindale Way
Mississauga, Ontario L5V 1J2
Canada

Jones and Bartlett Publishers
International
Barb House, Barb Mews
London W6 7PA
United Kingdom

Jones and Bartlett's books and products are available through most bookstores and online booksellers. To contact Jones and Bartlett Publishers directly, call 800-832-0034, fax 978-443-8000, or visit our website www.jbpub.com.

Production Credits
Publisher: Kevin Sullivan
Acquisitions Editor: Emily Ekle
Acquisitions Editor: Amy Sibley
Associate Editor: Patricia Donnelly
Editorial Assistant: Rachel Shuster
Associate Production Editor: Sarah Bayle
Associate Marketing Manager: Ilana Goddess
Manufacturing and Inventory Control Supervisor: Amy Bacus
Composition: diacriTech, Chennai, India
Cover Design: Kristin E. Ohlin
Cover Image: © Lana Langlois/Dreamstime.com
Printing and Binding: Malloy, Inc.
Cover Printing: Malloy, Inc.

Library of Congress Cataloging-in-Publication Data
Contemporary issues in women's cancers / [edited by] Suzanne Lockwood.
    p. ; cm.
Includes bibliographical references and index.
ISBN-13: 978-0-7637-2602-7 (alk. paper)
ISBN-10: 0-7637-2602-8 (alk. paper)
   1. Cancer in women–United States. 2. Generative organs, Female–Cancer–United States. 3. Breast–Cancer–United States. 4. Women–Diseases–United States. I. Lockwood, Suzanne.
   [DNLM: 1. Genital Neoplasms, Female–United States. 2. Breast Neoplasms–United States. 3. Women's Health–United States. WP 145 C761 2009]
   RC281.W65C67 2009
   616.99′40082–dc22

2008029743

6048
Printed in the United States of America
12 11 10 09 08   10 9 8 7 6 5 4 3 2 1

Contents

Chapter 5: Nonepithelial Ovarian Malignancies **99**

Margaret M. Fields, MSN, ANP-BC, AOCNP®

Chapter 6: Preinvasive Cervical Cancer *119*

Margaret Fischer, RN, MSN, ANP-BC

Chapter 7: Invasive Cervical Cancer *133*

Connie L. Birk, RN, BSN, OCN®

Chapter 8: Vulvar and Vaginal Cancers 155

Amber Door, RN, BSN, OCN®

Chapter 9: Gynecologic Sarcomas 173

Amber Door, RN, BSN, OCN®

Chapter 10: Cancer Genetics *183*

Sheri Babb, MS, CGC

Judith A. Parham, RN, MSN

Chapter 11: Sexuality Issues *205*

Evelyn H. Larrison, RN, BSN

Chapter 14: The Sequelae of Cancer and its Treatment 245

Susan J. McIntyre, RN, MN, ANP-BC, AOCN®

Chapter 15: The Impact of Gynecologic Cancer on the Family 279

Suzanne Lockwood, PhD, RN, OCN®, CHPN

Preface

Why a textbook about contemporary issues in women's cancer? This is a question we asked ourselves when we were asked to write the preface for this book. As two of the original gyn-oncology nurses in this country, we found a relatively easy answer. In the early years of our clinical practice there were no texts written for nurses by nurses. Our knowledge was gleaned from the medical literature and later nursing texts written on cancers in general; none specifically addressed gynecologic cancer in depth. The Society of Gynecologic Nurse Oncologists (SGNO) published the first complete nursing text on women's cancers in 1997. The SGNO members wrote the previous version of this text, *Women and Cancer: A Gynecologic Oncology Nursing Perspective*, because it was recognized that there was not an in-depth text for use in clinical practice by this population of nurses. This text has detailed information on anatomy and physiology, treatment options, and symptom management of all disease sites. Due to the many years of struggle without a text, we embraced this text and thought how very fortunate the new nurses in gyn-oncology were to be able to have a comprehensive, up-to-date, ready reference to enhance their clinical practice.

The answer to the question WHY became very clear: Why not?

Recognizing that there are gaps in the scientific knowledge that underlie clinical practice and that medical and nursing practice has been changed by greater emphasis on the central role the patients play in the process, it is timely to create a text that addresses these contemporary issues. This text is conceived in the midst of healthcare system changes in the United States and changes in treatment and diagnosis of cancers that are affecting healthcare delivery to women.

Contemporary Issues in Women's Cancers addresses these new concerns in a way that will bring together cultural issues, the woman within the community, family issues, and the impact on the family and resources available to the nurses and health providers who work with women who have cancer. One can see that the focus of this text is different than the more traditional text and therefore will be a timely addition to *Women and Cancer: A Gynecologic Oncology Nursing Perspective*.

Contemporary Issues in Women's Cancers is the result of many individuals' gifts and talents. All of the contributors are members of SGNO, a nonprofit organization and dedicated group of health providers who credit their patients with enriching their lives and contributing to their professional growth. These authors give of their time and talent daily as they care for women with cancer and are committed to sharing their expertise with other health providers in the field. They represent a diverse group of clinical specialists, researchers, and educators who live in geographically expanded communities ranging all around the United States. Credit must also be given to the various authors' family members because they patiently tolerated the time taken to produce this book.

It is the goal of the authors as members of the SGNO to disseminate current knowledge with the hope that every health provider that uses this text will grow and expand in their loving care and service to their patients.

Mary Lou Cullen, RNP, MS
Dorothy C. Donahue, RN

Contributors

Marylou S. Anton, MSN, RN, OCN®
Clinical Administrative Director
University of Texas
M.D. Anderson Cancer Center
Houston, Texas

Sheri Babb, MS, CGC
Genetic Counselor
Department of Obstetrics and Gynecology
Division of Gynecologic-Oncology
Washington University School of Medicine
St. Louis, Missouri

Connie L. Birk, RN, BSN, OCN®
Oncology Nursing Manager
Gynecologic Oncology Associates
Newport Beach, California

Lynn Cloutier, RN, MSN, AOCN®, ACNP-BC
Inpatient Nurse Practitioner
Department of Gynecologic Oncology
University of Texas
M.D. Anderson Cancer Center
Houston, Texas

Mary Lou Cullen, RNP, MS
Nurse Practitioner—Retired
Pittsford, New York

Dorothy C. Donahue, RN
Retired
Southampton, New York

Amber Door, RN, BSN, OCN®
Gynecologic Nurse Oncologist
Gynecologic Oncology of West Michigan
Grand Rapids, Michigan

Margaret M. Fields, MSN, ANP-BC, AOCNP®
University of Texas
M.D. Anderson Cancer Center
Houston, Texas

Margaret Fischer, RN, MSN, ANP-BC
Nurse Practitioner
Stony Brook University Medical Center
Stony Brook, New York

Sheryl Redlin Frazier, RN, BSN, OCN®
Clinical Learning Consultant
Nursing Education and Development
Vanderbilt University Medical Center
Nashville, Tennessee

Wendy Holt, RN, BSN, OCN®
Oncology Research Nurse
St. Vincent's Medical Center
Jacksonville, Florida

Evelyn H. Larrison, RN, BSN
Gynecologic Oncology Nurse Consultant
DeForest, Wisconsin

Carol Larson, RN, MSN
Manager of Oncology Services
Sutter Medical Center of Santa Rosa
Santa Rosa, California

Suzanne Lockwood, PhD, RN, OCN®, CHPN
Associate Professor, Nursing and Director, Center
    for Oncology Education and Research
Texas Christian University
Fort Worth, Texas

Susan J. McIntyre, RN, BSN, MN,
    ANP-BC, AOCN®
Nurse Practitioner
Minnesota Oncology Hematology
St. Paul, Minnesota

Judith A. Parham, RN, MSN
Clinical Coordinator
Barnes Hospital
St. Louis, Missouri

Barbara C. Poniatowski, MS, RN-BC, AOCN®
Senior Clinical Educator
GlaxoSmithKline Pharmaceuticals
Lutherville, Maryland

Lois Anaya Winkelman, MS, RN, AOCN®
Rush University Medical Center Department
    OB/GYN
Section of Gynecologic Oncology
Chicago, Illinois

Chrisann Accario Winslow, RN, MSN, AOCN®
Clinical Nurse Specialist/Research Coordinator
Division of Gynecologic Oncology
Washington University School of Medicine
St. Louis, Missouri

Chapter 1

Overview and Epidemiology

Chrisann Accario Winslow, RN, MSN, AOCN®

Introduction

In 2008, an estimated 1,437,180 people in the United States will be diagnosed with cancer, and 565,650 will die of cancer. An estimated 244,210 new cases of cancer will be attributed to breast and gynecological malignancies in women. An estimated 97,460 women will die of breast and gynecological malignancies.[1] Estimates of premature deaths that could have been avoided through cancer screening vary from 3% to 35% depending on a variety of assumptions. The aim of this chapter is to focus on the epidemiological factors associated with breast and gynecological malignancies, as well as screening and prevention strategies.

Breast Cancer

With 182,460 cases expected, invasive breast cancer will be the most frequently diagnosed nonskin malignancy in 2008 for women in the United States.[1] In the same year, breast cancer will kill approximately 40,480 women, second only to lung cancer as a cause of cancer mortality in women.[1] From 2001–2005, the median age at diagnosis for cancer of the breast was

61 years of age. Approximately 0.0% were diagnosed under age 20; 1.9% between 20 and 34; 10.6% between 35 and 44; 22.4% between 45 and 54; 23.3% between 55 and 64; 19.8% between 65 and 74; 16.5% between 75 and 84; and 5.5% at 85+ years of age. Despite a prior long-term trend of gradually increasing breast cancer incidence, data from the Surveillance, Epidemiology, and End Results Program shows a decrease from 1990 to 2002 in breast cancer mortality of 2.3% per year.[2] From 2001–2005, the median age at death for cancer of the breast was 69 years of age. Approximately 0.0% died under age 20; 1.0% between 20 and 34; 6.4% between 35 and 44; 15.3% between 45 and 54; 19.6% between 55 and 64; 20.1% between 65 and 74; 22.9% between 75 and 84; and 14.7% at 85+ years of age.

In addition to invasive breast cancer, 67,770 new cases of in situ breast cancer are expected to occur among women in 2008. Approximately 85% will be ductal carcinoma in situ (DCIS), a result of increased use of screening with mammography.[1]

The overall 5-year relative survival rate for 1996–2004 was 88.7%. Five-year relative survival rates by race were: 89.9% for white women; 77.1% for black women. Sixty-one percent of breast cancer cases are diagnosed while the cancer is still confined to the primary site (localized stage); 31% are diagnosed after the cancer has spread to regional lymph nodes or directly beyond the primary site; 6% are diagnosed after the cancer has already metastasized (distant stage); and for the remaining 2% the staging information was unknown. The corresponding 5-year survival rates were: 98.1% for localized; 83.8% for regional; 27.1% for distant; and 56.9% for unstaged.[2]

Etiology

Breast cancer generally develops with a series of genetic changes that contribute to the dynamic process known as carcinogenesis.[3] An accumulation of genetic changes is thought to correspond to the phenotypic changes associated with the evolution of malignancy. The carcinogenesis sequence is a series of histological changes, starting with tissue of normal appearance, followed by changes that lead to hyperplasia and dysplasia, of which the most severe forms are difficult to distinguish from carcinoma in situ.[4]

Risk Factors

Identified risk factors for breast cancer include age, reproductive and menstrual history, hormonal influences, radiation exposure, lifestyle factors, benign breast disease, and a history of familial risk. Cumulative risk of breast cancer increases with age, with most breast cancers occurring after age 50 years.[5] Breast cancer tends to occur at an earlier age in women with a genetic susceptibility than in sporadic cases. In cancer-prone families, the mean age of breast cancer diagnosis among women carrying BRCA1 or BRCA2 mutations is in the 40s.[6] Using the Claus model,

a statistical model based on data from the Cancer and Steroid Hormone Study, estimates of risk suggest an earlier age of onset in women who have a mother or sister affected with breast cancer at an early age.[7]

Many of the risk factors for breast cancer, including age at menarche, first birth, and menopause, suggest hormonal influences for the development of the disease. Estrogen and progestin cause growth and proliferation of breast cells that may work through growth factors such as transforming growth factor (TGF)-alpha.[8] Women who develop breast cancer tend to have higher endogenous estrogen and androgen levels.[9] Following ovarian ablation, breast cancer risk may be reduced as much as 75% depending on age, weight, and parity, with the greatest reduction for young, thin, nulliparous women.[10–13] The removal of one ovary also reduces the risk of breast cancer, but to a lesser degree than the removal of both.[14]

Other hormonal changes also influence breast cancer risk. Childbirth is followed by a transient increase in risk and then a long-term reduction in risk, which is greater for younger women.[13,15,16] In one study, women who experienced a first full-term pregnancy before 20 years of age were half as likely to develop breast cancer as nulliparous women or women who underwent a first full-term pregnancy at 35 years or older.[17] Age at menarche also affects breast cancer risk. Women who experienced menarche at 11 years or younger have about a 20% greater chance of developing breast cancer than women who experienced menarche at 14 years or older.[18] Women with late menopause also experience increased risk. Reproductive risk factors may interact with more predisposing genotypes. In the Nurses' Health Study[6] the associations between age at first birth, menarche, and menopause and the development of breast cancer were observed only among women without a family history of breast cancer in a mother or sister. Breastfeeding is associated with a decreased risk of breast cancer.[7,8]

The use of oral contraceptives may slightly increase the risk of breast cancer among long-term users, but this appears to be a short-term effect. A meta-analysis of data from 54 studies noted a relative risk (RR) of 1.24 (95% confidence interval [CI], 1.15–1.33) for current users; however, 10 or more years after stopping no difference was seen.[19] Further, the cancers diagnosed in women who had ever used hormonal contraceptives were less advanced than those in nonusers, raising the possibility that the small excess among users was due to increased detection. Breast cancer risk associated with hormonal contraceptive use did not appear to vary with family history of breast cancer.[19]

Data exist from both observational and randomized clinical trials regarding the association between postmenopausal hormone replacement therapy (HRT) and breast cancer. A meta-analysis of data from 51 observational studies indicated a relative risk of breast cancer of 1.35 (95% CI, 1.21–1.49) for women who had used HRT for 5 or more years after menopause.[20] Another observational study, published after the meta-analysis, also observed a significant increased risk for long-term use in a nested case-control study from Puget Sound.[21]

The Women's Health Initiative (WHI), a randomized controlled trial of 160,000 postmenopausal women, investigated the risks and benefits of strategies that may reduce the incidence of heart disease, breast and colorectal cancer, and fractures, including dietary interventions and two trials of hormone therapy. The estrogen-plus-progestin arm of the study,

which randomized more than 16,000 women to receive combined hormone therapy or placebo, was halted early because health risks exceeded benefits.[15,16] One of the adverse outcomes prompting closure was a significant increase in both total (245 versus 185 cases) and invasive (199 versus 150 cases) breast cancers (RR = 1.24; 95% CI, 1.02–1.5, P <0.001) in women randomized to receive estrogen and progestin.[22] HRT-related breast cancers had adverse prognostic characteristics (more advanced stages and larger tumors) compared with cancers occurring in the placebo group, and HRT was also associated with a substantial increase in abnormal mammograms.[23]

Breast cancer incidence is greatly influenced by HRT use. After the 2002 WHI publication of the negative cardiovascular effect of HRT, HRT use in the United States dropped dramatically. With this decrease in HRT use, breast cancer incidence dropped by as much as 15% among postmenopausal women. The drop was observed in estrogen receptor–positive (ER+) disease.[24–26]

The association between HRT and breast cancer risk among women with a family history of breast cancer has not been consistent; some studies suggest risk is particularly elevated among women with a family history, while others have not found evidence for an interaction between these factors.[22,27–32]

Observations in survivors of the atomic bombings of Hiroshima and Nagasaki and in women who have received therapeutic radiation treatments to the chest and upper body document increased breast cancer risk as a result of radiation exposure.[33]

Several lifestyle factors are associated with breast cancer risk. These lifestyle factors include weight gain, obesity, fat intake, and level of physical activity. There is consistent evidence that increased body weight and weight gain during adulthood are associated with increased risk for breast cancer among postmenopausal (but not premenopausal) women.[34,35] This increased risk is likely due to the higher levels of estrogen produced by extra adipose tissue after menopause; the adverse effect of weight gain is not seen as readily among women taking postmenopausal hormone therapy (hormone replacement therapy) because it may be masked by higher levels of exogenous estrogens.

The Women's Health Initiative Observational Study observed 85,917 women aged 50 to 79 years and collected information on weight history as well as known risk factors for breast cancer. Height, weight, and waist and hip circumferences were measured. With a median follow-up of 34.8 months, 1030 developed invasive breast cancer. Among women who never used hormone replacement therapy/hormone therapy (HRT/HT), increased breast cancer risk was associated with weight at entry, body mass index (BMI) at entry, BMI at age 50, maximum BMI, adult and postmenopausal weight change, and waist and hip circumference. Weight was the strongest predictor, with a RR of 2.85 (95% CI, 1.81–4.49) for women weighing more than 82.2 kg, compared with those weighing less than 58.7 kg.[36]

Alcohol intake is also associated with an increase in risk.[37,38] particularly for women whose intake of folate is low. Many epidemiologic studies have shown an increased risk of breast cancer associated with alcohol consumption. Individual data from 53 case-control and cohort studies were included in a British meta-analysis. Compared with women who reported no alcohol consumption, the RR of breast cancer was 1.32 (95% CI, 1.19–1.45;

P <0.00001) for women consuming 35 to 44 g/day, and it was 1.46 (95% CI, 1.33–1.61; P <0.00001) for those consuming 45+ g/d. The RR of breast cancer increases by about 7% (95% CI, 5.5–8.7%; P <0.00001) for each 10 g (1 drink) per day. The same result was obtained, even after additional stratification for race, education, family history, age of menarche, height, weight, BMI, breastfeeding, oral contraceptive use, menopausal hormone use, and type and age of menopause.[39]

Another risk factor for developing breast cancer is benign breast disease (BBD).[39] The risk of developing breast cancer varies by the result of the breast biopsy (i.e., type of benign breast disease). The risk among women with atypical hyperplasia is 2.5 to 5.3 times that among women with nonproliferative BBD. Women who have proliferative disease without atypia are at a 1.6-fold to 1.9-fold risk.[40–42] Even among women with fibroadenomas who have no evidence of proliferative disease, breast cancer risk is increased 40% to 90% over an average of 22 years of follow-up.[43]

An increased risk of breast cancer has also been demonstrated for women who have increased density of breast tissue as assessed by mammogram.[39,40] This increased risk occurs in both premenopausal and postmenopausal women.[44] Compared with women with no visible breast density, a breast density of 75% or greater is associated with an approximately 5-fold increase in risk (95% CI, 3.6–7.1).[45] Some observational studies suggest the possibility of a genetic contribution to breast density.[46–48]

Women with a previous primary breast cancer have a 3-fold to 4-fold increase in risk of a second breast cancer in the contralateral breast.[49] Most studies report an annual risk of development of a second breast cancer of 0.5%

to 0.7%.[50] While the risk of contralateral breast cancer persists for up to 30 years after the original diagnosis, the median interval between primary breast cancer and contralateral disease is approximately 4 years.[51]

Although risk is similar following invasive and in situ ductal cancer, it is higher for women with a family history of breast cancer and for those with a lobular histology in the original cancer.[52] Lobular carcinoma in situ (LCIS), which is often an incidental finding in breast biopsies, is associated with an increased risk of subsequent invasive cancer. Long-term follow-up studies of women diagnosed with LCIS report relative risks of developing breast cancer ranging from 7 to 12. Risks are higher for women diagnosed at a younger age and for those with a family history of breast cancer. Subsequent breast cancers are most often of ductal histology and occur equally in either breast, suggesting that LCIS is a marker of risk rather than a precancerous lesion itself.[53]

In cross-sectional studies of adult populations, 5% to 10% of women have a mother or sister with breast cancer, and about 20% have either a first-degree relative or a second-degree relative with breast cancer.[54–57] In a pooled analysis of 38 studies, the relative risk of breast cancer conferred by a first-degree relative with breast cancer was 2.1 (95% CI, 2.0–2.2).[58] The level of risk varies with the age at which the affected relative was diagnosed: The younger the affected relative, the greater the risk posed to relatives.[54,55,57,58,60] This effect was noted to be strongest for women younger than 50 years who had a first-degree relative affected before age 50 years (RR = 3.3; 95% CI, 2.8–3.9).[58]

The number of affected relatives and the closeness of their biologic relationship are also important factors that must be taken into account.[55,56,58] The greater the number of affected relatives and the closer the biologic relationship, the greater the risk.[55,56,58] The number of female relatives in the family influences both the utility of the family history as a risk assessment tool and the significance of the family history. In families with few women, it may be difficult to identify a genetic susceptibility to breast or other female cancers. If a family has many female members, the proportion of affected relatives may be a more important indicator of risk than the number of affected relatives.

Studies of family history of ovarian cancer suggest an association with breast cancer risk. A first-degree relative with ovarian cancer confers a modest risk of breast cancer. The odds ratio (OR) derived from a case-control study based on the Utah Cancer Registry was 1.27 (95% CI, 0.91–1.77),[61] and other studies have found no evidence of increased risk.[59,62] The presence of both breast and ovarian cancer in a family increases the likelihood that a cancer-predisposing mutation is present.[63,64]

Screening

There are several different screening guidelines in place to screen women for breast cancer, including those published by the American Cancer Society (ACS), the National Cancer Institute (NCI), and the American College of Obstetrics and Gynecology (ACOG).

The 2008 ACS guidelines for the early detection of breast cancer in average-risk women emphasizes that for an average-risk woman, screening should begin at 20 years of age. Screening should consist of a combination of clinical breast examination every 3 years and annually after age 40, counseling to raise awareness of breast symptoms at health examinations, and regular mammography beginning at age 40.[65]

During discussions at health examinations, healthcare professionals can play a key role in raising awareness about the importance of recognizing symptoms of breast cancer and developing a heightened awareness about breast changes. Although the ACS no longer recommends that all women conduct regular breast self-examination (BSE), women should be informed about the potential benefits, limitations, and harms associated with BSE. Women may then choose to do BSE regularly, occasionally, or not at all. If a woman chooses to perform periodic BSE, she can receive instructions in the technique and/or have her performance reviewed.

When updated in 2008, the guidelines placed a strong emphasis on the healthcare professional's role in raising and regularly reinforcing awareness about breast cancer, early breast cancer detection, the importance of prompt reporting of any new symptoms, and most important, regular screening with mammography after age 40 years.[66] There is no set age at which mammography screening should be discontinued. Rather, the ACS recommends that the decision to stop mammography screening should be individualized, considering the potential benefits and risks of screening in the context of overall health status and anticipated longevity. As long as a woman is in good health and would be a candidate for breast cancer treatment, she should continue to be screened with mammography.[1]

Women at high risk (greater than 20% lifetime risk) should get an MRI and a mammogram every year. Women at moderately increased risk (15% to 20% lifetime risk) should talk with their doctors about the benefits and limitations of adding MRI screening to their yearly mammogram. Yearly MRI screening is not recommended for women whose lifetime risk of breast cancer is less than 15%.[66]

NCI recommends that women in their 40s should be screened every 1 to 2 years with mammography. Women aged 50 and older should be screened every 1 to 2 years with mammography. Women who are at higher-than-average risk of breast cancer should seek expert medical advice about whether they should begin screening before age 40 and the frequency of screening.[65]

ACOG recommends that women aged 40–49 years should have screening mammography every 1 to 2 years. Women aged 50 years and older should have annual screening mammography. Upon expert opinion, they also recommend that, despite a lack of definitive data for or against breast self-examination, breast self-examination has the potential to detect palpable breast cancer and can be recommended. All women should have clinical breast examinations annually as part of the physical examination.[67]

For women who carry BRCA1 or BRCA2 gene mutations, some cancer experts recommend annual or semi-annual clinical breast exams, along with annual mammography beginning at age 25-35 years.[67]

Prevention

There are several factors associated with reducing the risk of breast cancer by intervening in those behaviors that reduce risk. A low-fat diet might influence breast cancer risk through hormonal mechanisms. Ecologic studies show a positive correlation between international age-adjusted breast cancer mortality rates and the estimated per capita consumption of dietary fat.[68] A randomized controlled dietary modification study was undertaken among 48,835 postmenopausal women aged 50 to 79 years who were also enrolled in the Women's Health Initiative. The intervention promoted a goal of reducing total fat intake by 20%, using five servings per day of vegetables and fruit and six servings per day of grains. The intervention group accomplished a reduction of fat intake of approximately 10% over the 8.1 years' follow-up and was found to have lower estradiol and lower γ-tocopherol levels but no weight loss. The incidence of invasive breast cancer was slightly lower in the intervention group, with HR 0.91 (95% CI, 0.83–1.01).[69]

Fruit and vegetable consumption may be associated with reduced breast cancer risk.[70] Micronutrient intake may also play a role. Case-control studies show an inverse association between dietary beta-carotene intake and breast cancer risk. High intake of foods containing foliate, beta-carotene, and vitamins A and C may also reverse the increased risk associated with alcohol use.[71]

A vitamin analogue fenretinide has been shown to reduce breast carcinogenesis in preclinical studies.[72] A phase III Italian trial compared the efficacy of a 5-year intervention with fenretinide versus no treatment in 2972 women, aged 30 to 70 years, with surgically removed stage I breast cancer or DCIS. At a median observation time of 97 months, there were no statistically significant differences in the occurrence of contralateral breast cancer (P = 0.642), ipsilateral breast cancer (P = 0.177), incidence of distant metastases, nonbreast malignancies, and all-cause mortality.[73]

Active exercise may reduce breast cancer risk, particularly in young parous women.[74] There are numerous observational studies that have examined the relationship between physical activity and breast cancer risk.[75] Most of these studies have shown an inverse relationship between level of physical activity and breast cancer incidence. The average relative risk reduction is 30% to 40%. However, it is not known if or to what degree the observed association is due to confounding variables, such as diet or a genetic predisposition to breast cancer. A prospective study of over 25,000 women in Norway suggests that doing heavy manual labor or exercising 4 or more hours per week is associated with a decrease in breast cancer risk. This decrease is more pronounced in premenopausal women and in women of normal or less than normal body weight.[76]

Most breast cancer prevention research is based on evidence linking the development of this disease, in many cases, with exposure to the hormone estrogen. The focus of several recent breast cancer prevention studies has been on testing the effectiveness of drugs called selective estrogen receptor modulators (SERMs). SERMs are drugs that have some antiestrogen properties and some estrogen-like properties. Their antiestrogen activity may help reduce the risk of breast cancer by blocking the effects of estrogen on breast tissue. Their estrogen-like properties may help prevent the loss of bone density in postmenopausal women; however, SERMs may cause bone loss in premenopausal women.[77]

The Breast Cancer Prevention Trial (BCPT) was funded by NCI and conducted by the National Surgical Adjuvant Breast and Bowel Project (NSABP). The BCPT was designed to see whether tamoxifen, a SERM, can prevent breast cancer in women who are at an increased risk of developing this disease. The study began recruiting participants in April 1992 and closed enrollment in September 1997. This study involved 13,388 premenopausal and postmenopausal women. The data demonstrated 49% fewer diagnoses of invasive breast cancer in women who were randomized to take tamoxifen compared with women who were randomized to take a placebo. Women on tamoxifen also had 49% fewer diagnoses of noninvasive breast tumors.[77]

The National Surgical Adjuvant Breast and Bowel Project Study of Tamoxifen and Raloxifene (STAR) trial, a prospective, double-blind, randomized clinical trial conducted beginning July 1, 1999, initiated its final analysis after at least 327 invasive breast cancers were diagnosed. Patients were 19,747 postmenopausal women with a mean age of 58.5 years with increased 5-year breast cancer risk (mean risk, 4.03% [Standard Deviation (SD), 2.17%]). There were 163 cases of invasive breast cancer in women assigned to tamoxifen and 168 in those assigned to raloxifene (incidence, 4.30 per 1000 versus 4.41 per 1000; risk ratio [RR], 1.02; 95% confidence interval [CI], 0.82–1.28). There were fewer cases of noninvasive breast cancer in the tamoxifen group (57 cases) than in the raloxifene group (80 cases; incidence, 1.51 versus 2.11 per 1000; RR, 1.40; 95% CI, 0.98–2.00). There were 36 cases of uterine cancer with tamoxifen and 23 with raloxifene (RR, 0.62; 95% CI, 0.35–1.08). No differences were found for other invasive cancer sites, for ischemic heart disease events, or for stroke. Thromboembolic events occurred less often in the raloxifene group (RR, 0.70; 95% CI, 0.54–0.91). The number of osteoporotic fractures in the groups was similar. There were fewer cataracts (RR, 0.79; 95% CI, 0.68–0.92) and cataract surgeries (RR, 0.82; 95% CI, 0.68–0.99) in the women taking raloxifene. There was no difference in the total number of deaths (101 versus 96 for tamoxifen versus raloxifene) or in causes of death.[78]

Most breast cancer prevention trials involve women at increased risk of developing this disease. For example, it is clear that breast cancer occurs more often in women over age 60. Other factors associated with increased risk include a personal or family history of breast cancer and changes in certain genes, such as BRCA1 and BRCA2. Scientists at the NCI and the NSABP have developed a computer program (on CD-ROM) called the Breast Cancer Risk Assessment Tool. This tool can help women and their healthcare providers estimate a woman's chances of developing breast cancer based on several recognized risk factors. The Breast Cancer Risk Assessment Tool also provides information on tamoxifen.[79]

Doctors generally suggest that high-risk women be closely monitored and have regular medical checkups so that, if breast cancer develops, it is likely to be detected at an early stage.[80] These women may also consider participating in prevention studies, taking tamoxifen, or undergoing preventive surgery to reduce breast cancer risk. Preventive mastectomy is surgery to remove one or both breasts in an effort to prevent or reduce the risk of breast cancer.[81] Existing data suggest that preventive mastectomy may significantly reduce (by about 90%) the chance of developing breast cancer in moderate- and high-risk women.[82] Other data suggest that preventive oophorectomy (surgery to remove the ovaries of women at high risk of ovarian cancer because of BRCA1 or BRCA2 gene mutations) may reduce the risk of breast cancer by about 50%.[83]

The decision to join a study, take tamoxifen, or undergo preventive surgery is an individual one. With any medical procedure or intervention, both the benefits and the risks of the therapy must be considered. The balance of these factors will vary, depending on a woman's personal and family health history and how she weighs the benefits and risks.

Ovarian Cancer

Ovarian cancer is the fifth leading cause of cancer death among US women and has the highest mortality rate of all gynecologic cancers.[66] It is projected that 21,650 new cases of ovarian cancer will be diagnosed in the United States in 2008, and 15,520 women will die of this disease.[66] The incidence of epithelial ovarian cancer is age related, being generally a disease of postmenopausal women. Incidence increases after age 40 and peaks between 80 and 84 years of age. From 2001–2005, the median age at death for cancer of the ovary was 71 years of age. Approximately 0.1% died under age 20; 0.8% between 20 and 34; 3.1% between 35 and 44; 11.3% between 45 and 54; 19.2% between 55 and 64; 24.7% between 65 and 74; 28.4% between 75 and 84; and 12.4% at 85+ years of age. Nineteen percent of ovarian cancer cases are diagnosed while the cancer is still confined to the primary site (localized stage); 7% are diagnosed after the cancer has spread to regional lymph nodes or directly beyond the primary site; 67% are diagnosed after the cancer has already metastasized (distant stage); and for the remaining 7% the staging information was unknown. The corresponding 5-year relative survival rates were: 92.7% for localized; 71.1% for regional; 30.6% for distant; and 26.0% for unstaged.

Ovarian cancer survival is largely dependent upon the extent of disease at diagnosis.[3] The overall 5-year relative survival rate for 1996–2004 was 45.5%. Five-year relative survival rates by race were: 45.3% for white women and 38.4% for black women. The overall incidence of survival varies by age. Women who are younger than 65 years of age are more likely to survive 5 years (56%) following diagnosis than women aged 65 years or older (29%).[66] Based on rates from 2003–2005, 1.39% of women will be diagnosed with cancer of the ovary at some time during their lifetime. This number can also be expressed as 1 in 72 women will be diagnosed with cancer of the ovary during their lifetime.[3]

With improved therapies for ovarian cancer, 5-year overall survival may not represent a cure, and 10-year survival or disease-free survival may be a more meaningful endpoint. There are a significant number of women who are surviving with disease at 5 years who will probably die of their disease before reaching the point of 10 years after diagnosis.

Etiology

The pathogenesis of ovarian carcinoma remains unclear. Several theories have been proposed to explain the epidemiology of ovarian cancer. Fathalla's theory of "incessant ovulation" suggests that repeated ovulation traumatizes the ovarian epithelium, increasing the likelihood of errors occurring during DNA repair and the exposure of the epithelial cells to the estrogen-rich follicular fluid that is present during ovulation, thereby making the ovarian cells more susceptible to malignant change.[84]

The decreased risk of ovarian cancer associated with multiparity, pregnancy, lactation, and the oral contraceptive pill support Fathalla's theory and suggest that preventing ovulation can protect against ovarian cancer.[85] Persistent elevation of gonadotropins has also been proposed as an underlying mechanism leading to ovarian cancer.[86] The ovarian epithelium repeatedly invaginates throughout life to form clefts and inclusion cysts, leading to a theory that under excessive stimulation by gonadotropins (FSH and LH) and estrogen and its precursors, the ovarian epithelium may undergo malignant transformation. This theory would explain the decreased risk of ovarian cancer associated with pregnancy and oral contraceptive use. Another theory is that factors associated with excess androgenic stimulation of ovarian epithelial cells may be decreased by factors related to greater progesterone stimulation.[87] This third theory is supported by the findings that higher levels of androstenedione and dehydroepiandrosterone (DHEA) were associated with an increased risk of ovarian cancer and that an increased risk was also seen among women with polycystic ovary (PCO) syndrome.[88]

Risk Factors

The major risk factors for ovarian cancer are either reproductive or genetic. Reproductive factors include parity and oral contraceptive use. Women with a history of pregnancy have a 30%–60% reduction in the risk of developing ovarian cancer compared with nulliparous women. Three or more pregnancies can reduce the relative risk from 1.0 to 0.35–0.76. The use of combined estrogen and progesterone oral contraceptives reduces the risk of developing epithelial ovarian cancer by 30%–60%, with the greatest reduction in risk occurring in women with a history of oral contraceptive use for 5 or more years.[89,90]

In a prospective study of 329 ovarian cancer cases in the Breast Cancer Detection Demonstration Project, use of estrogen only was associated with a significant 60%

increased risk of ovarian cancer, and the risk increased with increasing duration of use.[91] In the WHI, 38 incident ovarian cancers were identified, and the hazard ratio for those taking estrogen plus progestin was 1.6 (95% CI, 0.8–3.2) compared with the placebo group.[92] Risk may also be increased among women who have used fertility drugs, especially those who remain nulligravid.[93] A small subset from a large retrospective cohort study did not confirm a strong link between infertility drugs and ovarian cancer risk.[94]

The single greatest ovarian cancer risk factor is a family history of the disease. Genetic factors in the development of ovarian cancer may result in a hereditary predisposition to ovarian carcinoma. Approximately 10% of ovarian cancer is hereditary, with the breast and ovarian cancer genes BRCA1 and BRCA2 accounting for the majority of that predisposition. A small percentage of the increased genetic risk appears to be related to the increased risk (10%–13% lifetime risk) in female members of the nonpolyposis colorectal cancer (Lynch II) syndrome.[95]

The lifetime risk of ovarian cancer in women with BRCA mutations is 28%–40%.[96] The incidence of BRCA mutations is quite high in Ashkenazi Jewish patients, and it has been estimated that the probability of finding a BRCA mutation in an Ashkenazi Jewish woman with ovarian or peritoneal cancer is approximately 40%.[97] Ovarian cancers arising in women with BRCA mutations are usually serous carcinomas and occur at a younger age. The median age for the diagnosis of ovarian cancer in patients with BRCA mutations is 48 years.[98] Some investigators have reported improved survival in BRCA mutation carriers, compared with non-BRCA mutation patients.[99] Three studies have shown a significant reduction in the risk of developing ovarian cancer if BRCA mutation carriers undergo prophylactic oophorectomy. There is also concern that women who have a BRCA mutation might develop a primary peritoneal carcinoma. In a recent study by Levine et al., BRCA mutation carriers had an 11.3-fold relative risk of developing carcinomas of the fallopian tube and a 37.7-fold relative risk of developing peritoneal cancer, compared with controls. However, the absolute incidence was only 0.6% for fallopian tube cancer and 1.3% for primary peritoneal cancer.[100]

The risk of acquiring ovarian cancer increases as a woman gets older. Before age 30 years, the risk of developing ovarian cancer is remote, even in hereditary cancer families; epithelial ovarian cancer is virtually nonexistent before age 20 years. Ovarian cancer incidence rises in a linear fashion from age 30 years to age 50 years and continues to increase, though at a slower rate, thereafter. The highest incidence is found in the eighth decade of life, with a rate of 57 cases per 100,000 women aged 75 to 79 years, compared with 16 cases per 100,000 women aged 40 to 44 years.[101]

Ovarian cancer incidence varies significantly depending on country of birth and ranges from a high of 14.9 cases per 100,000 women in Sweden to a low of 2.7 cases per 100,000 women in Japan.[102] Incidence in the United States is 13.3 cases per 100,000 women. Immigration appears to alter the risk to match that of the host country. Offspring of Japanese immigrants to the United States have an increased risk of developing ovarian cancer that approaches the rate among women born in the United States, indicating a possible role for dietary and environmental factors.

A woman's reproductive surgical history also may be an identifiable risk factor. Bilateral tubal ligation and hysterectomy have also been reported to be associated with reduced ovarian cancer risk.[103] A retrospective study and a prospective study have reported a > 90% reduction in risk of ovarian cancer in women with documented BRCA1 or BRCA2 mutations who chose prophylactic (risk-reducing) oophorectomy. In this same population, prophylactic removal of the ovaries also resulted in a nearly 50% reduction in the risk of subsequent breast cancer.[103]

Talc exposure is a controversial risk factor. An analysis of six case-control studies of talc and ovarian cancer found a statistically significant increase in risk (OR = 1.3; 95% CI, 1.1–1.6). A cohort study among nurses did not observe a risk of ovarian cancer associated with perineal talc use (RR = 1.09; 95% CI = 0.86–1.370).[104] Obesity has been associated with an increased mortality from ovarian cancer.[105] In cohort studies, height and body mass index, including high body mass index during adolescence, were associated with an increased risk of ovarian cancer, suggesting a role for diet and nutrition during the adolescent period.[106,107]

Associations with specific dietary factors and ovarian cancer are not consistent among case-control or cohort studies. Other case-control studies have shown a relationship between the consumption of milk, a primary source of dietary fat and lactose (a component of milk), and an increased risk for the development of ovarian cancer.[108,109] Another study, however, did not observe an association between consumption of lactose or free galactose and the risk of ovarian cancer.[110] A significant dose-response relationship between the intake of fat from animal sources and the risk of developing ovarian cancer has been reported.[111] A population-based case-control study observed an increased risk of ovarian cancer associated with saturated fat consumption and a decreased risk associated with vegetable fiber consumption.[112]

The association between serum cholesterol levels and the risk of ovarian cancer has been examined prospectively in two studies, but findings are inconsistent.[113,114] One study observed an increased risk with increasing cholesterol levels, but no association was observed in another study.[113,114] The Iowa Women's Study did not observe an association between dietary fat intake and ovarian cancer, but lactose and cholesterol were associated with a moderately increased risk.[115] Total vegetable intake, especially green leafy vegetables, was associated with a lower risk of ovarian cancer.[115]

The Nurses' Health Study did not observe an association between antioxidant nutrients from diet or supplements and ovarian cancer.[116] Higher levels of consumption of fruits and vegetables (more than 2.5 servings per day) during adolescence were associated with a decreased risk of ovarian cancer.[116] A protective association was also observed between serum selenium levels and the risk of ovarian cancer.[113] This finding differs from a report by the Nurses' Health Study, which failed to find an association between serum selenium levels and ovarian cancer.[116] Because of the small number of prospective studies and inconsistencies among case-control studies, these findings should be replicated.

Screening

Potential screening tests for ovarian cancer include vaginal ultrasound and the CA 125 antigen as a tumor marker. Bimanual pelvic examination as part of the routine pelvic examination plays a pivotal role in early detection.

The sensitivity and specificity of the pelvic examination are not characterized, but examination generally detects advanced disease.[117,118] Transvaginal ultrasonography (TVU) has been proposed as a screening method for ovarian cancer because of its ability to reliably measure ovarian size and detect small masses.[119] The benefit of ultrasonography for the early detection of ovarian cancer and reduction in mortality has not been evaluated in controlled studies.

The Prostate, Lung, Colorectal, and Ovarian (PLCO) cancer screening trial is an ongoing randomized clinical trial in the followup phase evaluating the efficacy of annual TVU in combination with CA 125 tests to reduce ovarian cancer mortality. An estimate of the false-positive rate associated with screening women aged 55 to 74 years is available from the baseline (prevalent) screening examination of women who participated in the PLCO trial and were randomized to be screened with TVU and serum CA 125 concentrations.[120] Among the 39,115 women randomized to the screening arm, at the initial TVU 1338 (4.7%) had an abnormal TVU examination; 1.9% of examinations were considered to be inadequate. The following TVU results were classified as abnormal (positive): "ovarian volume > 10 cm^3; cyst volume > 10 cm^3; any solid area or papillary projection extending into the cavity of a cystic ovarian tumor of any size; or any mixed (solid/cystic) component within a cystic ovarian tumor."[120]

Among women having both the TVU and CA 125 tests (28,506), 1703 had an abnormal result on at least one test; only 34 were abnormal on both screening tests. About 15% of women with at least one abnormal test did not undergo further evaluation. Of the 29 malignant neoplasms detected by follow-up procedures, 22 had an abnormal TVU. Nine of the neoplasms were of low malignant potential. Of the 21 invasive malignancies diagnosed, only two were stage I. Among women with an abnormal ultrasound, the number of surgeries performed per invasive cancer diagnoses was 41.2. The positive predictive value (PPV) for an abnormal TVU was 1%. This study provides a good assessment of the expected PPV for general population screening, compared with programs selectively screening high-risk groups where the PPV will be higher due to a higher prevalence of ovarian cancer.

CA 125 is a tumor-associated antigen that is used clinically to monitor patients with epithelial ovarian carcinomas.[121,122] The measurement of CA 125 levels, in combination with transvaginal ultrasonography, is the ovarian screening intervention being evaluated in the PLCO trial.[120,123,124] The most commonly reported CA 125 reference value that designates a positive screening test is 35 U/mL, and this was the reference value used in the PLCO trial to define an abnormal test result. Elevated CA 125 levels are not specific to ovarian cancer and have been observed in patients with nongynecological cancers and in the presence of certain other conditions, such as the first trimester of pregnancy or endometriosis.[122,125,126] Therefore its use as a general screening tool is not recommended or cost efficient.

The sensitivity of CA 125 for the detection of ovarian cancer was estimated in two nested case-control studies using serum banks.[128,129] The sensitivity for CA 125 levels of greater than or equal to 35 U/mL ranged from 20% to 57% for cases occurring within the first 3 years of follow-up; the specificity was 95%. Baseline (prevalent) screening from the PLCO trial obtained CA 125 measures on 28,803 (84.2%)

of women randomized to the screened arm.[130] Of these women, 402 (1.4%) had an abnormal level (CA 125 > 35 U/mL); 34 of these also had an abnormal TVU. Sixteen (55%) of the 29 women with ovarian cancer diagnosed had an abnormal CA 125. One of two women with invasive stage I disease had an elevated CA 125 level. Among women with an abnormal CA 125 measure only, 4.2 surgeries were performed per invasive cancer diagnosed. Among women with either an abnormal TVU or an abnormal CA 125 measure, 28.5 surgeries were performed per invasive cancer diagnosed.

A CA 125 screening program of 22,000 postmenopausal women with subsequent transabdominal ultrasound for those with elevated CA 125 levels (reference value of 30 U/mL) detected 11 of 19 cases of ovarian cancer occurring in the cohort for an apparent sensitivity of 58%.[130] The specificity for this screening study was 99.9%. Three of the 11 cases detected through screening were stage I disease. In one prospective screening study, the specificity of CA 125 levels of 35 U/mL was 97.6%.[131] Other Markers Proteomics has been used to identify patterns or specific serum markers that may be used in place of, or in conjunction with, CA 125 measures for the early detection of cancer.[132,133]

Proteomics is a new and exciting area on the horizon in ovarian cancer screening. It is the branch of genetics that studies the full set of proteins encoded by a genome. The idea behind proteomics is to compare the types and amounts of proteins in the sera of women known to be disease-free with those of women known to have ovarian cancer. The theory is based upon differences in specific proteins that may help to identify early-stage disease. Initial promising results were reported by the US Food and

Drug Administration and National Institutes of Health Clinical Proteomic team in 2002. Petricoin et al.[132] used sera from 50 women with ovarian cancer and 50 unaffected women as a training set. The researchers were able to identify five protein peaks in the ovarian cancer group that were not present in the unaffected group. The proteomic pattern completely discriminated cancer from no cancer. The identified pattern then was used to analyze 116 masked serum samples—50 from women with ovarian cancer and 66 from unaffected women and women with benign disorders. The established pattern correctly identified all 50 ovarian cancer cases, 18 of which were stage I. Sixty-three of the 66 nonmalignant samples were identified correctly. In the admittedly small sample, the test exhibited a sensitivity of 100%, specificity of 95%, and positive predictive value of 94%.[133] Of course, the high positive predictive value was in a highly preselected population that had an ovarian cancer prevalence of almost 50%.

Some questions have been raised regarding the test in the nonmalignant study population, which was performed with a specificity of 95%. Specificity in the general population is unknown.[134] Additionally, a specificity of 95% is inadequate for ovarian cancer screening in the general population because of the low prevalence of asymptomatic disease. Specificity greater than 99% is necessary to achieve the target positive predictive value of 10%. Perhaps the specificity of the test may reach acceptable levels as the data set grows, but that is not a certainty.[135]

The Pap test may occasionally detect malignant ovarian cells, but it is not sensitive (reported sensitivity of 10%–30%) and has not been evaluated for the early detection of ovarian cancer.[117] Another method of detection,

cytologic examination of peritoneal lavage obtained by culdocentesis, is technically difficult, uncomfortable to the patient, has low sensitivity for detecting early-stage disease, and has not been evaluated for screening.[117,136]

Prevention

Multiple studies have demonstrated a 40% to 50% decrease in ovarian cancer risk in women who take oral contraceptives.[137,138] The protective effect appears to increase with the duration of oral contraceptive use and to persist for 10 to 15 years after oral contraceptives have been discontinued. For example, a review of the literature demonstrated a 10% to 12% decrease in risk associated with use for 1 year and an approximate 50% decrease after 5 years of use. This reduced risk was present among both nulliparous and parous women.[139] In the general population, ovarian cancer risk is inversely associated with oral contraceptive use, tubal ligation, and childbearing. Among carriers of BRCA1 gene mutations, data study was done using women incidentally diagnosed with invasive epithelial ovarian cancer in the San Francisco Bay Area of California from March 1997 through July 2001. The contraceptive and reproductive histories of 36 carrier cases and 381 noncarrier cases with those of 568 controls identified by random digit dialing who were frequency matched to cases on age and race/ethnicity. In both carriers and noncarriers, reduced risk was associated with use of oral contraceptives (OR = 0.54; 95% CI: 0.26, 1.13) for carriers and 0.55 (95% CI: 0.41, 0.73) for noncarriers, duration of oral contraceptive use (risk reduction per year = 13%[p = 0.01]) for carriers and 6% (p < 0.001) for noncarriers, history of tubal ligation (OR = 0.68; 95%

CI: 0.25, 1.90) for carriers and 0.65 (95% CI: 0.45, 0.95) for noncarriers, and increasing parity (risk reduction per childbirth = 16% [p = 0.26]) for carriers and 24% (p < 0.001) for noncarriers. Results suggest that BRCA1 mutation carriers and noncarriers have similar risk reduction associated with oral contraceptive use, tubal ligation, and parity.[102]

In a prospective study, a 33% decrease in the risk of ovarian cancer among women who underwent tubal sterilization was observed after adjusting the data for oral contraceptive use, parity, and other ovarian cancer risk factors. This study also demonstrated a weaker, although statistically significant, decrease in risk associated with simple hysterectomy.[140]

Ovarian cancer is relatively uncommon, but it has a high mortality rate due to stage at diagnosis and lack of effective early detection methods. As a result, most women present with extensive abdominal carcinomatosis, and therapy is generally aimed at achieving remission rather than cure. The strategy of performing risk-reducing salpingo-oophorectomy (RRSO) in BRCA mutation carriers has the potential to significantly decrease ovarian cancer mortality in these individuals. In the past, RRSO was performed in women with a strong family history of ovarian cancer, whereas currently the decision to proceed with RRSO is based primarily on the results of BRCA mutational analysis.[141]

Women with a deleterious mutation in the BRCA1 or BRCA2 genes have a marked increase in the risk of ovarian cancer compared with the general population. Prophylactic oophorectomy is a potential option to reduce the risk of developing ovarian cancer. A family-based study among women with BRCA1 or BRCA2 mutations found that of the 259 women who had undergone bilateral prophy-

lactic oophorectomy, two (0.8%) developed subsequent papillary serous peritoneal carcinoma, and six (2.8%) had stage I ovarian cancer at the time of surgery. Twenty percent of the 292 matched controls who did not have prophylactic surgery developed ovarian cancer. Prophylactic surgery was associated with a greater than 90% reduction in the risk of ovarian cancer, (RR = 0.04; 95% CI, 0.01–0.16) with an average follow-up of 9 years.[142]

Some factors may bias the estimate of benefit. Prophylactic surgical removal of the ovaries has been offered for many years as a potential preventative of ovarian cancer in women deemed to be at increased hereditary risk for this disease. Now it is possible to test for specific mutations of the BRCA1 and BRCA2 genes that render members of hereditary breast ovarian cancer (HBOC) syndrome families susceptible to cancer. Widespread intra-abdominal carcinomatosis, which mimics metastatic ovarian serous carcinoma, has been reported following oophorectomy in individuals at increased hereditary risk.

A study was conducted to examine and report the occurrence of intra-abdominal carcinomatosis, as well as other cancers, following prophylactic oophorectomy in patients who carry cancer susceptibility mutations of BRCA1 and BRCA2 and to assess the cumulative risks for this disease. The study goal was to assist in development of appropriate surgical interventions, based on currently available information, and to counsel patients who choose prophylactic surgery on potential long-term prognosis. From 72 HBOC syndrome families that carried either BRCA1 or BRCA2 cancer-associated mutations, 238 individuals who had undergone prophylactic oophorectomy were recorded between

January 1985 and December 2002. During a mean follow-up of 9.3 years, cancers were diagnosed in 27 subjects, including 16 individuals with breast cancer and five patients with intra-abdominal carcinomatosis. Histological review of the prophylactically removed ovaries found borderline lesions in two cases, one with possible early stromal invasion. A 3.5% cumulative risk for all mutation carriers and a 3.9% cumulative risk for BRCA1 mutation carriers were calculated through 20 years of follow-up after prophylactic oophorectomy. Calculated cumulative risk of developing intra-abdominal carcinomatosis after prophylactic oophorectomy in members of HBOC syndrome families, specifically those who carry deleterious mutations, are well below the estimated risks of ovarian cancer published in the literature for similar patients.[143]

The degree of risk for ovarian cancer, potential morbidity and mortality of surgery, and the risks associated with early menopause should be taken into account when considering prophylactic oophorectomy for high-risk women. Underlying ovarian cancer risk can be assessed through accurate pedigrees and/or genetic markers of risk. Because of uncertainties about cancer risks associated with specific gene mutations, genetic information may be difficult to interpret outside of families with a high incidence of ovarian cancer. Three inherited ovarian cancer susceptibility syndromes have been described: (1) familial site-specific ovarian cancer; (2) familial breast/ovarian cancer; and (3) the Lynch II syndrome, which is a combination of breast, ovarian, endometrial, gastrointestinal, and genitourinary cancers.[144,145] Considering family history in the absence of specific information on BRCA1/2 mutation status, unaffected women who have two or three relatives with

ovarian cancer have a cumulative ovarian cancer risk of about 7%.[144] Women who have a mother or sister with ovarian cancer have a cumulative lifetime risk of ovarian cancer of about 5%.

Cervical Cancer

An estimated 11,070 new cervical cancers and 3870 cervical cancer deaths will occur in the United States in 2008.[66] An additional 1,250,000 women will be diagnosed with precancers annually by cytology using the Papanicolaou (Pap) smear. From 2001–2005, the median age at diagnosis for cancer of the cervix uteri was 48 years of age. Approximately 0.1% were diagnosed under age 20 years; 15.2% between age 20 and 34 years; 25.9% between age 35 and 44 years; 23.4% between age 45 and 54 years; 15.5% between age 55 and 64 years; 10.4% between age 65 and 74 years; 6.8% between age 75 and 84 years; and 2.5% at 85+ years of age.[2]

Fifty-one percent of cervix uteri cancer cases are diagnosed while the cancer is still confined to the primary site (localized stage); 35% are diagnosed after the cancer has spread to regional lymphnodes or directly beyond the primary site; 10% are diagnosed after the cancer has already metastasized (distant stage) and for the remaining 5% the staging information was unknown. The corresponding 5-year relative survival rates were: 91.7% for localized; 55.9% for regional; 16.6% for distant; and 59.4% for unstaged. From 2001–2005, the median age at death for cancer of the cervix uteri was 57 years of age. Approximately 0.0% died under age 20 years; 5.4% between age 20 and 34 years; 16.5% between age 35 and 44 years; 23.0% between age 45 and 54 years; 19.5% between age 55 and 64 years; 15.0% between age 65 and 74 years;

13.5% between age 75 and 84 years; and 7.0% at 85+ years of age.

The overall 5-year relative survival rate for 1996–2004 was 71.2%. Five-year relative survival rates by race were: 72.5% for white women and 61.8% for black women.[2] Based on rates from 2003–2005, 0.69% of women born today will be diagnosed with cancer of the cervix uteri at some time during their lifetime. This number can also be expressed as 1 in 145 women will be diagnosed with cancer of the cervix uteri during their lifetime. The incidence of cervical cancer has decreased dramatically with the advent and widespread adoption of screening via gynecological examinations and Pap smears.

Etiology

A continuum of pathologic changes of the cervix uteri may be diagnosed, ranging from atypical squamous cells of undetermined significance to low-grade squamous intraepithelial lesions (LSIL) to high-grade squamous intraepithelial lesions (HSIL) to invasive cancer. The precancerous conditions LSIL and HSIL are also referred to as cervical intraepithelial neoplasia (CIN) 1, 2, and 3. Lesions can regress, persist, or progress to an invasive malignancy, with LSIL (CIN 1) more likely to regress spontaneously and HSIL (CIN 2/CIN 3) more likely to persist or progress. The average time for progression of CIN 3 to invasive cancer has been estimated to be 10 to 15 years.[146]

Risk Factors

Nearly all cases of cervical cancer are associated with human *Papillomavirus* (HPV) infection,[147,148] which is transmitted during sexual activity. Therefore, cervical cancer is seen more frequently in women with sexual activity at an early age and with multiple partners.

Epidemiologic studies to evaluate risk factors for the development of squamous intraepithelial lesions (SIL) and cervical malignancy demonstrate conclusively a sexual mode of transmission of a carcinogen.[1] HPV-associated genital tract disease is now the most commonly diagnosed sexually transmitted disease in the United States. It is now widely accepted that human *Papillomavirus* (HPV) is the primary etiologic infectious agent.[148] The finding of HPV viral DNA integrated in the majority of cellular genomes of invasive cervical carcinomas supports epidemiologic data linking this agent to cervical cancer; however, direct causation has not been demonstrated.[149] Other sexually transmitted factors, including herpes simplex virus 2, may play a cocausative role.[1]

HPVs belong to a family of small (8-kb pairs) double-stranded circular DNA viruses that infect squamous epithelia of the genital tract, anal and perianal areas, and mucosal epithelium of the larynx. Approximately 20 million people in the United States at any given time are infected with HPV and are able to transmit it to others. Low-risk HPVs, such as HPV-6 and HPV-11, cause benign genital warts, whereas high-risk types, such as HPV-16 and HPV-18, are associated with the development of high-grade squamous intraepithelial lesions and cervical cancer. It is estimated that HPV-16 accounts for approximately 60% of cervical cancers, with HPV-18 adding another 10%–20%. Infection in both women and men is clearly related to sexual activity as well as environmental factors such as birth control pills and smoking. For women, the most striking risk factors for HPV infection and the development of detectable pathology are numerous lifetime sexual partners and early onset of sexual activity.[150,151]

HPV infects the basal cells of human epithelial surfaces. Infected basal cells divide; some progeny remain as infected basal cells, while others move away from the basement membrane, differentiate, and become epithelial cells. Virus replication and assembly is tightly linked to the differentiation program of epithelial cells. Infectious virions are produced only in the terminally differentiated cell and are shed as virus-laden squamous cells. This explains why HPV cannot grow in tissue culture.[150,151]

By infecting only the basal layer cells and executing viral replication and assembly only in a fully differentiated cell, HPV avoids the immune system of the host. The success of this strategy is documented by very poor immune response (humoral as well as cell mediated) to HPV infection. The nature of this response is under investigation; nevertheless, most women who are infected spontaneously resolve their infection in less than 2 years. Infections that are not controlled and persist for prolonged periods can cause more severe pathologies and, ultimately, cancer.[150,152]

Cigarette smoking places a woman at an increased risk for squamous cell carcinoma of the cervix.[153,154,145] The longer the duration and intensity of smoking, the greater increase in the risk of developing cancer. Exposure to environmental tobacco smoke may increase a woman's risk to four times that of women who are nonsmokers and are not exposed to environmental smoking.[154] Case-control studies of women infected with HPV have examined the effect of various types and levels of tobacco exposure and found similar results.[145,155]

Long-term use of oral contraceptives has also been associated with cervical cancer. Compared to never-users, women who used oral contraceptives for fewer than 5 years did not have an increased risk of cervical cancer (OR = 0.73; 95% CI, 0.52–1.03). The OR for women who used oral contraceptives for 5 to 9 years was 2.82 (1.46–5.42), and for 10 or more years the OR was 4.03 (2.09–8.02).[156]

Women with HIV infection are approximately five times more likely than uninfected women to have cervical squamous intraepithelial lesions (SIL), the precursor to invasive cervical cancer.[157–160] Invasive cervical cancer is found about three times more frequently in HIV-infected versus uninfected women.[161] HIV-infected black and Hispanic women in the United States may have a 4- to 7-fold increased risk of invasive cervical cancer.[162] The underlying causes for the association remain unclear.[158–164]

Screening

Cervical cancer screening guidelines have been recommended by several organizations, although each are somewhat different. Most recommend initial Papanicolaou (Pap) test screening 3 years after the onset of vaginal intercourse or by the age of 21, whichever comes first. Annual screening is recommended by most organizations, although ACS and ACOG make a distinction between women younger than and older than age 30 years. According to ACS and ACOG, women older than age 30 years may be tested every 2 or 3 years if they have three negative Pap results on three consecutive occasions.[67,165]

ACS recommends that women older than age 70 years can stop screening if they have had normal results for the past 10 years, ACOG recommends that physicians make decisions based on individual patients, and the NCI recommends women aged 65 to 70 years who have had at least three normal Pap tests and no abnormal Pap tests in the past 10 years may decide, after speaking with their doctor, to stop cervical cancer screening.[166] Pap screening after hysterectomy generally is not recommended if the cervix was removed and if the hysterectomy was for benign disease.

The US Food and Drug Administration (FDA) approved HPV-DNA testing for adjunct surveillance with cytology testing either with conventional screening or with liquid-based technology. ACS recommends HPV screening, but not until women reach age 30 years. The recommendation is based on the relative frequency of HPV in sexually active women younger than age 30 years. ACS recommends screening every 3 years after age 30 years using conventional or liquid-based cytology combined with DNA testing, but DNA testing should not be performed more frequently than every 3 years.[167]

The Pap has never been examined in a randomized controlled trial. A large body of consistent observational data, however, supports its effectiveness in reducing mortality from cervical cancer. Both incidence and mortality from cervical cancer have sharply decreased in a number of large populations following the introduction of well-run screening programs.[168–171] Case-control studies have found that the risk of developing invasive cervical cancer is 3 to 10 times greater in women who have not been screened.[172–175] Risk also increases with long duration following the last normal Pap test, or similarly, with decreasing frequency of screening.[176,177] Screening every 2 to 3 years, however, has not been found to increase significantly the risk of finding invasive cervical cancer above the risk expected with annual screening.[177,178]

Since the development of the Pap test, a variety of devices have been implemented to obtain cells for cytological evaluation. They fall into two large categories: smear instruments and cervicovaginal lavage devices.[179] The conventional technique for Pap testing is to sample the cervical epithelium and the endocervical canal (including the transformation zone), usually with a combination of a spatula and endocervical brush. The sample is then smeared on a slide and immediately fixed. Between 6% and 65% of the cells are transferred from the collection device to the slide.[180]

More common liquid-based technologies include Thin Prep (Cytyc Corporation, Marlborough, Massachusetts) and AutoCyte Prep (TriPath Imaging, Burlington, North Carolina). Liquid-based preparation systems help prevent poor sampling, uneven cell distribution, and improper fixation on slides. Smears are obtained with either a cytobrush and Ayre spatula or a cervical broom device. Spatulas should be plastic rather than wooden.[181] Samples are not smeared directly onto glass slides but placed in small bottles containing fixative solution. At the laboratory, samples are filtered and centrifuged to remove excess blood and debris, and a thin layer of cells is transferred to a slide. Liquid-based or thin layer preparations improve the quality of the Pap test, decrease unsatisfactory smears, and often increase the number of precancerous lesions detected.[182] Generally, the techniques result in higher-quality smears for cytological review, and the residual material can be used for HPV testing.[183]

Unfortunately, 30% of cervical cancers are not detected early because of errors in sampling and interpretation.[183] The errors include incomplete sampling of the transformation zone, poorly prepared slides with drying artifacts or clumping of cells, and failure of pathologists or cytotechnologists to detect abnormal cells.

The overall false-negative rate of the Pap test for cervical cancer screening is estimated to be 15%–25%.[184] The overall sensitivity may range from 50%–77%.[185] A large meta-analysis suggested that extended tip spatulas used in conjunction with endocervical brushes are the most effective method for obtaining cervical cells.[186] Detection of endocervical cells suggests an adequate smear and is associated with earlier detection of the disease.

The major potential harm of screening for cervical cancer lies in the detection and treatment of many lesions, such as atypical squamous cells of undetermined significance (ASCUS) and low-grade squamous intraepithelial lesions (LSIL), that would never progress to cervical cancer. Women with LSIL or high-grade squamous intraepithelial lesions (HSIL) on Pap testing are usually referred for colposcopy and treated with cryotherapy or loop electrosurgical excision procedure. These procedures permanently alter the cervix and have unknown consequences on fertility and pregnancy. Because younger women are most likely to acquire human *Papillomavirus* infections and to be diagnosed with LSIL, they are thus most likely to suffer harms from interventions for a condition that often resolves spontaneously.[187]

Annually in the United States, 50 million women undergo screening; about 3.5 million (7%) will be referred for further evaluation. Of these, more than 2 million will be referred for further evaluation of ASCUS200.[188] Thus, Pap test screening results in a large number of colposcopies for benign conditions. Strategies to improve the specificity of the cervical cytopathology test are being evaluated by the ASCUS/LSIL Triage Study (ALTS).[189]

Ideally, determining the sensitivity and specificity of a screening test would involve a study that applies a "gold standard" test (such as colposcopy with appropriate biopsy) to all participants (whether the screening test is positive or negative). Sensitivity (the percentage of "true-positive" cases that are detected by the screening test) and specificity (the percentage of "true-negative" cases that are negative by the screening test) could be calculated. Such studies have rarely been done for any screening test for cervical cancer. Studies that compare the Papanicolaou (Pap) test with repeat Pap testing have found that the sensitivity of any abnormality on a single test for detecting high-grade lesions is 55% to 80%.[190,191] Because of the usual slow-growing nature of cervical cancer, the sensitivity of a program of regular Pap testing is likely higher.

To determine the sensitivity and specificity of the Pap smear, both a test threshold (i.e., the point at which the test will be considered to be "positive") and a reference-standard threshold (i.e., the point at which the reference standard is considered to be "positive") must be defined. In practice, ASCUS is often used as the test threshold and cervical intraepithelial neoplasia (CIN) 1 is often used as the reference threshold. This combination gives a sensitivity of about 68% and a specificity of about 75%. A more appropriate test threshold may be low-grade squamous intraepithelial lesions, with a reference threshold of CIN 2–3. This combination gives a sensitivity of 70% to 80%, with a specificity of about 95%.[192]

Prevention

Prevention strategies for cervical cancer should focus on encouraging women to receive screening, education on safe sexual practices, HPV vaccination, and smoking cessation. Given the etiologic role of HPV in the pathogenesis of cervical neoplasia, vaccines to immunize against HPV infection would offer a primary prevention strategy for cervical cancer. Users of barrier methods of contraception are associated with a reduced incidence of SIL presumptively secondary to protection from sexually transmitted disease.[193,194] Spermicides may be a contributing influence because they can have an antiviral action.[195] Barrier contraception may be incompletely effective because HPV can still be transmitted via skin or mucosal contact.

Persistent infection with oncogenic types of HPV such as HPV-16 and HPV-18 is associated with the development of cervical cancer.[148] Two viruslike particle (VLP) human *Papillomavirus* (HPV) vaccines have been shown to be nearly 100% effective in preventing type-specific persistent HPV infection.[196–201] These vaccines have an almost identical external epitope structure to native HPV virions but are manufactured using recombinant biological techniques and contain no viral DNA so that they are neither infectious nor capable of inducing neoplasia. When administered parenterally in three doses over 6 months, these VLP vaccines induce neutralizing antibodies in humans that provide long-lasting HPV type-specific immunity. Severe adverse events directly related to HPV vaccines have been rare; specifically, the most commonly reported side effects are injection site inflammation and pain.[196–201] On June 8, 2006, the Food and Drug Administration (FDA) licensed the first vaccine developed to prevent cervical cancer and other diseases in females caused by certain types of genital human *Papillomavirus* (HPV). The quadrivalent vaccine, Gardasil®, protects against four HPV types (6, 11, 16, 18), which are responsible for 70% of cervical cancers and 90% of genital warts. On June 29, 2006, the Advisory Committee on Immunization

Practices (ACIP*) voted to recommend use of this vaccine in females, aged 9–26 years. Idiosyncratic reactions, such as neurodevelopmental delays, including autism, thought to be related to other childhood vaccines, have not been reported after vaccination against HPV. Importantly, the tested HPV vaccine preparations have been dispensed in single-dose vials to date. They have not contained preservatives required for multidose vials, such as thimerosal, a mercury-based preservative that has been inconsistently associated with developmental delays in epidemiological studies.

In a prospective, randomized trial of 12,167 16- to 26-year-old females, VLP vaccination against HPV type 16 and 18 provided 100% protection against high-grade HPV type 16–related and type 18–related cervical intraepithelial neoplasia, an important surrogate marker for protection against cancer.[201] Human *Papillomavirus* type 16 is the most common HPV type associated with high-grade cervical dysplasia as well as invasive cervical cancer and, together with HPV type 18, accounts for approximately 70% of cervical cancers.[196,198–201] Researchers followed young women (average age 23) who had received three doses of either an experimental HPV vaccine or a placebo between 2000 and 2003 while participating in an earlier study by the same researchers. The earlier study showed that the experimental vaccine prevented most infections with HPV-16 and HPV-18, the two types of HPV that cause most cases of cervical cancer.[202] The initial study followed 1113 women for about 2 years. The current follow-up study extended the follow-up period to 4.5 years for a subgroup of 776 women. More than 98% of the women who had been vaccinated continued to have antibodies against HPV-16 and HPV-18 in their blood throughout the extended follow-up period—a strong sign that the vaccine remained effective and was preventing them from becoming infected with those strains of HPV. In addition, none of the women in the vaccine group developed any abnormal changes in cells of the cervix of the type caused by HPV-16 or HPV-18. By contrast, women in the placebo group developed many precancerous abnormalities in the cells of the cervix.[202] The vaccine partly protected many women from two other strains of HPV, HPV-45, and HPV-31, which are the third and fourth most common HPV types associated with cervical cancer. None of the women vaccinated reported any serious side effects from the medication.[202]

A phase 3 trial was conducted to evaluate the efficacy of a prophylactic quadrivalent vaccine in preventing anogenital diseases associated with human *Papillomavirus* (HPV) types 6, 11, 16, and 18. The randomized, placebo-controlled, double-blind trial involved 5455 women between the ages of 16 and 24 years: 2723 were assigned women to receive vaccine and 2732 were assigned to receive placebo at day 1, month 2, and month 6. The women were followed for an average of 3 years after administration of the first dose. In the per-protocol population, those followed for vulvar, vaginal, or perianal disease included 2261 women (83%) in the vaccine group and 2279 (83%) in the placebo group. Those followed for cervical disease included 2241 women (82%) in the vaccine group and 2258 (83%) in the placebo group. Vaccine efficacy was 100% for each of the coprimary end points. In an intention-to-treat analysis, including those with prevalent infection or disease caused by vaccine-type and non-vaccine-type HPV, vaccination reduced the rate of any vulvar or vaginal perianal lesions regardless of the causal HPV

type by 34% (95% CI, 15 to 49), and the rate of cervical lesions regardless of the causal HPV type by 20% (95% CI, 8 to 31).[203] HPV vaccination does not substitute for routine cervical cancer screening (Pap tests) and is not intended to treat cervical cancers.[204]

In support of the Food and Drug Administration (FDA), Centers for Disease Control (CDC), NIP, and ACIP, CDC's Division of Cancer Prevention and Control offers the following statement about HPV and cervical cancer:

- Regular cervical cancer screening (Pap test) is recommended for all women (starting within 3 years of when a woman begins sexual activity or at age 21 years, whichever comes first).
- HPV vaccination for girls and women aged 9–26 years is supported.
- HPV vaccination for women aged 27 years or older is not supported.
- All women receiving the HPV vaccine should continue to receive regular cervical cancer screening (Pap tests) according to established screening recommendations.

The American College of Obstetricians and Gyencologists reccomends that all girls ages 11-12 years should be routinely given the HPV vaccine.

Endometrial Cancer

Endometrial cancer is the most common invasive gynecologic cancer in US women, with 40,100 new cases projected to occur in 2008.[1] This disease primarily affects postmenopause women at an average age of 60 years at diagnosis.[2] About

70% of all cases are found in women between the ages of 45 and 74 years, with the highest number diagnosed in the 55 to 64 age group. Only 8% occur in younger women. The chance of any woman being diagnosed with this cancer during her lifetime is about 1 in 41. There are over 500,000 women who are survivors of this cancer. Although this cancer is 40% more common in white women, black women are nearly twice as likely to die from it.[66]

Although it is estimated that approximately 7470 women will die of endometrial cancer in 2008, the mortality rate has declined in the United States about 25% from 1974 to the present. From 2001–2005, the median age at diagnosis for cancer of the endometrium was 62 years of age. Approximately 0.0% were diagnosed under age 20 years; 1.5% between age 20 and 34 years; 6.4% between age 35 and 44 years; 18.9% between age 45 and 54 years; 28.8% between age 55 and 64 years; 22.8% between age 65 and 74 years; 16.5% between age 75 and 84 years; and 5.1% at 85+ years of age.

From 2001–2005, the median age at death for cancer of the corpus and uterus, NOS was 73 years of age.[4] Approximately 0.0% died under age 20; 0.4% between age 20 and 34 years; 2.2% between age 35 and 44 years; 8.1% between age 45 and 54 years; 18.4% between age 55 and 64 years; 26.4% between age 65 and 74 years; 28.7% between age 75 and 84 years; and 15.9% at 85+ years of age.

The stage distribution based on historic stage shows that 69% of corpus and uterus, NOS cancer cases are diagnosed while the cancer is still confined to the primary site (localized stage); 17% are diagnosed after the cancer has spread to regional lymphnodes or directly beyond the primary site; 9% are diagnosed after the cancer

has already metastasized (distant stage); and for the remaining 4% the staging information was unknown. The corresponding 5-year relative survival rates were: 95.5% for localized; 67.5% for regional; 23.6% for distant; and 56.1% for unstaged.

The stage distribution based on histologic stage shows that 70% of corpus and uterus cancer cases are diagnosed while the cancer is still confined to the primary site (localized stage); 17% are diagnosed after the cancer has spread to regional lymph nodes or directly beyond the primary site; 9% are diagnosed after the cancer has already metastasized (distant stage); and for the remaining 4% the staging information was unknown. The corresponding 5-year relative survival rates were: 95.5% for localized; 67.5% for regional; 23.6% for distant; and 56.1% for unstaged. Based on rates from 2001–2005, 2.48% of women born today, or 1 in 40, will be diagnosed with cancer of the corpus and uterus at some time during their lifetime.[2]

In the interval from 1973 to 1978, there was a transient increase in the incidence of endometrial cancer without an associated increase in mortality. This phenomenon corresponded with increased use of estrogen replacement therapy at that time. Endometrial cancer rates across the board would be somewhat higher if they were adjusted for the portion of the female population who have undergone hysterectomy. One study estimated that adjustment for age-specific hysterectomy would yield a uterine cancer incidence rate that was approximately 20% higher.[205] In the mid-1970s, the diagnosis of approximately 15,000 cases of postmenopausal endometrial cancers in excess of those expected on the basis of the underlying secular trend has been related to the use of exogenous estrogen therapy.[206]

Etiology

Endometrial cancer is usually preceded by endometrial hyperplasia. Adenocarcinoma accounts for > 80% of endometrial cancers. Other types include papillary serous, clear cell, squamous, and mucinous carcinoma. The cancer may spread from the surface of the uterine cavity to the cervical canal; through the myometrium to the serosa and into the peritoneal cavity; via the lumen of the fallopian tube to the ovary, broad ligament, and peritoneal surfaces; via the bloodstream, leading to distant metastases; or via the lymphatics. The higher (more undifferentiated) the grade of the tumor, the greater is the likelihood of deep myometrial invasion, pelvic or para-aortic lymph node metastases, or extrauterine spread.[207]

Risk Factors

Major differences exist between black and white women with respect to stage of endometrial cancer at detection and subsequent survival. Even though the incidence of endometrial cancer is lower among black women, mortality is higher. The National Cancer Institute initiated a Black/White Cancer Survival Study and found that black women with endometrial cancer had higher-grade and more aggressive histology than white women.[208–210] It is difficult to disentangle the effects that biology and socioeconomic status may have on the lower survival rates of African American women with endometrial cancer. Evidence suggests that lower income is associated with advanced-stage disease, lower probability of receiving a hysterectomy, and lower survival rates.[209] Other studies, however, have not found a black/white difference in the interval from patient-reported symptom recognition to initial medical consultation and

concluded that it is unlikely that patient delay after onset of symptoms could explain much of the excess of advanced-stage disease found in black women.[211] Further research is necessary to understand why black women tend to be diagnosed with more aggressive disease and have a higher probability of dying than white women, despite their lower incidence of endometrial cancer.

In addition to the risk of developing endometrial cancer in association with the use of estrogen replacement therapy unaccompanied by progesterone, a number of additional risk factors have been identified and often appear to be related to estrogenic effects. Among these factors are obesity, a high-fat diet, reproductive factors like nulliparity, early menarche and late menopause, polycystic ovarian syndrome, and tamoxifen use.

The first report of an association between estrogen replacement therapy and endometrial cancer appeared at the end of 1975.[212] These results were soon confirmed by two similar studies.[213,214] A number of confirmatory studies indicated that the risk of developing endometrial cancer increased with duration of use (10-fold to 30-fold with 5 years or more of use), and that when estrogen replacement had been used for at least a year, the risk might persist for more than 10 years after discontinuation. Estrogen Replacement Therapy/HT unopposed by progesterone therapy is a cause of endometrial cancer in women with an intact uterus.[215–218] However, women taking combination estrogen-progesterone replacement therapy (HRT/HT) exhibit similar risk to women who do not take postmenopausal HT.[218,219]

The NSABP Breast Cancer Prevention Trial P-1 Study confirmed an increased incidence of endometrial cancer in women at high risk for invasive breast cancer who received tamoxifen, as compared with women who received placebo. The annual rate of endometrial cancer was 2.3 per 1000 among women who received tamoxifen and 0.91 per 1000 in the placebo group: a 2.53 greater risk for women taking chemopreventive tamoxifen (95% CI, 1.35-4.97). The increase in risk differed according to menopausal status; for women aged 49 years or younger RR was 1.21 (95% CI, 0.41–3.60) compared with 4.01 (95% CI, 1.70–10.90) for women aged 50 years and older. All of the invasive endometrial cancer cases that occurred among women taking tamoxifen were International Federation of Gynecology and Obstetrics (FIGO) stage I. Similarly, 14 out of 15 (93%) of the invasive endometrial cancer cases diagnosed among women taking placebo were FIGO stage I.[220]

Elevated body mass index (BMI) and obesity have been associated in several studies with increased risk of endometrial cancer. Studies have measured body fat in a variety of ways including body weight, BMI, waist-to-thigh circumference ratio, and waist-to-hip circumference ratio.[221] One of the possible mechanisms for the observed association is an increased level of serum estrone in obese women as a result of aromatization of androstenedione in adipose tissue, which increases the production of estrogen, a well-known cause of endometrial cancer.[222] Alternatively, obesity has been associated with a reduction in levels of sex hormone-binding globulin (SHBG), which can increase bioavailable estrogen.[223] Obesity has been associated with several factors known to increase the risk of endometrial cancer, including upper-body or central adiposity, polycystic ovarian syndrome, physical inactivity, and a diet high in saturated fat.[224]

A number of additional risk factors have been identified, and most appear to be related to estrogenic effects. Among these factors are high-fat diet, reproductive factors such as nulliparity, polycystic ovarian syndrome, early menarche, and late menopause. Women with hereditary nonpolyposis colorectal cancer (HNPCC) syndrome have a markedly increased risk of endometrial cancer compared to women in the general population. Among women who are HNPCC mutation carriers, the estimated cumulative incidence of endometrial cancer ranges from 20% to 60% by the age of 70 years. This risk appears to differ slightly based on the germline mutation; for MLH1 carriers the lifetime risk at age 70 years is 25%, while MSH2 mutation carriers have a 35% to 40% lifetime risk of endometrial cancer by age 70 years. The mean age of diagnosis for MLH1 or MSH2 carriers is 47 years, compared with 60 years for noninherited forms of endometrial cancer. The prognosis and survival are similar between HNPCC-related and noninherited forms of endometrial cancer.[225–229]

Screening

Routine screening of asymptomatic women for endometrial cancer has not been evaluated for its impact on endometrial cancer mortality.[230,231] Although high-risk groups can be identified, such as women with a uterus taking tamoxifen or using unopposed estrogens and women carrying genetic mutations for hereditary nonpolyposis colorectal cancer, the benefit of screening in reducing endometrial cancer mortality in these high-risk groups has not been evaluated. Published recommendations for screening certain groups of women at high risk for endometrial carcinoma are based on opinion regarding presumptive benefit.[66] Although risk factors include estrogen replacement therapy unopposed by progestins, tamoxifen therapy, and genetic mutations associated with hereditary nonpolyposis colon cancer, no controlled trials have been done to evaluate the effectiveness of screening for endometrial cancer in reducing mortality in these subpopulations.

Controversy exists among professional organizations regarding the need to screen for endometrial cancer. ACS and NCI do not recommend screening for endometrial cancer in most women because no scientific evidence proves that screening methods significantly reduce mortality rates and that the risks and costs of available screening methods outweigh the benefits.[232–234] ACS recommends that women at average risk should be counseled about the risks and symptoms of endometrial cancer, especially any abnormal or unexpected bleeding or spotting.

For women with or at risk for HNPCC, ACS recommends annual screening with endometrial biopsy and transvaginal ultrasound (TVU) starting at age 35.[232] For the same population, NCI (2005) recommends TVU and endometrial biopsy starting at age 25. The population includes women known to be carriers of an HNPCC gene mutation, women with a substantial likelihood for carrying the mutation (i.e., those who have a family member with the gene mutation), and women with a strongly suspected autosomal, dominant predisposition to colon cancer.[235]

For women at average risk for developing endometrial cancer, little consensus exists about the best way to screen. Most women present to their healthcare providers with complaints of abnormal uterine bleeding, a problem that accounts for as many as 33% of women referred to a gynecologist.[236] Abnormal uterine bleeding includes any change in the frequency or duration of menstrual cycles, the amount of bleeding, and bleeding between cycles.[237] About 90% of women diagnosed with endometrial cancer have abnormal uterine bleeding as a presenting symptom.[232]

TVU is used to measure endometrial thickness and to localize any lesions that should be sampled during biopsy. An endometrium thicker than 16 mm has been used as a predictor of abnormal pathology in premenopausal women with a sensitivity of 67%, specificity of 75%, and positive predictive value of 14%. In postmenopausal women, an endometrium thicker than 5 mm has a sensitivity of at least 82% and a specificity of 60% in predicting abnormal pathology.[238] An endometrium greater than 5 mm is the standard used for the diagnosis of endometrial cancer in postmenopausal women. TVU is a minimally invasive procedure that can be performed in a healthcare provider's office.[239]

Historically, dilatation and curettage (D & C) had been the accepted standard for diagnosing endometrial cancer. This is no longer true because of its risks, necessity to be performed in an operative setting, and cost.[236] In many cases, however, D & C is necessary to obtain endometrial tissue for pathologic examination. Currently, endometrial biopsy is the most commonly used method for diagnosis. Endometrial biopsy for the detection of abnormal endometrial pathology has a sensitivity ranging from 67%–96%.[240] Questions have been raised about the ability to get an accurate and adequate sample for testing; however, endometrial biopsy continues to be widely accepted as a first step in diagnostic evaluation because of its potential high sensitivity, minimal side effects, and ability to be performed in an office setting.[234]

Prevention

A protective effect on the endometrium of premenopausal women using combination oral contraceptives (COC) has been observed.[241] Combining estrogen and progestin COCs were used for 21 days of a 28-day cycle. On the days when the pill was not used, the endogenous estrogen levels remained low. With the use of COCs, the risk of developing endometrial cancer was decreased by approximately 40%, as demonstrated by case-control studies and supported by prospective cohort studies.[242–244] This decrease in risk was observed for at least 15 years after the women had ceased using COCs. Some evidence suggests that COCs must be used for up to a year before a decreased risk of endometrial cancer is observed.

Eight hundred and eighty eight postmenopausal women and 1111 population controls were enrolled in The Netherlands Cohort Study on Diet and Cancer. The study demonstrated a 46% reduction (RR = 0.54, 95% CI, 0.34–0.85, P trend = 0.002) in risk of endometrial cancer in women who were physically active 90 minutes or more per day, compared with less than 30 minutes each day.[245] When comparing women who exercised regularly with women who reported no exercise in the 2 years prior to diagnosis, the estimated risk of endometrial cancer was reduced by 38% (OR = 0.62, 95% CI, 0.51–0.76).[245]

In addition to the decreased risk of endometrial cancer recognized among parous women, lactation may also reduce risk. It has been hypothesized that inhibited ovulation during breastfeeding may suppress the risk of endometrial cancer. A case-control study conducted in Mexico City among low-risk women indicates a 58% to 72% reduction in risk of endometrial cancer associated with increasing duration of lactation, with a statistically significant trend. A similar trend was reported for an increase in the number of children who were breastfed.[246] A population-based case-control study conducted among Wisconsin women reported a statistically nonsignificant reduction in risk for parous women who breastfed for at least 2 weeks compared with those who did not breastfeed, OR = 0.90 (95% CI, 0.72–1.13). Increasing duration of lactation was not associated with a decrease in disease risk. However, breastfeeding within the past 3 decades was associated with a reduced risk of disease, OR = 0.58 (95% CI, 0.36–0.96). The risk of endometrial cancer was reduced by 50% (95% CI, 0.28–0.90) for women who breastfed for the first time at the age of 30 or older.[247]

A limited number of studies, mostly observational, have described a relationship association between dietary factors and risk of endometrial cancer. However, findings are consistent that a diet low in saturated fats and high in fruit and vegetable intake is associated with a reduced risk of developing endometrial cancer.[248–250] There is case-control evidence suggesting that regular consumption of soy products reduces the risk of endometrial cancer.[251,252]

Vaginal Cancer

In the United States in 2008 there will be an estimated 2,210 new cases and 760 deaths from vaginal cancer.[1] Carcinomas of the vagina are uncommon tumors comprising 1% to 2% of gynecologic malignancies. They can be effectively treated, and when found in early stages, they are often curable. The histological distinction between squamous cell carcinoma and adenocarcinoma is important because the two types represent distinct diseases, each with a different pathogenesis and natural history. Squamous cell vaginal cancer (approximately 85% of cases) initially spreads superficially within the vaginal wall and later invades the paravaginal tissues and the parametria. Distant metastases occur most commonly in the lungs and liver.[253] Adenocarcinoma (approximately 15% of cases) has a peak incidence between 17 and 21 years of age and differs from squamous cell carcinoma by an increase in pulmonary metastases and supraclavicular and pelvic node involvement.[254] Rarely, melanoma and sarcoma are described as primary vaginal cancers. Adenosquamous carcinoma is a rare and aggressive mixed epithelial tumor comprising approximately 1% to 2% of cases.

Prognosis depends primarily on the stage of disease, but survival is reduced in patients who are greater than 60 years of age, are symptomatic at the time of diagnosis, have lesions of the middle and lower third of the vagina, or have poorly differentiated tumors.[255,256] In addition, the length of vaginal wall involvement has been found to be significantly correlated to survival and stage of disease in squamous cell carcinoma patients.[257]

Etiology

Most vaginal cancers occur in the upper one-third of the posterior vaginal wall. They may spread by direct extension (into the local paravaginal tissues, bladder, or rectum), through inguinal lymph nodes from lesions in the lower vagina, through pelvic lymph nodes from lesions in the upper vagina, or hematogenously.[258]

Risk Factors

Particular factors appear to make a woman more likely to develop vaginal cancer. Even if a woman does have one or more risk factors

for vaginal cancer, it is impossible to know for sure how much that risk factor contributed to causing the cancer. Many women with vaginal cancer do not have any apparent risk factors.

Squamous cell cancer of the vagina occurs mainly in older women. Over two-thirds of women are 60 years old or older when they are diagnosed. Clear cell adenocarcinomas are rare and occur most often in patients less than 30 years of age who have a history of in utero exposure to diethylstilbestrol (DES). The incidence of this disease, which is highest for those exposed during the first trimester, peaked in the mid-1970s, reflecting the use of DES in the 1950s.[254] Young women with a history of in utero DES exposure should be followed carefully to diagnose vaginal cancer at an early stage. In women who have been carefully followed and well managed, the disease is highly curable.

Vaginal adenosis is most commonly found in young women who had in utero exposure to DES and may coexist with a clear cell adenocarcinoma, although it rarely progresses to adenocarcinoma. Adenosis is replaced by squamous metaplasia, which occurs naturally and requires follow-up but not removal. The natural history, prognosis, and treatment of other primary vaginal cancers (sarcoma, melanoma, lymphoma, and carcinoid tumors) may be different, and specific references should be sought.[259]

About 65% to 80% of vaginal intraepithelial neoplasia (VAIN) or vaginal cancers contain the HPV virus. Certain types of HPV have been strongly associated with vaginal cancers. These types, namely types 16 and 18, are also associated with cervical cancer. These are different than the types that cause genital warts. Certain types of sexual behavior increase a woman's risk of getting HPV infection. These high-risk sexual behaviors include intercourse at an early age, having many sexual partners, having sex with a person who has had many partners, and having unprotected sex at any age.[260]

Having cervical cancer or cervical precancerous conditions (cervical intraepithelial neoplasia or cervical dysplasia) increases a woman's risk of developing vaginal squamous cell cancer. This is because cervical and vaginal cancers have similar risk factors, such as HPV infection. In fact, a recent study found that in women who had a vaginal cancer after treatment for cervical cancer, the DNA changes in the vaginal cancer cells were the same as those in the previous cervical cancer cells.[260]

Some studies suggest that women whose cervical cancers were treated with radiation therapy have an increased risk of vaginal cancer, possibly because the radiation damaged the DNA of vaginal cells. However, other studies have not supported this conclusion, and the issue remains unresolved.[258,261] Some studies suggest that long-term (chronic) irritation of the vagina in women using a pessary may slightly increase the risk of squamous cell vaginal cancer. However, this association is extremely rare, and no studies have conclusively proven that pessaries actually cause vaginal cancer.[258,261]

Tobacco use may also play a role in this disease, particularly in younger women, as it does for cervical cancer. One clue is that women with vaginal cancer have a high chance of developing lung cancer, and lung cancer is highly correlated with smoking.[258]

Screening

There are no standardized screening guidelines for vaginal cancers. Most vaginal squamous cell cancers are believed to develop from pre-cancerous changes, called vaginal intraepithelial neoplasia (VAIN), that may be present for years before a true cancer forms. Detection of these pre-cancers by regular Pap tests permits treatment to prevent a true cancer from developing.[1] Biopsies and coloposcopies should be performed in areas of suspicion.[261]

Prevention

The best way to reduce the risk of vaginal cancer is to avoid known risk factors whenever possible. But because many women with vaginal cancer have no known risk factors, it is not possible to completely prevent this disease.[261] Avoiding HPV infection may reduce a woman's vaginal cancer risk. However, many vaginal cancers do not have evidence of HPV infections, so this approach will not entirely prevent the disease.[261] Although there are no studies as to whether the cervical cancer vaccine will prevent vaginal cancer, there is hope that many cases will be prevented through the use of this vaccine.[261]

Avoiding tobacco use may also reduce the risk of vaginal cancer, in addition to obvious benefits of greatly reducing risk of developing far more common cancers of the lungs, mouth, throat, bladder, kidneys, and several other organs.[261]

Most vaginal squamous cell cancers are believed to develop from precancerous changes, called vaginal intraepithelial neoplasia (VAIN), that may be present for years before a true cancer forms. Detection of these precancers by regular Pap testing allows for early diagnosis and treatment, reducing the opportunity for a true cancer to develop.[261] Cells of the vaginal lining are usually picked up unintentionally (by chance) by the spatula during the procedure. Therefore, many cases of VAIN are found in women whose vaginal lining is not intentionally scraped. Of course, in women whose cervix has been removed by surgery, Pap test samples are purposely taken from the lining of the upper vagina.[261]

As already noted, many women with VAIN may also have a similar condition involving their cervix (cervical intraepithelial neoplasia or CIN). If a Pap test finds CIN, the next step in evaluation (colposcopy) will be to thoroughly examine the cervix, the vagina, and at times the vulva.[261]

Vulvar Cancer

ACS estimates that 3740 women will be diagnosed with and 880 women will die of vulvar cancer.[1] In 2008 there will be 3740 new cases and 880 deaths from vuvlar cancer.[1]

From 2001–2005, the median age at diagnosis for cancer of the vulva was 69 years of age. Approximately 0.2% were diagnosed under age 20 years; 2.6% between age 20 and 34 years; 8.5% between age 35 and 44 years; 15.9% between age 45 and 54 years; 16.1% between age 55 and 64 years; 17.7% between age 65 and 74 years; 24.8% between age 75 and 84 years; and 14.2% at 85+ years of age.[2]

From 2001–2005, the median age at death for cancer of the vulva was 79 years of age.[4] Approximately 0.0% died under age 20; 0.7% between age 20 and 34 years; 2.5% between age 35 and 44 years; 6.5% between age 45 and 54 years; 9.8% between age 55 and 64 years; 17.3% between age 65 and 74 years; 34.1% between age 75 and 84 years; and 29.1% at 85+ years of age.

The overall 5-year relative survival rate for 1996–2004 from 17 SEER geographic areas was 76.9%. Five-year relative survival rates by race were: 77.1% for white women and 72.3% for black women.[2]

Sixty-one perecent of vulva cancer cases are diagnosed while the cancer is still confined

to the primary site (localized stage); 29% are diagnosed after the cancer has spread to regional lymphnodes or directly beyond the primary site; 4% are diagnosed after the cancer has already metastasized (distant stage); and for the remaining 6% the staging information was unknown. The corresponding 5-year relative survival rates were: 91.5% for localized; 56.1% for regional; 15.9% for distant; and 61.6% for unstaged.

The stage distribution based on histologic stage shows that 61% of vulva cancer cases are diagnosed while the cancer is still confined to the primary site (localized stage); 29% are diagnosed after the cancer has spread to regional lymph nodes or directly beyond the primary site; 4% are diagnosed after the cancer has already metastasized (distant stage); and for the remaining 6% the staging information was unknown. The corresponding 5-year relative survival rates were: 91.5% for localized; 56.1% for regional; 15.9% for distant; and 61.6% for unstaged.[2]

Vulvar cancer is primarily a disease of elderly women but has been observed in premenopausal women as well. It is most commonly squamous cell carcinoma in type, although other histological types do occur. Vulvar cancer is highly curable when diagnosed in an early stage.

Etiology

In many cases, the development of vulvar cancer is preceded by condyloma or squamous dysplasias. Prevailing evidence favors human Papillomavirus (HPV) as a causative factor in genital tract carcinomas. The labia majora is the most common site of involvement and accounts for about 50% of cases. The labia minora accounts for 15% to 20% of cases. The clitoris and Bartholin's glands are less frequently involved.[262]

Risk Factors

Several risk factors increase the odds of developing vulvar cancer, although most women with these risks do not develop it. And some women without any apparent risk factors develop vulvar cancer. When a woman develops vulvar cancer or precancerous changes, it is usually not possible to say with certainty that a particular risk factor was the cause.

Behavioral and other risk factors have been linked to the development of vulvar cancer. HPV type 16 HSVII, multiple sex partners, venereal warts, and smoking place women at an increased risk. Over the past decade, the prevalence of Vulvar Intrepithelial Neoplasm in young women has increased significantly.[263] VIN is clearly a premalignant finding and is associated with HPV infection, particularly subtypes 16 and 18. One study evaluated tissue samples from 48 patients with vulvar cancer. These patients ranged in age from 45 to 88 years. HPV DNA was detected by polymerase chain reaction in 48 percent of the specimens, of which 96% were from subtypes 16 and 18. HPV detection was not associated with age, but 71% were associated with coexisting severe (grade 3) VIN.[264]

A retrospective review of women with vulvar cancer found a statistically significant correlation between patients younger than age 45 years and HPV (RR, 11.34), cigarette smoking (RR, 2.83), having more than two sexual partners (RR, 2.87), sexual initiation before age 19 years (RR, 2.43), and low economic status (RR, 1.77). In patients older than age 45 years, there was a statistically significant correlation between VIN and vulvar cancer and VNED (RR, 23.6), residence in a rural area (RR, 2.17), low economic status (RR, 1.89), menopause

before age 45 (RR, 1.84), poor hygiene (RR, 1.76), endocrine disorders (RR, 1.94), and low serum vitamin A levels (RR, 1.78).[265]

Another study[266] of women with vulvar cancer identified an OR for vulvar cancer of 18.8 (CI 11.9 to 29.8) among current smokers who were HPV-16 seropositive, compared with women who had never smoked and were HPV-16 seronegative.

Lichen sclerosis, a type of VNED, is thought to be a predisposing factor in the development of HPV-negative vulvar cancer. According to the "itch-scratchlichen sclerosis hypothesis," lichen sclerosis, by causing a severe pruritus, sets up an itch-scratch cycle that over time causes the development of squamous cell hyperplasia. Further progression results in atypia formation, followed by VIN and eventual invasive squamous cell cancer. This hypothesis suggests that treatment of lichen sclerosis with topical steroids would prevent vulvar cancer in these patients, and some early research supports this suggestion.[267] Aggressive evaluation and treatment of VNEDs could have a dramatic impact on the incidence of vulvar cancer in this subgroup of patients. A history of chronic vulvar disease and breast cancer also increases risk.[265]

HIV is the virus that causes the acquired immunodeficiency syndrome (AIDS). Because this virus damages the body's immune system, it makes women more susceptible to persistent HPV infections, which may, in turn, increase the risk of precancerous vulvar changes and vulvar cancer. Scientists also believe that the immune system plays a role in destroying cancer cells and slowing their growth and spread.[268]

Women with vulvar cancer also have a higher risk of cervical cancer. The likely reason for this association is the role of HPV infection in causing both of these cancers. Smoking is associated with an increased risk of cervical cancer. Because of the smoking, women also have a higher risk of other smoking-related cancers.[268]

Women with a family history of melanoma or dysplastic nevi (atypical moles) elsewhere on the body are at risk for developing a melanoma on the vulva.[268] Hypertension, diabetes mellitus, and obesity have been found to coexist in up to 25% of patients, although they are not considered to be independent risk factors.[3] In the past, syphilis and other granulomatous diseases have been associated with vulvar cancer.[3] This association is unlikely, given the significant decline in incidence of syphilis since 1992.

Screening

There are no standardized guidelines for screening of vulvar cancers. It is recommended that Pap smear and pelvic examination be utilized. Biopsies and coloposcopies should be performed in areas of suspicion.[261] Vulvar self-exam provides an easy self-care technique. Because neoplasm in the genital tract is multifocal, evaluation of the vagina and cervix should be performed on women with vulvar cancer.[259]

Prevention

HPV infection is a vulvar cancer risk factor that can be reduced by avoiding certain sexual practices outlined in the section on risk factors and by delaying onset of sexual activity.[268] The earlier sexual contact with others is begun, the more likely it is that a person will become infected with HPV, and the more time any HPV infection will have to progress to cancer. For these reasons, postponing the beginning of sexual activity in life and limiting the number of sexual partners are two ways to reduce the risk of developing HPV infection and vulvar cancer.[268]

A new vaccine has been approved by the FDA that will protect against infection with HPV types 16 and 18. It is currently recommended for use in young females before they become sexually active (to prevent cervical cancers and precancers), and it is being looked at for possible use in males. While studies have not yet been done, the hope is that this may eventually help prevent other cancers linked to HPV, including vulvar cancers.[268]

Not smoking is another way to lower vulvar cancer risk, in addition to obvious benefits of greatly reducing the risk of developing far more common cancers of the lungs, mouth, throat, bladder, kidneys, and several other organs.[268]

Conclusion

Gynecologic cancer incidence and prevalence has increased over the last several decades; however, survival rates have improved as a direct result of improved screening and early detection. Nurses who provide care to these patients must be educated in identified risk factors, which can be used in educating women about risk reduction behaviors and the importance of knowing their family history.

References

1. American Cancer Society. (2008a). *Cancer facts and figures 2008*. Atlanta, GA: Author. Retrieved June 9, 2008.

2. Ries LAG, Melbert D, Krapcho M, et al, eds. *SEER Cancer Statistics Review, 1975–2005*. Bethesda, MD: National Cancer Institute, 2008. http://seer.cancer.gov/csr/1975_2005/. Based on November 2007 SEER data submission, published on the SEER web site 2008. Accessed June 5, 2008.

3. Boone, CW, Kelloff, GJ, Freedman, LS. Intraepithelial and postinvasive neoplasia as a stochastic continuum of clonal evolution, and its relationship to mechanisms of chemopreventive drug action. *J Cell Biochem.* 1993;Suppl 17G:14–25.

4. Kelloff, GJ, Boone, CW, Steele, VE, et al. Progress in cancer chemoprevention: Perspectives on agent selection and short-term clinical intervention trials. *Cancer Res.* 1994;54(Suppl 7):2015s-2024s.

5. Brinton LA, Schairer C, Hoover RN, et al. Menstrual factors and risk of breast cancer. *Cancer Invest.* 1988;6(3):245–254.

6. Furberg H, Newman B, Moorman P, et al. Lactation and breast cancer risk. *Int J Epidemiol.* 1999;28(3):396–402.

7. Knabbe C, Lippman ME, Wakefield LM, et al. Evidence that transforming growth factor-beta is a hormonally regulated negative growth factor in human breast cancer cells. *Cell.* 1987;48(3):417–428.

8. Collaborative Group on Hormonal Factors in Breast Cancer. Breast cancer and breastfeeding: collaborative reanalysis of individual data from 47 epidemiological studies in 30 countries, including 50,302 women with breast cancer and 96,973 women without the disease. *Lancet.* 2002;360(9328):187–195.

9. Smith PG, Doll R. Late effects of x irradiation in patients treated for metropathia haemorrhagica. *Br J Radiol.* 1976;49(579):224–232.

10. Trichopoulos D, MacMahon B, Cole P. Menopause and breast cancer risk. *J Natl Cancer Inst.* 1972;48(3):605–613.

11. Feinleib M. Breast cancer and artificial menopause: a cohort study[abstract]. *J Natl Cancer Inst.* 1968;41(2):315–329.

12. Kampert JB, Whittemore AS, Paffenbarger RS Jr. Combined effect of childbearing, menstrual events, and body size on age-specific breast cancer risk[abstract]. *Am J Epidemiol.* 1988;128(5):962–979.

13. Hirayama T, Wynder EL. A study of the epidemiology of cancer of the breast, II: the influence of hysterectomy. *Cancer.* 1962;15(1):28–38.

14. Pike MC, Krailo MD, Henderson BE, et al. 'Hormonal' risk factors, 'breast tissue age' and the age-incidence of breast cancer. *Nature.* 1983;303(5920):767–770.

15. Lambe M, Hsieh C, Trichopoulos D, et al. Transient increase in the risk of breast cancer after giving birth. *N Engl J Med.* 1994;331(1):5–9. http://www.ncbi.nlm.nih.gov/entrez/query.fcgi?cmd=Retrieve&db=PubMed&list_uids=8202106&dopt=Abstract

16. Henderson BE, Pike MC, Ross RK, et al. Epidemiology and risk factors. In: Bonadonna G, ed. *Breast Cancer: Diagnosis and Management.* Chichester, NY: John Wiley & Sons; 1984:15–33.

17. Collaborative Group on Hormonal Factors in Breast Cancer. Breast cancer and hormonal contraceptives: collaborative reanalysis of individual data on 53,297 women with breast cancer and 100,239 women without breast cancer from 54 epidemiological studies. *Lancet.* 1996;347(9017):1713–1727.

18. Colditz GA, Rosner BA, Speizer FE; Nurses' Health Study Research Group. Risk factors for breast cancer according to family history of breast cancer. *J Natl Cancer Inst.* 1996;88(6):365–371.

19. Collaborative Group on Hormonal Factors in Breast Cancer. Breast cancer and hormone replacement therapy: collaborative reanalysis of data from 51 epidemiological studies of 52,705 women with breast cancer and 108,411 women without breast cancer. *Lancet.* 1997;350(9084):1047–1059.

20. Chen CL, Weiss NS, Newcomb P, et al. Hormone replacement therapy in relation to breast cancer. *JAMA.* 2002;287(6):734–741.

21. Writing Group for the Women's Health Initiative Investigators. Risks and benefits of estrogen plus progestin in healthy postmenopausal women: principal results from the Women's Health Initiative randomized controlled trial. *JAMA.* 2002;288(3):321–333.

22. Steinberg KK, Thacker SB, Smith SJ, et al. A meta-analysis of the effect of estrogen replacement therapy on the risk of breast cancer. *JAMA.* 1991;265(15):1985–1990.

23. Chlebowski RT, Hendrix SL, Langer RD, et al. Influence of estrogen plus progestin on breast cancer and mammography in healthy postmenopausal women: The Women's Health Initiative Randomized Trial. *JAMA.* 2003;289(24):3243–3253.

24. Glass AG, Lacey JV Jr, Carreon JD, et al. Breast cancer incidence, 1980–2006: combined roles of menopausal hormone therapy, screening mammography, and estrogen receptor status. *J Natl Cancer Inst.* 2007;99(15):1152–1161.

25. Robbins AS, Clarke CA. Regional changes in hormone therapy use and breast cancer incidence in California from 2001 to 2004. *J Clin Oncol.* 2007;25(23): 3437–3439.

26. Kerlikowske K, Miglioretti DL, Buist DS, et al. Declines in invasive breast cancer and use of postmenopausal hormone therapy in a screening mammography population. *J Natl Cancer Inst.* 2007;99(17):1335–1339.

27. Schuurman AG, van den Brandt PA, Goldbohm RA. Exogenous hormone use and the risk of postmenopausal breast cancer: results from The Netherlands Cohort Study. *Cancer Causes Control.* 1995;6(5):416–424.

28. Sellers TA, Mink PJ, Cerhan JR, et al. The role of hormone replacement therapy in the risk for breast cancer and total mortality in women with a family history of breast cancer. *Ann Intern Med.* 1997;127(11):973–980.

29. Stanford JL, Weiss NS, Voigt LF, et al. Combined estrogen and progestin hormone replacement therapy in relation to risk of breast cancer in middle-aged women. *JAMA.* 1995;274(2):137–142.

30. Colditz GA, Egan KM, Stampfer MJ. Hormone replacement therapy and risk of breast cancer: results from epidemiologic studies. *Am J Obstet Gynecol.* 1993;168(5):1473–1480.

31. Gorsky RD, Koplan JP, Peterson HB, et al. Relative risks and benefits of long-term estrogen. *Obstetrics and Gynecology.* 1994 Feb;83(2):161–166.

32. Helzlsouer KJ, Harris EL, Parshad R, et al. Familial clustering of breast cancer: possible interaction between DNA repair proficiency and radiation exposure in the development of breast cancer. *Int J Cancer.* 1995;64(1):14–17.

33. Radimer KL, Ballard-Barbash R, Miller JS, et al. Weight change and the risk of late-onset breast cancer in the original Framingham cohort. *Nutr Cancer.* 2004;49:7–13.

34. Trentham-Dietz A, Newcomb PA, Egan KM, et al. Weight change and risk of postmenopausal breast cancer (United States). *Cancer Causes Control.* 2000;11:533–542.

35. Hamajima N, Hirose K, Tajima K, et al. Alcohol, tobacco and breast cancer—collaborative reanalysis of individual data from 53 epidemiological studies, including 58,515 women with breast cancer and 95,067 women without the disease. *Br J Cancer.* 2002;87:1234–1245.

36. Smith-Warner SA, Spiegelman D, Yaun SS, et al. Alcohol and breast cancer in women: a pooled analysis of cohort studies. *JAMA.* 1998;279:535–540.

37. Morimoto LM, White E, Chen Z, et al. Obesity, body size, and risk of postmenopausal breast cancer: The Women's Health Initiative (United States). *Cancer Causes Control.* 2002;13(8):741–751.

38. Gail MH, Brinton LA, Byar DP, et al. Projecting individualized probabilities of developing breast cancer for white females who are being examined annually. *J Natl Cancer Inst.* 1989;81(24):1879–1886.

39. Dupont WD, Page DL. Risk factors for breast cancer in women with proliferative breast disease. *N Engl J Med.* 1985;312(3):146–151.

40. Carter CL, Corle DK, Micozzi MS, et al. A prospective study of the development of breast cancer in 16,692 women with benign breast disease. *Am J Epidemiol.* 1988;128(3):467–477.

41. London SJ, Connolly JL, Schnitt SJ, et al. A prospective study of benign breast disease and the risk of breast cancer. *JAMA.* 1992;267(7):941–944.

42. Dupont WD, Page DL, Parl FF, et al. Long-term risk of breast cancer in women with fibroadenoma. *N Engl J Med.* 1994;331(1):10–15.

43. Boyd NF, Byng JW, Jong RA, et al. Quantitative classification of mammographic densities and breast cancer risk: results from the Canadian National Breast Screening Study. *J Natl Cancer Inst.* 1995;87(9):670–675.

44. Byrne C, Schairer C, Wolfe J, et al. Mammographic features and breast cancer risk: effects with time, age, and menopause status. *J Natl Cancer Inst.* 1995;87(21):1622–1629.

45. Pankow JS, Vachon CM, Kuni CC, et al. Genetic analysis of mammographic breast density in adult women: evidence of a gene effect. *J Natl Cancer Inst.* 1997;89(8):549–556.

46. Boyd NF, Lockwood GA, Martin LJ, et al. Mammographic densities and risk of breast cancer among subjects with a family history of this disease. *J Natl Cancer Inst.* 1999;91(16):1404–1408.

47. Vachon CM, King RA, Atwood LD, et al. Preliminary sibpair linkage analysis of percent mammographic density. *J Natl Cancer Inst.* 1999;91(20):1778–1779.

48. Kelsey JL, Gammon MD. The epidemiology of breast cancer. *CA Cancer J Clin.* May-June 1991;41(3):146–165.

49. Singletary SE, Taylor SH, Guinee VF, et al. Occurrence and prognosis of contralateral carcinoma of the breast. *J Am Coll Surg.* 1994;178(4):390–396.

50. Cook LS, White E, Schwartz SM, et al. A population-based study of contralateral breast cancer following a first primary breast cancer (Washington, United States). *Cancer Causes Control.* 1996;7(3):382–390.

51. Habel LA, Moe RE, Daling JR, et al. Risk of contralateral breast cancer among women with carcinoma in situ of the breast. *Ann Surg.* 1997;225(1):69–75.

52. Bodian CA, Perzin KH, Lattes R. Lobular neoplasia. Long term risk of breast cancer and relation to other factors. *Cancer.* 1996;78(5):1024–1034.

53. Yang Q, Khoury MJ, Rodriguez C, et al. Family history score as a predictor of breast cancer mortality: prospective data from the Cancer Prevention Study II, United States, 1982–1991. *Am J Epidemiol.* 1998;147(7):652–659.

54. Colditz GA, Willett WC, Hunter DJ, et al. Family history, age, and risk of breast cancer. Prospective data from the Nurses' Health Study. *JAMA.* 1993;270(3):338–343.

55. Slattery ML, Kerber RA. A comprehensive evaluation of family history and breast cancer risk. The Utah Population Database. *JAMA.* 1993;270(13): 1563–1568.

56. Johnson N, Lancaster T, Fuller A, et al. The prevalence of a family history of cancer in general practice. *Fam Pract.* 1995;12(3):287–289.

57. Pharoah PD, Day NE, Duffy S, et al. Family history and the risk of breast cancer: a systematic review and meta-analysis. *Int J Cancer.* 1997;71(5):800–809.

58. Negri E, Braga C, La Vecchia C, et al. Family history of cancer and risk of breast cancer. *Int J Cancer.* 1997;72(5):735–738.

59. Hemminki K, Vaittinen P. Familial breast cancer in the family—cancer database. *Int J Cancer.* 1998;77(3):386–391.

60. Kerber RA, Slattery ML. The impact of family history n ovarian cancer risk. The Utah Population Database. *Arch Med.* 1995;155(9):905–912.

61. Auranen A, Pukkala E, Mäkinen J, et al. Cancer incidence in the first-degree relatives of ovarian cancer patients. *Br J Cancer.* 1996;74(2):280–284.

62. Couch FJ, DeShano ML, Blackwood MA, et al. BRCA1 mutations in women attending clinics that evaluate the risk of breast cancer. *N Engl J Med.* 1997;336(20):1409–1415.

63. Shattuck-Eidens D, Oliphant A, McClure M, et al. BRCA1 sequence analysis in women at high risk for susceptibility mutations. Risk factor analysis and implications for genetic testing. *JAMA.* 1997;278(15):1242–1250.

64. Smith RA, Saslow D, Sawyer KA, et al. American Cancer Society guidelines for breast cancer screening: update 2003. *CA Cancer J Clin.* 2003;53:141–169.

65. National Cancer Institute. *Breast cancer PDQ.* Bethesda, MD: Author; 2008.

66. American Cancer Society. *Endometrial (Uterine Cancer).* Atlanta, GA: Author; 2008.

67. American College of Obstetricians and Gynecologists. Protect and detect: what women should know about cancer. Accessed June 5, 2008.

68. Prentice RL, Caan B, Chlebowski RT, et al. Low-fat dietary pattern and risk of invasive breast cancer: The Women's Health Initiative Randomized Controlled Dietary Modification Trial. *JAMA.* 2006;295(6): 629–642.

69. Smith-Warner SA, Spiegelman D, Yaun SS, et al. Intake of fruits and vegetables and risk of breast cancer: a pooled analysis of cohort studies. *JAMA.* 2001;285(6):769–776.

70. Zhang S, Hunter DJ, Forman MR, et al. Dietary carotenoids and vitamins A, C, and E and risk of breast cancer. *J Natl Cancer Inst.* 1999;91(6):547–556.

71. Bohlke K, Spiegelman D, Trichopoulou A, et al. Vitamins A, C and E and the risk of breast cancer: results from a case-control study in Greece. *Br J Cancer.* 1999;79(1):23–29.

72. Veronesi U, De Palo G, Marubini E, et al. Randomized trial of fenretinide to prevent second breast malignancy in women with early breast cancer. *J Natl Cancer Inst.* 1999;91(21):1847–1856.

73. Bernstein L, Henderson BE, Hanisch R, et al. Physical exercise and reduced risk of breast cancer in young women. *J Natl Cancer Inst.* 1994;86(18):1403–1408.

74. Friedenreich CM. Physical activity and cancer prevention: from observational to intervention research. *Cancer Epidemiol Biomarkers Prev.* 2001;10(4): 287–301.

75. Thune I, Brenn T, Lund E, et al. Physical activity and the risk of breast cancer. *N Engl J Med.* 1997;336(18):1269–1275.

76. National Cancer Institute. *Breast Cancer Prevention Studies 2008*. Bethesda, MD: Author; 2008.

77. Fisher B, Costantino JP, Wickerham DL, et al. Tamoxifen for prevention of breast cancer: report of the National Surgical Adjuvant Breast and Bowel Project P–1 Study. *J Natl Cancer Inst.* 1998;90(18):1371–1388.

78. Victor G, Vogel JP, Costantino DL, et al. National Surgical Adjuvant Breast and Bowel Project (NSABP). Effects of tamoxifen vs raloxifene on the risk of developing invasive breast cancer and other disease outcomes: the NSABP study of tamoxifen and raloxifene (STAR) P-2 trial. *JAMA.* June 21, 2006;295:2727–2741.

79. Thull DL, Vogel VG. Recognition and management of hereditary breast cancer syndromes. *Oncologist.* 2004;9(1):13–24.

80. Stefanek M, Hartmann L, Nelson W. Risk-reduction mastectomy: clinical issues and research needs. *J Natl Cancer Inst.* 2001;93(17):1297–1306.

81. Hartmann LC, Schaid DJ, Woods JE, et al. Efficacy of bilateral prophylactic mastectomy in women with a family history of breast cancer. *N Engl J Med.* 1999;340(2):77–84.

82. Rebbeck TR, Lynch HT, Neuhausen SL, et al. Prophylactic oophorectomy in carriers of BRCA1 or BRCA2 mutations. *N Engl J Med.* 2002;346(21):1616–1622.

83. Yancik R, Ries LG, Yates JW. Ovarian cancer in the elderly: an analysis of surveillance, epidemiology, and end results program data. *Am J Obstet Gynecol.* 1986;154:639–647.

84. Riman T, Persson I, Nilsson S. Hormonal aspects of epithelial ovarian cancer: review of epidemiological evidence. *Clin Endocrinol.* 1998;49(6):695–707.

85. Fathalla, MF. Incessant Ovulation—A factor in ovarian neoplasia? *Lancet.* 1971; 2(7716), 163.

86. Cramer DW, Welch WR. Determinants of ovarian cancer risk. II. Inferences regarding pathogenesis. *J Natl Cancer Inst.* 1983;71(4):717–721.

87. Risch HA. Hormonal etiology of epithelial ovarian cancer, with a hypothesis concerning the role of androgens and progesterone. *J Natl Cancer Inst.* 1998;90(23):1774–1786.

88. Helzlsouer KJ, Alberg AJ, Gordon GB, et al. Serum gonadotropins and steroid hormones and the development of ovarian cancer. *JAMA.* 1995;274(24): 1926–1930.

89. Daly M, Obrams GI. Epidemiology and risk assessment for ovarian cancer. *Semin Oncol.* 1998;25:255–264.

90. Greene MH, Clark JW, Blayney DW. The epidemiology of ovarian cancer. *Semin Oncol.* 1984;11:209–211.

91. Stratton JF, Pharoah P, Smith SK, et al. A systematic review and meta-analysis of family history and risk of ovarian cancer. *Br J Obstet Gynaecol.* 1998;105(5):493–499.

92. Lacey JV Jr, Mink PJ, Lubin JH, et al. Menopausal hormone replacement therapy and risk of ovarian cancer. *JAMA.* 2002;288(3):334–341.

93. Anderson GL, Judd HL, Kaunitz AM, et al. Effects of estrogen plus progestin on gynecologic cancers and associated diagnostic procedures: The Women's Health Initiative randomized trial. *JAMA.* 2003;290(13):1739–1748.

94. Whittemore AS, Harris R, Itnyre J; Collaborative Ovarian Cancer Group. Characteristics relating to ovarian cancer risk: collaborative analysis of 12 US case-control studies. II. Invasive epithelial ovarian cancers in white women. *Am J Epidemiol.* 1992;136(10): 1184–1203.

95. Ozols RF, Rubin SC, Thomas GM, Robboy SJ. Epithelial ovarian cancer. In: Hoskins WJ, et al, eds. *Principles and Practice of Gynecologic Oncology.* 4th ed. Philadelphia, PA: Lippincott, Williams and Wilkins; 2005:895–988.

96. Boyd J. Molecular genetics of hereditary ovarian cancer. *Oncol.* 1998;12:399–406.

97. Rubin SC, Benjamin I, Behbakht K, et al. Clinical and pathological features of ovarian cancer in women with germ-line mutations of BRACA1. *N Engl J Med.* 1996;335:1413–1416.

98. Boyd J, Rubin SC. Hereditary ovarian cancer: molecular genetics and clinical implications. *Gynecol Oncol.* 1997;64:196–206.

99. Levine DA, Argenta PA, Yee CJ, et al. Fallopian tube and primary peritoneal carcinomas associated with BRCA mutations. *J Clin Oncol.* 2003;21:4222–4227.

100. Amos CI, Struewing JP. Genetic epidemiology of epithelial ovarian cancer. *Cancer.* 1993;71(Suppl 2):566–572.

101. Heintz AP, Hacker NF, Lagasse LD. Epidemiology and etiology of ovarian cancer: a review. *Obstet Gynecol.* 1985;66(1):127–135.

102. Tortolero-Luna G, Mitchell MF. The epidemiology of ovarian cancer. *J Cell Biochem.* 1995;Suppl. 23: 200–207.

103. Hankinson SE, Hunter DJ, Colditz GA, et al. Tubal ligation, hysterectomy, and risk of ovarian

cancer. A prospective study. *JAMA*. 1993;270(23):2813–2818.

104. Gertig DM, Hunter DJ, Cramer DW, et al. Prospective study of talc use and ovarian cancer. *J Natl Cancer Inst*. 2003;92(3):249–252.

105. Schouten LJ, Goldbohm RA, van den Brandt PA. Height, weight, weight change, and ovarian cancer risk in the Netherlands cohort study on diet and cancer. *Am J Epidemiol*. 2003;157(5):424–433.

106. Engeland A, Tretli S, Bjørge T. Height, body mass index, and ovarian cancer: A follow-up of 1.1 million Norwegian women. *J Natl Cancer Inst*. 2003;95(16):1244–1248.

107. Mettlin CJ, Piver MS. A case-control study of milk-drinking and ovarian cancer risk. *Am J Epidemiol*. 1990;132(5):871–876.

108. Cramer DW, Harlow BL, Willett WC, et al. Galactose consumption and metabolism in relation to the risk of ovarian cancer. *Lancet*. 1989;2(8654):66–71.

109. Risch HA, Jain M, Marrett LD, et al. Dietary lactose intake, lactose intolerance, and the risk of epithelial ovarian cancer in southern Ontario (Canada). *Cancer Causes Control*. 1994;5(6):540–548.

110. Shu XO, Gao YT, Yuan JM, et al. Dietary factors and epithelial ovarian cancer. *Br J Cancer*. 1989;59(1):92–96.

111. Risch HA, Jain M, Marrett LD, et al. Dietary fat intake and risk of epithelial ovarian cancer. *J Natl Cancer Inst*. 1994;86(18):1409–1415.

112. Helzlsouer KJ, Alberg AJ, Norkus EP, et al. Prospective study of serum micronutrients and ovarian cancer. *J Natl Cancer Inst*. 1996;88(1):32–37.

113. Hiatt RA, Fireman BH. Serum cholesterol and the incidence of cancer in a large cohort. *J Chronic Dis*. 1986;39(11):861–870.

114. Kushi LH, Mink PJ, Folsom AR, et al. Prospective study of diet and ovarian cancer. *Am J Epidemiol*. 1999;149(1):21–31.

115. Fairfield KM, Hankinson SE, Rosner BA, et al. Risk of ovarian carcinoma and consumption of vitamins A, C, and E and specific carotenoids: a prospective analysis. *Cancer*. 2001;92(9):2318–2326.

116. Garland M, Morris JS, Stampfer MJ, et al. (1995). Prospective study of toenail selenium levels and cancer among women. *J Natl Cancer Inst*. 1995;87(7):497–505.

117. Smith LH, Oi RH. Detection of malignant ovarian neoplasms: a review of the literature. I. Detection of the patient at risk; clinical, radiological and cytological detection. *Obstet Gynecol Surv*. 1984;39(6):313–328.

118. Hall DJ, Hurt WG. (1982). The adnexal mass. *J Fam Pract*. 1982;14(1):135–140.

119. Keettel WC, Pixley EE, Buchsbaum HJ. Experience with peritoneal cytology in the management of gynecologic malignancies. *Am J Obstet Gynecol*. 1974;120(2):174–182.

120. Buys SS, Partridge E, Greene MH, et al. Ovarian cancer screening in the Prostate, Lung, Colorectal and Ovarian (PLCO) cancer screening trial: findings from the initial screen of a randomized trial. *Am J Obstet Gynecol*. 2005;193(5):1630–1639.

121. Bast RC Jr, Feeney M, Lazarus H, et al. Reactivity of a monoclonal antibody with human ovarian carcinoma. *J Clin Invest*. 1981;68(5):1331–1337.

122. Bast RC Jr, Klug TL, St John E, et al. A radioimmunoassay using a monoclonal antibody to monitor the course of epithelial ovarian cancer. *N Engl J Med*. 1983;309(15):883–887.

123. Jacobs I, Stabile I, Bridges J, et al. Multimodal approach to screening for ovarian cancer. *Lancet*. 1988;1(8580):268–271.

124. Gohagan JK, Levin DL, Prorok JC, et al, eds. The Prostate, Lung, Colorectal and Ovarian (PLCO) cancer screening trial. *Control Clin Trials*. 2000;21(Suppl 6):249S–406S.

125. Niloff JM, Knapp RC, Schaetzl E, et al. CA125 antigen levels in obstetric and gynecologic patients. *Obstet Gynecol*. 1984;64(5):703–707.

126. Haga Y, Sakamoto K, Egami H, et al. Evaluation of serum CA125 values in healthy individuals and pregnant women. *Am J Med Sci*. 1986;292(1):25–29.

127. Jacobs I, Bast RC Jr. The CA 125 tumour-associated antigen: a review of the literature. *Hum Reprod*. 1989;4(1):1–12.

128. Helzlsouer KJ, Bush TL, Alberg AJ, et al. Prospective study of serum CA-125 levels as markers of ovarian cancer. *JAMA*. 1993;269(9):1123–1126.

129. Jacobs I, Davies AP, Bridges J, et al. Prevalence screening for ovarian cancer in postmenopausal women by CA 125 measurement and ultrasonography. *BMJ*. 1993;306(6884):1030–1034.

130. Einhorn N, Sjövall K, Knapp RC, et al. Prospective evaluation of serum CA 125 levels for early detection of ovarian cancer. *Obst Gynecol*. 1992;80(1):14–18.

131. Zhang Z, Bast RC Jr, Yu Y, et al. Three biomarkers identified from serum proteomic analysis for the detection of early stage ovarian cancer. *Cancer Res*. 2004;64(16):5882–5890.

132. Petricoin EF, Ardekani AM, Hitt BA, et al. Use of proteomic patterns in serum to identify ovarian cancer. *Lancet.* 2002;359(9306):572–577.

133. Lafky JM, Maihle NJ. The parable of the proteome: cancer biomarkers. *Trends Cell Biol.* 2002;12:358.

134. Daly MB, Ozols RF. The search for predictive patterns in ovarian cancer: proteomics meets bioinformatics. *Cancer Cell.* 2002;1(2):111–112.

135. Hankinson SE, Colditz GA, Hunter DJ, et al. A quantitative assessment of oral contraceptive use and risk of ovarian cancer. *Obstet Gynecol.* 1992;80(4):708–714.

136. Higgins RV, van Nagell JR Jr, Woods CH, et al. Interobserver variation in ovarian measurements using transvaginal sonography. *Gynecol Oncol.* 1990;39(1):69–71.

137. Centers for Disease Control and the National Institute of Child Health and Human Development. The reduction in risk of ovarian cancer associated with oral-contraceptive use. *N Engl J Med.* 1987;316(11):650–655.

138. McGuire V, Feldberg A, Mills M, et al. Relation of contraceptive and reproductive history to ovarian cancer risk in carriers and noncarriers of BRCA1 gene mutations. *Am J Epidemiol.* 2004;160(7):613–618.

139. Narod SA, Risch H, Moslehi R, et al; Hereditary Ovarian Cancer Clinical Study Group. Oral contraceptives and the risk of hereditary ovarian cancer. *N Engl J Med.* 1998;339(7):424–428.

140. Guillem JG, Wood WC, Moley JF, et al. ASCO/SSO review of current role of risk-reducing surgery in common hereditary cancer syndromes. *J Clin Oncol.* 2006;24(28):4642–4660.

141. Casey MJ, Snyder C, Bewtra C, Narod SA, Watson P, Lynch HT. Intra-abdominal carcinomatosis after prophylactic oophorectomy in women of hereditary breast ovarian cancer syndrome kindreds associated with BRCA1 and BRCA2 mutations. *Gynecol Oncol.* 2005;99(2):520–521.

142. Trimble EL, Karlan BY, Lagasse LD, et al. Diagnosing the correct ovarian cancer syndrome. *Obstet Gynecol.* 1991;78(6):1023–1026.

143. Committee on Gynecologic Practice. Genetic risk and screening techniques for epithelial ovarian cancer. ACOG Committee Opinion: Committee on Gynecologic Practice. (Number 117). *Intl J Gynaecol Obstet.* 1992;41(3):321–323.

144. Kerlikowske K, Brown JS, Grady DG. Should women with familial ovarian cancer undergo prophylactic oophorectomy? *Obstet Gynecol.* 1992;80(4):700–707.

145. National Cancer Institute. *Cervical cancer PDQ.* Health professional version. Bethesda, MD: Author. Accessed June 5, 2008.

146. zur Hausen H, de Villiers EM. Human papillomaviruses. *Annu Rev Microbiol.* 1994;48:427–447.

147. Schiffman MH, Bauer HM, Hoover RN, et al. Epidemiologic evidence showing that human papillomavirus infection causes most cervical intraepithelial neoplasia. *J Natl Cancer Inst.* 1993;85(12):958–964.

148. Mahdavi A, Monk BJ. Vaccines against human papillomavirus and cervical cancer: promises and challenges. *Oncologist.* 2005;10:528–538.

149. Goldstone SE, Winkler B, Ufford LJ, et al. High prevalence of anal squamous intraepithelial lesions and squamous-cell carcinoma in men who have sex with men as seen in a surgical practice. *Dis Colon Rectum.* 2001;44:690–698.

150. Nobbenhuis MA, Walboomers JM, Helmerhorst TJ, et al. Relation of human papillomavirus status to cervical lesions and consequences for cervical-cancer screening: a prospective study. *Lancet.* 1999;354:20–25.

151. Brinton LA. Epidemiology of cervical cancer—overview. *IARC Sci Pub.* 1992;119:3–23.

152. Hellberg D, Nilsson S, Haley NJ, et al. Smoking and cervical intraepithelial neoplasia: nicotine and cotinine in serum and cervical mucus in smokers and nonsmokers. *Am J Obstet Gynecol.* 1988;158(4):910–913.

153. Brock KE, MacLennan R, Brinton LA, et al. Smoking and infectious agents and risk of in situ cervical cancer in Sydney, Australia. *Cancer Res.* 1989;49(17):4925–4928.

154. Ho GY, Kadish AS, Burk RD, et al. HPV 16 and cigarette smoking as risk factors for high-grade cervical intra-epithelial neoplasia. *Intl J Cancer.* 1998;78(3):281–285.

155. Muñoz N, Franceschi S, Bosetti C, et al. Role of parity and human papillomavirus in cervical cancer: The IARC multicentric case-control study. *Lancet.* 2002;359(9312):1093–1101.

156. Mandell GL, Mildvan D, eds. *Atlas of Infectious Diseases.* 2nd ed. Edinburgh, Scotland: Churchill Livingstone; 1997.

157. Kreiss JK, Kiviat NB, Plummer FA, et al. Human immunodeficiency virus, human papillomavirus,

and cervical intraepithelial neoplasia in Nairobi prostitutes. *Sex Transm Dis.* 1992;19:54–59.

158. Wright TC Jr, Ellerbrock TV, Chiasson MA, et al. The New York Cervical Disease Study. Cervical intraepithelial neoplasia in women infected with human immunodeficiency virus. *Obstet Gynecol.* 1994;84:591–597.

159. Laga M, Icenogle JP, Marsella R, et al. Genital papillomavirus infection and cervical dysplasia. *Intl J Cancer.* 1992;50:45–48.

160. Marte C, Kelly P, Cohen M, et al. Papanicolaou smear abnormalities in ambulatory care sites for women infected with the human immunodeficiency virus. *Am J Obstet Gynecol.* 1992;166:1232–1237.

161. Chiasson M, Kelley K, Vazquez F, et al. Incidence of invasive cervical cancer in HIV seropositive women in New York City. Second AIDS and Malignancy Conference; April 1998; Bethesda, MD.

162. Chin KM, Sidhu JS, Janssen RS, Weber JT. Invasive cervical cancer in human immunodeficiency virus-infected and uninfected hospital patients. *Obstet Gynecol.* 1998;92:83–87.

163. Maiman M, Fruchter RG, Serur E, Boyce JG. Prevalence of human immunodeficiency virus in a colposcopy clinic. *JAMA.* 1988;260:2214–2215.

164. Smith RA, Cokkinides V, Eyre HJ. American Cancer Society guidelines for the early detection of cancer, 2006. *CA Cancer J Clin.* 2006;56:11–25.

165. National Cancer Institute. *Cervical cancer PDQ: Prevention.* Health professional version. Bethesda, MD: Author. Accessed June 5, 2008.

166. Saslow D, Runowicz CD, Solomon D, et al. American Cancer Society guideline for the early detection of cervical neoplasia and cancer. *CA Cancer J Clin.* 2002;52:342–362.

167. Lǎǎrǎ E, Day NE, Hakama M. Trends in mortality from cervical cancer in the Nordic countries: association with organised screening programmes. *Lancet.* 1987;1(8544):1247–1249.

168. Christopherson WM, Lundin FE Jr, Mendez WM, et al. Cervical cancer control: a study of morbidity and mortality trends over a twenty-one-year period. *Cancer.* 1976;38(3):1357–1366.

169. Miller AB, Lindsay J, Hill GB. Mortality from cancer of the uterus in Canada and its relationship to screening for cancer of the cervix. *Intl J Cancer.* 1976;17(5):602–612.

170. Johannesson G, Geirsson G, Day N. The effect of mass screening in Iceland, 1965–74, on the inci-

dence and mortality of cervical carcinoma. *Intl J Cancer.* 1978;21(4):418–425.

171. Aristizabal N, Cuello C, Correa P, et al. (1984). The impact of vaginal cytology on cervical cancer risks in Cali, Colombia. *Intl J Cancer.* 1984;34(1):5–9.

172. Clarke EA, Anderson TW. Does screening by "Pap" smears help prevent cervical cancer? A case-control study. *Lancet.* 1979;2(8132):1–4.

173. La Vecchia C, Franceschi S, Decarli A, et al. "Pap" smear and the risk of cervical neoplasia: quantitative estimates from a case-control study. *Lancet.* 1984;2(8406):779–782.

174. Herrero R, Brinton LA, Reeves WC, et al. Screening for cervical cancer in Latin America: a case-control study. *Intl J Epidemiol.* 1992;21(6):1050–1056.

175. Celentano DD, Klassen AC, Weisman CS, et al. Duration of relative protection of screening for cervical cancer. *Prev Med.* 1989;18(4):411–422.

176. IARC Working Group on Evaluation of Cervical Cancer Screening Programmes. Screening for squamous cervical cancer: duration of low risk after negative results of cervical cytology and its implication for screening policies. Clinical research edition. *Br Med J.* 1986;293(6548):659–664.

177. Kleinman JC, Kopstein A. Who is being screened for cervical cancer? *Am J Public Health.* 1981;71(1):73–76.

178. Bidus MA, Zahn CM, Maxwell GL, Rodriguez M, Elkas JC, Rose GS. The role of self-collection devices for cytology and human papillomavirus DNA testing in cervical cancer screening. *Clin Obstet Gynecol.* 2005;48:127–132.

179. Nuovo J, Melnikow J, Howell LP. New tests for cervical cancer screening. *Am Fam Physician.* 2001;64:780–786.

180. Bundrick JB, Cook DA, Gostout BS. Screening for cervical cancer and initial treatment of patients with abnormal results from Papanicolaou testing. *Mayo Clin Proc.* 2005;80:1063–1068.

181. O'Meara AT. Present standards for cervical cancer screening. *Curr Opin Oncol.* 2002;14:505–511.

182. Raffle AE, Alden B, Quinn M, et al. Outcomes of screening to prevent cancer: analysis of cumulative incidence of cervical abnormality and modelling of cases and deaths prevented. *BMJ.* 2003;326(7395):901.

183. Farley J, McBroom JW, Zahn CM. Current techniques for the evaluation of abnormal cervical cytology. *Clin Obstet Gynecol.* 2005;48:133–146.

184. Andy C, Turner LF, Neher JO. Clinical inquiries. Is the ThinPrep better than conventional Pap smear at detecting cervical cancer? *J Fam Prac.* 2004;53: 313–315.

185. Schooff M, Lawlor A. What is the best collection device for screening cervical smears? *Am Fam Physician.* 2004;69:1661–1662.

186. Russell J, Crothers BA, Kaplan KJ, Zahn CM. Current cervical screening technology considerations: liquid-based cytology and automated screening. *Clin Obstet Gynecol.* 2005;48:108–119.

187. Solomon D, Schiffman M, Tarone R, et al. Comparison of three management strategies for patients with atypical squamous cells of undetermined significance: baseline results from a randomized trial. *J Natl Cancer Inst.* 2001;93(4):293–299.

188. Schiffman M, Adrianza ME. ASCUS-LSIL Triage Study. Design, methods and characteristics of trial participants. *Acta Cytol.* 2000;44(5):726–742.

189. Soost HJ, Lange HJ, Lehmacher W, et al. The validation of cervical cytology. Sensitivity, specificity and predictive values. *Acta Cytol.* 1991;35(1):8–14.

190. Benoit AG, Krepart GV, Lotocki RJ. Results of prior cytologic screening in patients with a diagnosis of Stage I carcinoma of the cervix. *Am J Obstet Gynecol.* 1984;148(5):690–694.

191. Nanda K, McCrory DC, Myers ER, et al. Accuracy of the Papanicolaou test in screening for and follow-up of cervical cytologic abnormalities: a systematic review. *Ann Intern Med.* 2000;132(10):810–819.

192. Martin-Hirsch P, Lilford R, Jarvis G, et al. Efficacy of cervical-smear collection devices: a systematic review and meta-analysis. *Lancet.* 1999;354(9192): 1763–1770.

193. Hildesheim A, Brinton LA, Mallin K, et al. Barrier and spermicidal contraceptive methods and risk of invasive cervical cancer. *Epidemiol.* 1990;1(4): 266–272.

194. Celentano DD, Klassen AC, Weisman CS, et al. The role of contraceptive use in cervical cancer: The Maryland Cervical Cancer Case-Control Study. *Am J Epidemiol.* 1987;126(4):592–604.

195. Miller BE, Flax SD, Arheart K, et al. The presentation of adenocarcinoma of the uterine cervix. *Cancer.* 1993;72(4):1281–1285.

196. Koutsky LA, Ault KA, Wheeler CM, et al. A controlled trial of a human papillomavirus type 16 vaccine. *N Engl J Med.* 2002;347:1645–1651.

197. Villa LL, Costa RL, Petta CA, et al. Prophylactic quadrivalent human papillomavirus (types 6,

11, 16, and 18) L1 virus-like particle vaccine in young women: a randomised double-blind placebo-controlled multicentre phase II efficacy trial. *Lancet Oncol.* 2005;6:271–278.

198. Harper DM, Franco EL, Wheeler C, et al. Efficacy of a bivalent L1 virus-like particle vaccine in prevention of infection with human papillomavirus types 16 and 18 in young women: a randomised controlled trial. *Lancet.* 2004;364:1757–1765.

199. Harper DM, Franco EL, Wheeler CM, et al. Sustained efficacy up to 4.5 years of a bivalent L1 virus-like particle vaccine against human papillomavirus types 16 and 18: follow-up from a randomised control trial. *Lancet.* 2006;367:1247–1255.

200. Merck. Merck's investigational vaccine GARDASIL™ prevented 100 percent of cervical pre-cancers and non-invasive cervical cancers associated with HPV types 16 and 18 in new clinical study. http://www.merck.com/newsroom/press_releases/research_and_development/2005_1006.html. Published 2006. Accessed May 16, 2006.

201. Monk BJ, Wiley DJ. Will widespread human papillomavirus prophylactic vaccination change sexual practices of adolescent and young adult women in America? *Obstet Gynecol.* 2006;108:420–424.

202. Centers for Disease Control and Prevention. Advisory committee on immunization practices (ACIP) of the Centers for Disease Control and Prevention. http://www.cdc.gov/nip/ACIP/. Accessed May 16, 2006.

203. Garland SM, Hernandez-Avila M, Wheeler CM, et al. Quadrivalent vaccine against human papillomavirus to prevent anogenital diseases. *N Engl J Med.* 2007;356(19):1928–1943.

204. Howe HL. Age-specific hysterectomy and oophorectomy prevalence rates and the risks for cancer of the reproductive system. *Am J Public Health.* 1984;74(6):560–563.

205. Jick H, Walker AM, Rothman KJ. The epidemic of endometrial cancer: a commentary. *Am J Public Health.* 1980;70(3):264–267.

206. The Merck Manual for Health Care Professionals online. Endometrial cancer. Accessed October 29, 2006.

207. National Cancer Institute. *Endometrial cancer PDQ: Prevention.* Health professional version. Accessed June 5, 2008.

208. Barrett RJ 2nd, Harlan LC, Wesley MN, et al. Endometrial cancer: stage at diagnosis and associated factors in black and white patients. *Am J Obstet Gynecol.* 1995;173(2):414–423.

209. Coates RJ, Click LA, Harlan LC, et al. Differences between black and white patients with cancer of the uterine corpus in interval from symptom recognition to initial medical consultation (United States). *Cancer Causes Control.* 1996;7(3):328–336.

210. Madison T, Schottenfeld D, James SA, et al. Endometrial cancer: socioeconomic status and racial/ethnic differences in stage at diagnosis, treatment, and survival. *Am J Public Health.* 2004;94(12):2104–2111.

211. Smith DC, Prentice R, Thompson DJ, et al. Association of exogenous estrogen and endometrial carcinoma. *N Engl J Med.* 1975;293(23):1164–1167.

212. Mack TM, Pike MC, Henderson BE, et al. Estrogens and endometrial cancer in a retirement community. *N Engl J Med.* 1976;294(23):1262–1267.

213. Ziel HK, Finkle WD. Increased risk of endometrial carcinoma among users of conjugated estrogens. *N Engl J Med.* 1975;293(23):1167–1176.

214. Walker AM, Jick H. Cancer of the corpus uteri: increasing incidence in the United States, 1970–1975. *Am J Epidemiol.* 1979;110(1):47–51.

215. Gray LA Sr, Christopherson WM, Hoover RN. Estrogens and endometrial carcinoma. *Obstet Gynecol.* 1977;49(4):385–389.

216. McDonald TW, Annegers JF, O'Fallon WM, et al. Exogenous estrogen and endometrial carcinoma: case-control and incidence study. *Am J Obstet Gynecol.* 1977;127(6):572–580.

217. Antunes CM, Strolley PD, Rosenshein NB, et al. Endometrial cancer and estrogen use. Report of a large case-control study. *N Engl J Med.* 1979;300(1):9–13.

218. Shapiro S, Kelly JP, Rosenberg L, et al. Risk of localized and widespread endometrial cancer in relation to recent and discontinued use of conjugated estrogens. *N Engl J Med.* 1985;313(16):969–972.

219. Fisher B, Costantino JP, Redmond CK, Fisher ER, Wickerham DL, Cronin WM. Endometrial cancer in tamoxifen-treated breast cancer patients: findings from the National Surgical Adjuvant Breast and Bowel Project (NSABP) B-14. *J Natl Cancer Inst.* 1994;86:527–537.

220. Purdie DM, Green AC. Epidemiology of endometrial cancer. *Best Pract Res Clin Obstet Gynaecol.* 2001;15(3):341–354.

221. Enriori CL, Reforzo-Membrives J. Peripheral aromatization as a risk factor for breast and endometrial cancer in postmenopausal women: a review. *Gynecol Oncol.* 1984;17(1):1–21.

222. Davidson BJ, Gambone JC, Lagasse LD, et al. Free estradiol in postmenopausal women with and without endometrial cancer. *J Clin Endocrinol Metab.* 1981;52(3):404–408.

223. Troisi R, Potischman N, Hoover RN, et al. Insulin and endometrial cancer. *Am J Epidemiol.* 1997;146(6):476–482.

224. Watson P, Vasen HF, Mecklin JP, et al. The risk of endometrial cancer in hereditary nonpolyposis colorectal cancer. *Am J Med.* 1994;96(6):516–520.

225. Aarnio M, Mecklin JP, Aaltonen LA, et al. Life-time risk of different cancers in hereditary non-polyposis colorectal cancer (HNPCC) syndrome. *Int J Cancer.* 1995;64(6):430–433.

226. Aarnio M, Sankila R, Pukkala E, et al. Cancer risk in mutation carriers of DNA-mismatch-repair genes. *Int J Cancer.* 1999;81(2):214–218.

227. Berends MJ, Wu Y, Sijmons RH, et al. Toward new strategies to select young endometrial cancer patients for mismatch repair gene mutation analysis. *J Clin Oncol.* 2003;21(23):4364–4370.

228. Boks DE, Trujillo AP, Voogd AC, et al. Survival analysis of endometrial carcinoma associated with hereditary nonpolyposis colorectal cancer. *Int J Cancer.* 2002;102(2):198–200.

229. Pritchard KI. Screening for endometrial cancer: is it effective? *Ann Intern Med.* 1989;110(3):177–179.

230. Eddy D. ACS report on the cancer-related health checkup. *CA Cancer J Clin.* 1980;30(4):193–240.

231. Burke W, Petersen G, Lynch P, et al; Cancer Genetics Studies Consortium. Recommendations for follow-up care of individuals with an inherited predisposition to cancer. I. Hereditary nonpolyposis colon cancer. *JAMA.* 1997;277(11):915–919.

232. Tiffen JM, Mahon SM. Educating women regarding the early detection of endometrial cancer—what is the evidence? *Clin J Oncol Nurs.* 2006;10(1):102–104.

233. National Cancer Institute. *Endometrial cancer PDQ: Screening.* Health professional version. http://www.nci.nih.gov/cancertopics/pdq/screening/endometrial/healthprofessional. Accessed June 5, 2008.

234. Smith RA, von Eschenbach AC, Wender R, et al. American Cancer Society guidelines for the early detection of cancer: update of early detection guidelines for prostate, colorectal, and endometrial cancers. *CA Cancer J Clin.* 2001;51:38–75.

235. Cooper J, Stegmann BJ. Clinical evaluation of abnormal uterine bleeding. In: Coukos G, Rubin

SC, eds. *Cancer of the Uterus.* New York, NY: Marcel Dekker; 2005:195–223.

236. Livingstone M, Fraser IS. Mechanisms of abnormal uterine bleeding. *Hum Reprod Update.* 2002;8:60–67.

237. Thurmond A, Mendelson E, Bohm-Velez M, et al, eds. *Role of Imaging in Abnormal Vaginal Bleeding.* Reston, VA: American College of Radiology; 1996. Accessed September 8, 2005.

238. Medverd JR, Dubinsky TJ. Cost analysis model: US versus endometrial biopsy in evaluation of peri- and postmenopausal abnormal vaginal bleeding. *Radiol.* 2002;222:619–627.

239. Society of Obstetricians and Gynaecologists of Canada. *SOGC Clinical Practice Guidelines: Diagnosis of Endometrial Cancer in Women with Abnormal Vaginal Bleeding.* Ottowa, Ontario, Canada: Author; 2000.

240. Centers for Disease Control and the National Institute of Child Health and Human Development. Combination oral contraceptive use and the risk of endometrial cancer. *JAMA.* 1987;257(6):796–800.

241. Ramcharan S, Pellegrin FA, Ray R, et al. (1981). *The Walnut Creek Contraceptive Drug Study: A Prospective Study of the Side Effects of Oral Contraceptives.* Bethesda, MD: US Government Printing Office; Vol 3, NIH Publication No. 81-564.

242. Beral V, Hannaford P, Kay C. Oral contraceptive use and malignancies of the genital tract. Results from the Royal College of General Practitioners' Oral Contraception Study. *Lancet.* 1988;2(8624):1331–1335.

243. Schouten LJ, Goldbohm RA, van den Brandt PA. Anthropometry, physical activity, and endometrial cancer risk: results from the Netherlands Cohort Study. *J Natl Cancer Inst.* 2004;96(21):1635–1638.

244. Littman AJ, Voigt LF, Beresford SA, et al. Recreational physical activity and endometrial cancer risk. *Am J Epidemiol.* 2001;154(10):924–933.

245. Salazar-Martinez E, Lazcano-Ponce EC, Gonzalez Lira-Lira G, et al. Reproductive factors of ovarian and endometrial cancer risk in a high fertility population in Mexico. *Cancer Res.* 1999;59(15):3658–3662.

246. Newcomb PA, Trentham-Dietz A. Breast feeding practices in relation to endometrial cancer risk, USA. *Cancer Causes Control.* 2000;11(7):663–637.

247. Littman AJ, Beresford SA, White E. The association of dietary fat and plant foods with endometrial cancer (United States). *Cancer Causes Control.* 2001;12(8):691–702.

248. McCann SE, Freudenheim JL, Marshall JR, et al. Diet in the epidemiology of endometrial cancer in western New York (United States). *Cancer Causes Control.* 2000;11(10):965–974.

249. Trichopoulou A, Lagiou P, Kuper H, et al. Cancer and Mediterranean dietary traditions. *Cancer Epidemiol Biomarkers Prev.* 2000;9(9):869–873.

250. Zheng W, Kushi LH, Potter JD, et al. Dietary intake of energy and animal foods and endometrial cancer incidence. The Iowa women's health study. *Am J Epidemiol.* 1995;142(4):388–394.

251. Xu WH, Zheng W, Xiang YB, et al. Soya food intake and risk of endometrial cancer among Chinese women in Shanghai: population based case-control study. *BMJ.* 2004;328(7451):1285.

252. Gallup DG, Talledo OE, Shah KJ, et al. Invasive squamous cell carcinoma of the vagina: a 14-year study[abstract]. *Obstet Gynecol.* 1987;69(5):782–785.

253. Herbst AL, Robboy SJ, Scully RE, et al. Clear-cell adenocarcinoma of the vagina and cervix in girls: analysis of 170 registry cases[abstract]. *Am J Obstet Gynecol.* 1974;119(5):713–724.

254. Kucera H, Vavra N. Radiation management of primary carcinoma of the vagina: clinical and histopathological variables associated with survival[abstract]. *Gynecol Oncol.* 1991;40(1):12–16.

255. Eddy GL, Marks RD Jr, Miller MC 3rd, et al. Primary invasive vaginal carcinoma[abstract]. *Am J Obstet Gynecol.* 1991;165(2):292–298.

256. Dixit S, Singhal S, Baboo HA. Squamous cell carcinoma of the vagina: a review of 70 cases[abstract]. *Gynecol Oncol.* 1993;48(1):80–87.

257. Perez CA, Gersell DJ, McGuire WP, Morris M. In: Hoskins W, Perez C, Young R, eds. *Principles and Practice of Gynecologic Oncology.* Philadelphia, PA: Lippencott and Raven; 1997:919–986.

258. Sulak P, Barnhill D, Heller P, et al. Nonsquamous cancer of the vagina. *Gynecol Oncol.* 1988;29(3):309–320.

259. Hicks M. Vaginal cancer. In: Piver M, ed. *Handbook of Gynecologic Oncology.* Boston, MA: Little, Brown and Company; 1997:214–225.

260. American Cancer Society. *Detailed Guide: Vaginal Cancer.* Atlanta, GA: Author. Accessed July 21, 2006.

261. Macnab JC, Walkinshaw SA, Cordiner JW, et al. Human papillomavirus in clinically and histologically normal tissue of patients with genital cancer. *N Engl J Med.* 1986;315(17):1052–1058.

262. Burke T. Vulvar cancer. In: Barakat RR, Bevers MV, Gershenson CM, Hoskins WJ, eds. *Handbook of Gynecologic Oncology.* London, England: Martin Dunitz; 2000:207–215.

263. Joura EA, Losch A, Haider-Angeler MG, Breitenecker G, Leodolter S. Trends in vulvar neoplasia. Increasing incidence of vulvar intraepithelial neoplasia and squamous cell carcinoma of the vulva in young women. *J Reprod Med.* 2000;45:613–615.

264. Crum CP. Carcinoma of the vulva: epidemiology and pathogenesis. *Obstet Gynecol.* 1992;79:448–454.

265. Madeleine MM, Daling JR, Carter JJ, et al. Cofactors with human papillomavirus in a population-based study of vulvar cancer. *J Natl Cancer Inst.* 1997;89:1516–1523.

266. Scurry J. Does lichen sclerosus play a central role in the pathogenesis of human papillomavirus negative vulvar squamous cell carcinoma? The itch-scratch-lichen sclerosus hypothesis. *Int J Gynecol Cancer.* 1999;9:89–97.

267. American Cancer Society. *Detailed Guide: Vulvar Cancer.* Atlanta, GA: Author; 2008.

268. Hacker NF. Vulvar cancer. In: Berek JS, Hacker NF, eds. *Practical Gynecologic Oncology.* 3rd ed. Philadelphia, PA: Williams & Wilkins; 2000: 553–596.

Chapter 2

Breast Cancer

Wendy Holt, RN, BSN, OCN®

Breast cancer remains the most common cancer among women. In America it is the second leading cause of death for women, with lung cancer being the first.[1] For women ages 40 to 55 years, it is the leading cause of death in the United States and accounts for 15% of all cancer deaths.[2] Although the numbers remain high, the overall mortality rate from 1990 to 2004 decreased 2.2% annually.[1] For women under age 50 years, the annual death rate from 1990 to 2004 decreased 3.3%, and it decreased by 2.0% for women age 50 years and older.[1] The improved mortality rate in breast cancer since 1990 has been credited to both early detection and improved treatments.[1] However, with an overall 5-year survival rate of 87%, many women are long-term survivors of the disease.[2] Whether a woman is a long-time survivor or newly diagnosed, there are many complex issues for her to consider. These issues may not only pertain to the women themselves but also to the nurses who care for them.

Diagnosis

Several tools are used to diagnose breast cancer; one of the most popular is the mammogram.

Over the years, there have been several population-based evaluations and randomized studies looking at mammography as a screening tool for early diagnosis of breast cancer. The results of these studies have all clearly favored the use of mammography for early detection, and because of its capability to find cancer several years prior to any physical symptoms, mammography is considered to be the most effective tool available for early detection.[1] For women who have average risk and no symptoms, mammograms are used as screening; these are usually scheduled annually starting at age 40.[3]

For women who have high risk (e.g., BRCA1 or BRCA2 carriers), have a previous history of breast cancer, or have a questionable finding on a screening mammogram, a diagnostic mammogram may be used.[3] This is done using the same machine as the screening mammogram; the difference is that the diagnostic mammogram is done in "real time." In real time, the radiologist is present at the time of screening and looks at each view as it is taken to determine if further imaging may be needed for better evaluation. Immediately following the completion of the procedure, the radiologist will meet with the woman to discuss the results.[3]

Other imaging methods that may be used, if needed, are the ultrasound or magnetic resonance imaging (MRI). Ultrasound is not routinely used, but may be helpful when used in addition to mammography to determine the difference between a solid mass and a fluid-filled cyst.[3] MRI is more expensive than mammography and therefore is not used routinely.[3] In 2007, the American Cancer Society (ACS) reported new recommendations regarding the use of MRI for women who are considered high risk (20%–25% or greater lifetime risk) for breast cancer.[3] For these women, it is recommended that they have annual screening using both MRI and mammography.[3]

When an abnormality has been confirmed by mammography or other measures, a biopsy is necessary to confirm a malignancy.[3] There are several different biopsy techniques; choosing one is dependent upon the characteristics and size of the mass.[2] The procedures vary from invasive to less invasive. The less-invasive procedures include fine-needle aspiration (FNA) and core needle biopsy. These are used for those findings that are considered to be below to moderate risk for malignancy. An excisional or incisional biopsy is a more invasive procedure typically used for highly suspicious findings.[3]

FNA is used when it is thought that fluid is present in a palpable mass. A fluid-filled mass is often consistent with a cyst, which is usually mobile and rubbery in feel.[3] FNA is usually done in the office by using a 10–20 cc syringe with a small gauge needle. The needle is placed into the mass and fluid is withdrawn (**Figure 2-1**). The consistency and color may vary, the fluid may be very thin to very thick, and the color can range from light yellow to brown. In women who have had previous aspirations and a history of benign cysts, the fluid

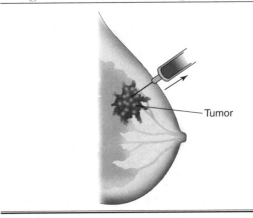

Figure 2-1 Fine-needle aspiration.

Tumor

may not be sent off to cytology each time.[3] If this is the case, a 1- to 2-month follow-up is recommended. If the fluid has returned, another FNA with cytology or an excisional biopsy may be indicated.[4]

A core-cutting needle biopsy is different from the previous technique in that it still involves a needle, but it also removes a core of histological material. With this method, the diagnosis is more definitive than that of the FNA.[3] The false-negative results are fewer due to a larger number of cells being obtained for evaluation.[3] The procedure uses a 14-gauge needle in combination with a spring-loaded device.[3] This device is trigger activated and places the needle into the mass.[3] This method allows one or more samples to be collected.[4] Because the spring-loaded device may cause a loud "pop" when used, it is important for the nurse to prepare the patient ahead of time.[3]

The more invasive procedures include both the excisional and the incisional biopsy. An excisional biopsy may also be referred to as an open biopsy (**Figure 2-2**). This procedure is performed by a surgeon when there is a single palpable

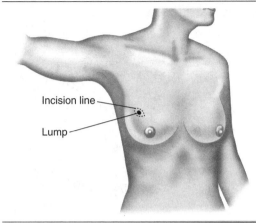

Figure 2-2 Excisional biopsy.

Incision line —

Lump —

mass that is highly suspicious for malignancy.[3] The goal is to excise the total mass, leaving no residual cancer. When the biopsy is completed and margins are found to be clear, no further surgery is needed.[2] An incisional biopsy is used for diagnostic purposes and may be done when a complete removal of the mass is not necessary or possible.[2] Here only a small section of the mass is removed for pathology.[2]

There are no surgical procedures without risk. Complications that may arise from breast biopsies include bleeding, slow healing, and infection. It is important for nurses to know these risks and instruct the patient properly. Patient instruction should include keeping the site clean and dry and calling the provider at any sign of complication.[3] In addition, specific signs of infection should be described to the patient, such as fever, redness, or drainage.[3] It is also important for the nurse to discuss pain following the procedure and how best to manage it. In most cases, acetaminophen or acetaminophen with codeine is sufficient; patients should be instructed to avoid nonsteroi-

dal anti-inflammatory drugs due to associated bleeding.[3]

Treatment

The treatment phase begins once a diagnosis has been confirmed. The type and length of treatment is dependent on the diagnosis. For some women this may be surgery alone, whereas others may require a combination of treatment.

Surgery

When the diagnosis of breast cancer has been confirmed, for most women the next step will include surgery. The goal of surgery is to remove all the cancer, leaving clear margins of healthy tissue. There are two options: a lumpectomy followed by radiation, or a mastectomy, with or without immediate reconstruction. Results of a long-term study comparing the two procedures have shown that these two methods are equal when it comes to survival.[5] Often the decision on what type of procedure to have can be very difficult and overwhelming for women. Nurses can play an important role by making sure women have what they need to make an informed decision.

A lumpectomy, sometimes called a segmental mastectomy, is the most conservative option a woman can choose. With this procedure, only the tumor and the surrounding area are removed (**Figure 2-3**). The amount of breast tissue removed is determined by the size of the tumor and the distance needed for clear margins. This procedure is most often followed by radiation therapy to the rest of the breast to remove any errant cancer cells that may exist. The risk for recurrence with a lumpectomy and radiation is 3% to 19%.[2] This combination is the standard

Figure 2-3 Segmental mastectomy.

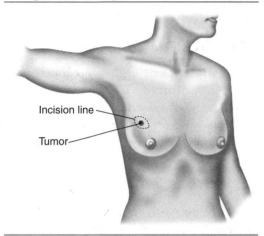

Incision line

Tumor

Figure 2-4 Modified radical mastectomy.

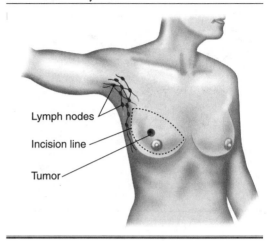

Lymph nodes

Incision line

Tumor

treatment for women with stage I and II breast cancer.[2] It is important for the woman to know all that is involved, and an initial consultation with a radiation oncologist prior to surgery can be very helpful with this.

A mastectomy is used as the primary treatment to reduce tumor size, and in addition it allows for systemic therapy to be more effective.[2] The likelihood of a poor cosmetic outcome resulting from conservative surgery and/or radiation, large or bulky tumors, multiple areas of involvement, and personal choice are all indications for a mastectomy.[2] There are two types: a modified radical mastectomy (MRM) and a total mastectomy. The MRM is the most common surgery used in the United States for the treatment of breast cancer.[2] The procedure involves removal of the entire breast, including the nipple, areola, and pectoral fascia while preserving the pectoralis major; in addition, axillary lymph nodes are removed (**Figure 2-4**).

A total mastectomy involves the same procedure, with the difference being preservation of the axillary lymph nodes and pectoral muscles. This is commonly used for high-risk

women who choose to have prophylactic surgery or women who have a recurrence following a lumpectomy and radiation (**Figure 2-5**).[2]

Complications following either type of mastectomy are very similar, and, as with any surgery, there is risk for infection. Early presentation following surgery may be cellulitis, whereas formation of an abscess is typically seen farther out from surgery.[2] Following the removal of a breast, it is not uncommon for women to experience phantom pain or sensation; these may include tenderness, nipple sensation, erotic sensation, itching, and pain.[2] As many as 50% of women experience these symptoms.[2] These can appear immediately after surgery or they may not be apparent until weeks following surgery. This can be even more disturbing for a woman who is not prepared with this information; therefore, it is important for the nurse to include this as part of each patient's education.

Axillary lymph node dissection (ALND) is routinely done with a MRM. The axillary nodes are the primary ones connected to the breast and obtain 85% of lymphatic drainage.[2] The

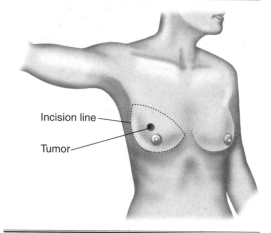

Figure 2-5 Total mastectomy.

Incision line

Tumor

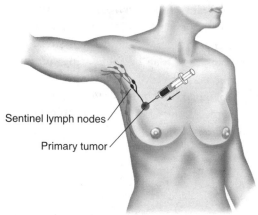

Figure 2-6 Sentinal node biopsy.

Sentinel lymph nodes

Primary tumor

prognosis for breast cancer is determined by the number of lymph nodes involved, making this an important part of the surgery.[2] The presence of lymphatic invasion, the size of the tumor, and histologic grade are all indicators that the axillary lymph nodes are likely to be involved.[2] Morbidities associated with breast cancer are often related to ALND. Nurses who care for these women should be aware of this because it is an important part of the education needed both before and after surgery. The major morbidities include lymphedema, injury or thrombosis of the axillary vein, and injury to motor nerves located in the axillary.[2] Less common may be seroma formation, shoulder dysfunction, and loss of sensation in the area of the intercostobrachial nerve.[2] The procedure may be optional for women with the following conditions: those with favorable tumors, those who have a related morbidity, the elderly, and those whose treatment would not be affected by nodal status.[2]

The sentinel node biopsy (SNB) is a simple procedure and involves less surgery than the traditional ALND. It is a relatively new advancement in the treatment of breast cancer and can

be very useful for staging and determining treatment in early breast cancer.[6] The sentinel nodes obtain lymphatic fluid from a breast tumor prior to the axillary nodes and are known as the "gatekeepers."[6] If there are no cancer cells in the sentinel nodes, further node dissection may not be indicated; if the sentinel node is positive for cancer cells, further ALND would be necessary to determine the spread of the disease and treatment needed[6] (**Figure 2-6**).

Drains are placed at the wound site during surgery to collect excess fluid that occurs following surgery, and the drains are in place for approximately 10 days.[6] The site where the drain enters the skin should be cleaned every day, and the fluid should be emptied twice a day.[6] Drain care instruction for both the woman and her caretakers should be a priority for nurses in charge of these patients. Instruction can be done before or after the surgery, keeping in mind that if done before, reinforcement should be done prior to discharge. In many instances it is the patient's husband, or someone else who is close to the patient, who assumes responsibility for the drain. This involvement allows the caretaker to take part in the care giving and be supportive. The drain will be removed as an outpatient procedure when there is minimal drainage for 2 consecutive days.[6] The woman should be told that there may be some stinging when the tube is removed, but there should not be any prolonged discomfort.[6] Women should be instructed to start range-of-motion exercises immediately following removal of the drains; this will ensure a full recovery.[6]

Following surgery, most women are able to leave the hospital the next day. For most, pain and discomfort is minimal and can be relieved with oral pain medication after the first 24 hours.[6] In most cases, women who have had a mastectomy with ALND should be able to return to normal activity 3 to 4 weeks following surgery.[6]

For women who have disfiguring surgery, such as a mastectomy, reconstruction surgery may be an option. This may be done at the time of initial surgery, or it may be done at a later date. Many factors determine the timing and procedure involved for reconstruction surgery. Women who consider this should be encouraged to discuss their options with their physician prior to surgery.

If immediate reconstruction is not an option, a temporary prosthetic is used in combination with a surgical bra at the time of discharge. When the drains have been removed and sufficient healing has occurred, a prescription may be given for a permanent prosthesis. This is a silicone-filled shell that fits into a special pocket within the bra. These come in a variety of shapes, sizes, weights, and skin tones. In addition to cosmetics, the prosthesis also aides in restoring balance in the chest and shoulder region.

Radiation

Radiation therapy works by the use of high-energy rays that injure the ability for cancer cells to multiply and therefore destroy the cells.[6] It is most commonly used for early stage breast cancer in combination with a lumpectomy; however, in the United States, less than 50% of stage I or II breast cancer is treated with radiation.[2] Having radiation as a treatment option allows women with early local disease to choose breast conservation. Using the option of breast conservation with radiation has been shown to be equal to that of a mastectomy for control of local disease.[2] It may also be used following a full mastectomy for women with advanced primary tumors and multiple node involvement.[2] This is considered to be adjuvant therapy, and the radiation is given to the chest wall and the nearby lymph nodes.[2]

Radiation treatments are typically given 5 days a week over a 5- to 6-week period; each treatment is approximately 2 to 5 minutes.[6] Prior to the initial treatment, the woman will be scheduled for a simulated treatment. The purpose of this visit is to mark the specific areas intended for treatment. This allows for accuracy in the radiation field and helps to maximize the radiation to the area where it is most needed. This is done by having the woman lie on a table where she will be positioned under the radiation machine. Ink markings are placed on the areas where the radiation is to be directed. These marks will remain in place for the duration of treatment.

For most women, the thought of radiation can be very scary. Proper education by the nurse can help to alleviate much of the fear and apprehension. As part of the teaching process, it is important to include what the patient can expect and to rule out any myths about radiation. Examples of the type of information that nurses should tell patients are that there may be some warmth and tingling in the local area being treated, but radiation itself is not painful; and that the treatment will not make the patient radioactive.[6] For comfort during the weeks of treatment, women are best advised to wear loose-fitting cotton clothing and no bra.[6] The patient should be told that redness may occur locally, which may be more noticeable for women with fair skin. Other side effects may include fatigue, arm and/or breast edema, and darkening of the skin in the local area.[2]

Adjuvant Therapy

Adjuvant therapy consists of either systemic chemotherapy and/or hormonal therapy. The main goal for adjuvant therapy is to prevent the spread of disease by eliminating any undetected cancer cells outside the breast.[7] Systemic therapy consists of various chemotherapy regimens that can last 3–6 months, although the type of regimen and schedule may vary; most women will receive treatment for part of each month followed by a short rest period.[6] Chemotherapy can be given by injection or orally, and this will vary with the type of regimen prescribed by the oncologist. The standard class of drugs used for breast cancer is the anthracyclines (e.g., Adriamycin or epirubicin). These are commonly used in combination with other drugs, such as 5-fluorouracil or cyclophosphamide.[6] As an added benefit for those women with node-positive breast cancer, a taxane may be added to the regimen.[2] With the many choices, treatment decisions may be difficult for some women; therefore, communication with the entire healthcare team is essential. Women can also access the National Comprehensive Cancer Network (NCCN) at

www.nccn.org/professionals/physician_gls/PDF/breast.pdf for further help.

Despite the many choices for adjuvant treatment, the side effects are very similar, and it is important for women to know the potential side effects prior to treatment. Chemotherapy damages any cell that is active and involves the entire body; therefore, it produces a number of side effects.[6] The most dreaded is nausea and vomiting. Fortunately, however, with the many types of effective medication available, these side effects are usually minimal.[6] Other common side effects include hair loss, risk for bleeding and infection, mucositis, anemia, myalgia, and weight gain.[6] Management of symptoms should include both medical and nursing support. Initial education on side effects that may occur during treatment can be very beneficial in reducing some of the anxiety associated with diagnosis and treatment. It is also important to have continued support and reinforcement available throughout the course of treatment. An available list of resources can be helpful with this.

Immunological therapy—the use of antibodies that target specific proteins in cancer cells—is a new approach in treating breast cancer.[6] HER2/neu makes a protein that regulates cell growth, and approximately 25% of women with breast cancer have an extra HER2/neu gene in their tumors.[6] Herceptin (trastuzumab) is an antibody that binds to these specific proteins and prevents growth of the cells. This is a treatment primarily used for women who have metastatic breast cancer and have not responded to other treatments. It is important for nurses to know that this drug has a potential to cause heart damage, and caution should be used if combined with other heart-damaging drugs (e.g., doxorubicin and epirubicin).[7] Other targeted therapy used for metastatic breast cancer includes such drugs as bevacizumab (Avastin) and lapatinib (Tykerb).

Bevacizumab is normally used in combination with other chemotherapy drugs such as paclitaxel. Its mechanism works by inhibiting growth of new blood vessels that enhance tumor growth. Side effects that nurses need to be aware of include slow wound healing, bleeding, kidney damage, and high blood pressure.

Lapatinib is a targeted therapy that is taken orally and is normally combined with another oral drug called capecitabine. Lapatinib works by entering cells and interrupting the process that involves both the HER2 and HER1 receptors.[7] Two important side effects to be aware of with this drug include acne and diarrhea.[7]

Hormonal therapy (antiestrogen drugs) is used in those women whose tumors test positive for estrogen. Estrogen is a known hormone that can cause increased cell growth in breast cancer.[6] The main production of this hormone stems from the ovaries, but it is also produced by the adrenal glands and fat tissue.[7] Not all tumors are sensitive to estrogen; therefore, an estrogen receptor, or ER, test is done at the time of surgery to determine the benefit of hormonal therapy. Estrogen-positive tumors are more likely to respond to antiestrogen drugs.[6] These drugs are not intended to lower estrogen levels but to block the effect that estrogen has on cancer cells and therefore limit growth of the breast cancer cells.[7] Tamoxifen, toremifene, fulvestrant, and raloxifene are all anitiestrogen drugs. Although these drugs are all in the same category, the indications for each may vary; therefore, it is important for the woman to discuss her options with a healthcare provider.[7] Of these drugs, tamoxifen is the most commonly used and the drug of choice for premenopausal women.[7] Common side effects of tamoxifen include hot flashes, mood swings, and vaginal discharge;

less common side effects are blood clots and an increased risk for endometrial cancer and uterine sarcoma.[7]

Aromatase inhibitors are another class of hormonal therapy drugs. There are three approved drugs in this category: anastrozole (Arimidex), letrozole (Femara), and exemestane (Aromasin). These drugs work by blocking the enzyme aromatase. Aromatase is responsible for estrogen production in postmenopausal women. It is not capable of stopping the ovaries from producing estrogen, so it is used only for women who are postmenopausal.[7] In a comparison done with tamoxifen, these drugs have been shown to have fewer of the side effects, which include uterine cancer and blood clots.[7] Other side effects that women need to know about with this drug are loss of calcium, bone fractures, hot flashes, and joint pain.[7] Women should be encouraged to discuss these potential side effects with their healthcare provider prior to starting therapy.[7]

Long-Term Follow-Up

Despite the type of treatment, the continuum of care for all women diagnosed with breast cancer should include long-term follow-up. This is important for both cancer surveillance and evaluation of any latent effects that can occur following treatment. During this time each woman's needs may differ; issues can range from very complex to very simple, but regardless each one is important. At the completion of treatment, each woman should discuss with her healthcare provider her individual needs for long-term follow-up.

Survivorship

Unfortunately, the effects and concerns of breast cancer do not end at the completion of treatment. For some women, there may be chronic or latent side effects from treatment, such as pain or fatigue. In addition, the fear of possible recurrence can weigh heavily following treatment. It is important that when treatment is complete the woman has a chance to discuss her concerns. A nurse can play an important role in preparing the woman for this transition. This can be done by validating her concerns and providing information on what she might expect when her treatment is finished.

Pain following treatment can be attributed to any number of things. If a woman has had radiation, there may be delayed pain that can show up as late as 3 to 6 months following treatment.[8] This pain is generally caused from inflammation in the pectoralis major muscle related to the radiation done in this area. Another type of discomfort that may show up later is stiffness in the shoulder. This is usually related to surgery and can cause much concern for women—quite often, they are fearful that the cancer is back. Nurses can help by reassuring them that pain after treatment is normal, even if it is delayed. In addition, women may have a tendency to pamper or protect the side with pain, and this can cause more problems. If not used, the arm and muscles will continue to weaken, and if they become worse, surgery may be required to repair them.[8] It is important for women to be instructed that exercise and use of the affected arm is the best therapy, and in some cases, physical therapy would be a good option. This option can be discussed with their healthcare providers.

Fatigue after treatment can become worse before it gets better. One study showed that 61% of women who had chemotherapy experienced more fatigue than the women who did not have treatment.[8] The three most common methods of treating the fatigue are exercise, blood transfusions, and medication. Erythropoietin is a common injection used to help produce more red blood cells in the bone marrow. This may take several injections over a period of time before a difference is noted. There have been several studies showing success with exercise, but if the fatigue is severe, this may be neither easy nor appealing.[8]

One of the greatest difficulties for women following treatment can be the fear of recurrence, and any bodily changes that occur may cause alarm. Close follow-up with their healthcare providers can help to alleviate some of these concerns and fears. However, some women may be so frightened of a recurrence that their compliance for medical follow-up is negatively affected.[3] For these women, individual counseling or involvement with a support group may be helpful.[3] It is important for nurses not only to recognize the issues that women may encounter long after treatment but to also advocate for them. In doing so, the nurse should recognize the need for careful psychosocial assessment at the time of follow-up.[3] The guidelines for follow-up vary between invasive and noninvasive breast cancer, and it is important for women to know what is recommended for their particular diagnosis. For women with an invasive breast cancer, the risk for recurrence depends on many factors, such as the stage of cancer and the type of cancer cells that were found at the time of diagnosis.[6] These women are at a greater risk for recurrence in the first 2 years following treatment, with a decreased risk once they have surpassed 5 years.[6] Follow-up care for women with invasive breast cancer should include a physical exam every 4 months for the first 2 years, decreasing to every 6 months for 3 years, and then decreasing to annually at the 5-year mark.[6] In addition, women should also be encouraged to do monthly breast self-exams and annual mammograms. If a woman has had reconstructive surgery following a mastectomy, it is important to inform her that mammograms are not necessary for the reconstructed breast.[6] Unlike invasive breast cancer patients, women with noninvasive or very early breast cancer are at a much lower risk for recurrence; therefore, follow-up care is usually less assertive.[6] Follow-up may be individualized based on needs, and it is important that women discuss this with their healthcare providers following treatment.

The nurse should be aware that each woman may handle her experience with breast cancer very differently. Women will come to realize that life as it was will never be again. This is a time of healing, and emotions can range from sadness to joy and back again. Working through this healing process may move very quickly for some, and not so quickly for others, and support and understanding can make all the difference for these women as they move through their individual journey of recovery.

Issues After Treatment

The complexity of issues following treatment is many and can vary throughout the lifespan; they can range from physical to psycho-social. There are many factors that may contribute to this, such as family history, diagnosis, type of treatment, and age. Not all issues are going to affect every woman; therefore it is important that each woman be given the information that she may need. Women should be encouraged

to discuss these topics with their healthcare provider as needed.

Genetics

Genetics play an important role in cancer today, and over the past several years much knowledge has been gained in this area. BRCA1 (Breast Cancer Gene 1), the first gene related to genetic breast cancer, was discovered in 1990; in 1991 this same gene was also linked to ovarian cancer.[8] In addition, there is a higher occurrence of breast cancer bilaterally and at a younger age.[8] Less common is the BRCA2 (Breast Cancer Gene 2), which was discovered in 1994.[8] This gene mutation has a lower incidence of ovarian cancer, and men as well as women can be affected by the BRCA2.[8]

Approximately 20% of all familiar breast cancer has no genetic connection.[8] However, for women who have the BRCA1 or BRCA2 mutation, the risk for breast cancer is 50% to 80%.[8] Because of the low incidence of hereditary breast cancer, genetic testing is not recommended for all women but should be offered for women who are considered to be high risk. This would generally include those women who are at a 10% or higher risk for a genetic mutation.[8] Factors that determine a woman to be at higher risk include having one or more first-degree relatives or two or more first- and second-degree relatives with one of the following:[8]

- A diagnosis of breast cancer alone prior to age 50 years
- Breast cancer prior to age 50 years and ovarian cancer at any age
- Breast and ovarian cancer at any age
- Ovarian cancer alone
- Ashkenazi Jewish ancestry in combination with breast cancer

Genetic testing may involve many choices and decisions; therefore, it may not be for everyone. If a woman is in a high-risk category for having the BRCA1 or BRCA2, it is important for nurses to connect them with the proper resources to receive the correct information regarding testing. When a woman is tested and the results are positive, this no longer just affects her but may also involve other family members, such as siblings or her own children. Prior to any testing, a woman should meet with a professional genetics counselor to discuss her risks and options. Included in the initial consultation will be a thorough family history. In addition, information about the test, including estimation of risk for both herself and other family members, accuracy of test, psychosocial issues, cost, risk management, surveillance, and screening is given.[2] Because of the in-depth information needed for a woman to make an informed decision regarding genetics testing, it is recommended that testing not be done with a gynecologist or primary care physician, but instead, it should be done at a research center where genetics counselors are available.[8]

Lymphedema

Lymphedema is a major problem that can occur at any time following breast cancer treatment. It results when there is a backup of lymphatic fluid that cannot be properly channeled through the remaining lymphatics in the axillary region, and this causes swelling of the affected arm. Although current use of less invasive procedures has decreased the incidence of lymphedema, it is reported that approximately 20% of women still suffer from this condition.[2] Studies comparing the sentinel biopsy and full axillary node dissection showed a sufficient decrease in lymphedema in women who had the sentinel biopsy. Lymphedema occurred 2% to 6% of the time in these women, whereas with full axillary dissection, it was 17% to 34%.[8]

Following surgery, women should be informed of the symptoms of lymphedema, as well as what they can do to reduce their risk for it. Symptoms can occur any time, from immediately following surgery to months or even years later.[9] There are three levels of severity, and these are categorized by grades. With grade I, there may be pitting edema, and the edema may subside with elevation of the arm; in grade II, the arm has increased edema with hardness noted instead of pitting; in grade III, the most severe changes of the skin occur, which are often described as "elephantiasis."[2] Although there are various degrees of lymphedema and different ways to manage the symptoms, it is important to know that it is not curable, and therefore prevention should be the main goal.

Avoiding injury to the extremity involved is an important measure in preventing lymphedema. Women should avoid having their blood pressure taken in the affected arm, in addition to injections or blood draws. Other things should include proper care of skin and nails, avoiding constrictive clothing, watching for infection, and elevating the arm above the heart whenever possible.[2] Swelling of any degree in the affected extremity should never be ignored. An excellent resource for both nurses and their patients who are at risk for lymphedema is the National Lymphedema Network. They can be accessed online at www.lymphnet.org.[2]

Fertility and Pregnancy

Although the number of women diagnosed with breast cancer prior to menopause is less than 20%, the concerns related to pregnancy and fertility following diagnosis for this small group is major.[2] In addition to the initial distress that most women feel when having to make treatment decisions, these young women may often have added distress if future pregnancy is wanted. It is important for nurses to recognize this as not only a health issue for these women; it also impacts their quality of life. Women who fall into this category should be encouraged to discuss their options fully with their oncologists prior to any treatment. A good resource for young women facing these issues is an organization called Fertile Hope, which can be accessed online at www.fertilehope.org.[3]

They have information regarding options prior to treatment, as well as during and following treatment.[3]

Long-Term Health Issues

It is important to note there are effects of treatment that may show up much later in life; they can occur from months to years following treatment. For women who have received treatment for breast cancer, some areas of concern for late effects might include menopause, heart disease, and osteoporosis. These are all things that not only affect a woman's health, but also her quality of life. It is important that women are aware of these risks and what they can do for themselves. The nurse should encourage women to discuss these risks fully with their healthcare provider early on in their care.

Menopause

Menopause is defined as 12 months without menstruation. This can take place as a natural process, with the average age being around 51 or 52 years.[2] It can also be induced by surgical removal of the ovaries or chemically with chemotherapy. Whether they are related to the natural process or induced, menopause symptoms remain the same. For most women, related symptoms tend to last 2 to 3 years on average and are usually transient.[8] It is important to note that symptoms can vary among women, and, therefore, so does the symptom management.

Although there are various symptoms that may accompany menopause, hot flashes are the most common, with 85% of women experiencing them.[2] The cause for these is unknown and can vary by individual. For women with breast cancer, these symptoms seem to be more intense than for those who experience menopause naturally. Women who experience hot flashes may have chills, sweats, increased heart rate, and anxiety. Flushing of the body may be noted.[2] This often occurs at night and may be a major interference with sleep. Things that may help with this include avoiding exercise around bedtime, keeping the bedroom cool, and avoiding caffeine and alcohol. There are several pharmacologic measures that are currently being used with success. Some of these require a prescription, whereas others may be over-the-counter remedies such as vitamins or herbal supplements. Because of the controversy of use for women with breast cancer, and because of the many available treatment options for hot flashes, a woman should first discuss these with her physician prior to taking anything.

In addition to hot flashes, women may also experience vaginal tissue changes. The vagina and lower urinary tract have more estradiol receptors than any other part of a woman's body; therefore, with cessation of estrogen production, the vaginal lining becomes thinner and more fragile, causing changes in pH. These vaginal tissue changes may increase the risk for vaginal infections; in addition, they can cause an increase in vaginal dryness. The dryness that occurs is related to a decrease in natural self-lubrication, which in turn may lead to pain and discomfort with sexual intercourse. In addition to vaginal changes, there may also be atrophic changes involving the urinary system. When this occurs, symptoms may include frequent urinary tract infections, nocturia, dysuria, frequency, and urgency of urination, as well as stress incontinence.[2]

There are several options that may be used for management of these symptoms. For vaginal dryness, lubricants that may help include Replens, K-Y liquid or jelly, and Astroglide.[2] These may be especially helpful in reducing painful intercourse. For urinary symptoms, increasing fluid intake may be beneficial; in addition, voiding at regular intervals and Kegel exercises may also be helpful (**Table 2-1**).

Table 2-1 INSTRUCTIONS FOR KEGEL EXERCISES.

1. To understand the principle of this exercise, go to the bathroom, begin to urinate, and in midstream stop the flow of urine.
2. Develop a routine doing this away from the toilet by contracting the muscles, holding them, and releasing them.
3. Over time, increase the time of holding the contraction (e.g., start with three counts, increase to five counts, and then in time hold for 10 counts).
4. Do three sets of 10, three times a day.
5. These exercises can be done anytime, anywhere, without recognition by others that they are being done.

Heart Disease

The leading cause of death for women in the United States is cardiovascular disease, and the risk for this is increased when a woman enters menopause.[2] The cause for this is related to the decreased levels of estrogen. Estrogen works as a protection mechanism for the heart by helping to keep the low density lipoprotein (LDL) and the high density lipoprotein (HDL) at healthy levels.[2] Other well-known risk factors for heart disease include obesity, diabetes, lack of exercise, high blood pressure, and cigarette smoking.[2] Although many women with breast cancer have limited options with regards to estrogen supplements, it is important for them to know that there are things they can do to help reduce their risk for cardiovascular disease. If smoking is an issue, and knowing the risk associated with heart disease, the woman should consider that giving up smoking is very important, although it may be difficult. The nurse should direct women to resources that can help them with this. Both the American Lung Association and the American Cancer Society are well-known sources. Regular exercise is very important and should be done at least three times a week for 30-minute intervals.[2] Diet is also very important and should consist of a lower fat intake; this will aid in maintaining healthy LDL and HDL levels.

Osteoporosis

Osteoporosis is defined as softening of the bone and bone loss.[8] This results from lower estrogen levels, making women who have reached menopause higher risk. Women diagnosed with breast cancer may be at even higher risk for osteoporosis than the average woman. This is related to early menopause induced by chemotherapy and women who are not able to take estrogen supplements following menopause.[2]

Table 2-2 INTERNET INFORMATION SOURCES FOR WOMEN WHO ARE DIAGNOSED WITH BREAST CANCER.

- American Cancer Society: w ww.cancer.org
- National Cancer Institute: www.cancer.gov
- National Comprehensive Cancer Network: www.nccn.org
- WebMD: www.webmd.com
- Cancer Information Service: www.cis.nci.nih. gov
- Living Beyond Breast Cancer: www.lbbc.org
- National Coalition for Cancer Survivorship: www.canceradvocacy.org
- American Medical Association: www. ama-assn.org
- American Institute for Cancer Research: www.aicr.org
- American Medical Women's Association: www.amwa-doc.org

Women who are unable to take estrogen supplements for chemotherapy-induced menopause may lose as much as 30% of their bone mass within the first year.[2]

There are several pharmacologic measures that may be prescribed for menopause management, including estrogen replacement. Because of the contraindications of estrogen therapy in many women with breast cancer, estrogen replacement may not be an option. It is important for women to discuss their options with their healthcare providers prior to taking anything.

Nonpharmacologic interventions include such things as diet and exercise. Weight-bearing exercises are needed to help maintain bone mass; regular exercise is recommended three times a week at 30-minute intervals.[2] In addition to regular exercise, diet is also very important and should

include a high intake of calcium. It is recommended that women take 1500 mg of calcium divided into three 500 mg doses, with an added 200 to 400 IU of vitamin D to aid in calcium absorption.[2] Caffeine interferes with the absorption of calcium; therefore, nurses should instruct women to avoid taking their calcium supplements with caffeine.[2] Other means of increasing calcium include dairy products, fruits, and vegetables.

Resources

There are numerous resources for women who are diagnosed with breast cancer (**Table 2-2**).

References

1. American Cancer Society. *Breast Cancer Facts & Figures 2007–2008*. Atlanta, GA: Author.
2. Dow KH. *Pocket Guide to Breast Cancer*. 3rd ed. Sudbury, MA: Jones and Barlett; 2006.
3. Mahon SM. *Site-Specific Cancer Series: Breast Cancer*. Pittsburgh, PA: ONS Publishing Division; 2007.
4. Dimaggio C. State of the art of current modalities for the diagnosis of breast lesions. *Eur J Nucl Med Mol Imaging*. 2004; 31 (suppl 1): S56–S69.
5. Veronisi U, Cascinelli N, Mariani L, et al. Twenty-year follow-up of a randomized study comparing breast-conserving surgery with radical mastectomy for early breast cancer. *N Eng J Med*. 2002; 347(16): 1227–1232.
6. Singletary SE, Judkins AF. *Breast Cancer: Myths & Facts: What You Need to Know*. 4th ed. New York, NY: Oncology Publishing Group; 2005.
7. American Cancer Society & The National Comprehensive Cancer Network. *Breast Cancer Treatment Guidelines for Patients, Version IX*. Atlanta, GA: American Cancer Society; 2007.
8. Love SM, Lindsey K. *Dr. Susan Love's Breast Book*. 4th ed. Cambridge, MA: Da Capo Press; 2005.
9. Kaelin CM. *Living Through Breast Cancer*. New York, NY: McGraw-Hill; 2005.

Chapter 3

Endometrial Cancer

Lynn Cloutier, RN, MSN, AOCN®, ACNP-BC

Introduction

The American Cancer Society estimates that 40,100 new cases of endometrial cancer will be diagnosed in 2008, and 7470 women will die of the disease.[1] Endometrial cancer is the most common invasive gynecologic malignancy and the fourth most frequently diagnosed cancer among women.[2] Most cases are diagnosed at an early stage, when the opportunity for cure is high. Approximately 16% of patients with endometrial cancer have distant disease at time of diagnosis.[3] The outcome for women diagnosed with advanced-stage disease remains poor.

Epidemiology/Risk Factors

There are geographic and regional differences in epidemiology and risk factors. Caucasian women in America and Europe have a higher incidence than do women in Africa, South America, and Asia. However, within the United States, black and Asian women have a higher rate than their counterparts in other countries. Racial and geographical differences suggest genetic and environmental factors that influence the development of endometrial cancer.[4] Black women are more likely than white women to have papillary serous, advanced stage, higher tumor grade at diagnosis, and worse survival rates, despite receiving similar treatment.[5]

Who fits the profile of the woman at risk for endometrial cancer? The majority of patients, 75%, are postmenopausal, between the ages of 50–59 years.[6,7] Less than 5% of women who are diagnosed with endometrial cancer are less than 40 years of age. This disease is rare in childbearing years. When endometrial cancer occurs in younger women, it is usually associated with polycystic ovarian disease.[8] In a cohort study, women diagnosed earlier than age 50 years had a high incidence of obesity, nulliparity, irregular menses, and a high number of synchronous primary ovarian cancers.[9]

In the United States, rates are higher in whites; however, black women tend to present more often with a higher stage of disease, with regional or distant disease. Risk is related to the biologic behavior and aggressiveness of poorly differentiated carcinomas. Black women have a greater predisposition to a more aggressive type of endometrial cancer.[10] Black women with advanced endometrial cancer who receive similar therapy have a worse overall survival when compared with white women.[5] Only 52% of black women older than age 50 years have disease confined to the uterus at the time of original surgery, compared with 73% of white women age 50 years and older.[11] There is evidence to support a higher incidence in westernized populations, and higher rates are generally seen in urban than rural populations. Immigrant populations tend to assume the risks of native populations, highlighting the importance of environmental factors in the genesis of this disease.[12]

Risk factors are associated with extended periods of estrogenic stimulation (**Table 3-1**). These factors create an environment of prolonged or unopposed exposure to estrogen, either endogenous or exogenous. Examples of increased exogenous exposure include the use of unopposed estrogen as hormone replacement therapy or treatment with tamoxifen. Endogenous estrogen exposure may stem from obesity, anovulatory cycles, and estrogen-secreting tumors. In women over age 50 years, there is little ovarian production of progesterone, and the mitogenic effects of estrogen, either endogenous (i.e., adipose, tissue, skin) or exogenous (i.e., postmenopausal estrogen replacement), sources are largely unopposed.[13]

Some risk factors are related to reproductive cycle, such as menstrual cycle debut at an early age, having few children, late onset of menopause, and nulliparity. Other risk factors are more directly estrogen related, such as polycystic ovarian syndrome. Early age at menarche and late age at menopause resulting in prolonged, irregular menstrual span correlate with the development of endometrial cancer. A span longer than 39 years has a 4.2-fold risk

Table 3-1 Risk factors related to the development of endometrial cancer.

Factor Influencing Risk

Long-term use of high dosages of menopausal estrogens

Stein-Leventhal syndrome or estrogen-producing tumor

Residency in North America or Northern Europe

High cumulative doses of tamoxifen (Nolvadex)

Nulliparity

Obesity

History of infertility

Late age of natural menopause

Older age

White race

Early age at menarche

Higher level of education or income

Menstrual irregularities

History of diabetes, hypertension, gallbladder disease, or thyroid disease

Cigarette smoking

Long-term use of high dosages of combination oral contraceptives

Source: Adapted from Damlo, 2006.

over a span shorter than 25 years. Nulliparity is associated with a 2–3-fold increase in risk. The protective effect of parity has been hypothesized to be due to mechanical removal of premalignant and malignant cells with each delivery and the second describing a protective effect of high progesterone values during pregnancy.[14] Nulliparity is often a manifestation of infertility and is an independent risk factor for endometrial cancer. Conditions associated with infertility have also been linked to occurrence of endometrial cancer, such as Stein-Leventhal syndrome (polycystic ovary syndrome) and granulosa-thecal cell ovarian tumors.

The majority of conditions known to influence risk of endometrial cancer can be directly or indirectly associated with estrogen exposure. Use of unopposed estrogen replacement therapy is consistently associated with an increased risk. This risk is associated with years of use of estrogen therapy, and the risk continues years after estrogen therapy is stopped. The use of oral contraceptives is associated with decreased risk, and long-term use further reduces risk while the protective mechanism lasts for 20 years or longer.[4]

Endometrial cancer is a disease of postmenopausal women. However, 25% of cases occur in premenopausal patients, with 5% of cases developing in patients less than 40 years old.[12] Endometrial cancer is most commonly found between the ages of 50 and 65 years. As the population of the United States ages, endometrial cancer in elderly women is also increasing. Age remains a prognostic factor for endometrial cancer.[15]

A number of studies have shown that diets high in fat and low in complex carbohydrates and fiber increase a woman's risk of endometrial cancer. This association with diet persists after adjustment for body mass as well as other risk factors. Large body mass, in general and obesity in particular, places women at an increased risk of endometrial cancer.[16] An association with obesity is seen because obese women have higher endogenous estrogens than lean women. This difference is due to the aromatization of androstenedione to estrone in adipose tissues, as well as to the aromatization of androgens to estradiol, leading to a chronic low-level increase

in estrogen exposure.[17] This may be due to serum hormone-bound globulin (SHBG), which appears to be depressed in women with endometrial cancer. The level of SHBG is progressively depressed with increasing upper-body fat localization. With lower SHBG, there is a higher endogenous production of non-protein-bound estradiol[7] (**Figure 3-1**).

Phenotypically, the majority of women who develop endometrial cancer tend to be obese. Weight gain is associated with the development of endometrial cancer, and for each 5 kg weight gain, the risk for developing endometrial cancer increases by 21%. Cycling of weight also makes a woman at risk for endometrial cancer. A woman who loses 20 pounds and then regains at least half within a year has a 27% risk of developing the disease.[18] Women who are 30 pounds over ideal body weight have a 3-fold risk of developing endometrial cancer, while those 50 pounds or more over ideal body weight have a 10-fold increased risk.[12]

The diabetes–endometrial cancer association may be explained by the elevated estrogen levels, hyperinsulinemia or insulin-like growth factor 1 (IGF-1) in diabetic women. Adiponectin is a protein secreted by adipose cells and has been shown to be a surrogate marker for insulin resistance. Low levels of adinopectin correlates with hyperinsulinism and degree of insulin resistance. Low serum adiponectin is independently associated with endometrial cancer, and an association is found in obese and normal weight range women.[19]

Results from women in clinical trials for treatment of breast cancer have shown an increased risk in women who use tamoxifen. Tamoxifen therapy has an estrogenic proliferative effect on the endometrium.[14] Risk also increases depending on duration of treatment with tamoxifen

Figure 3-1 Relationship between postmenopausal hormones, obesity, and endometrial growth.

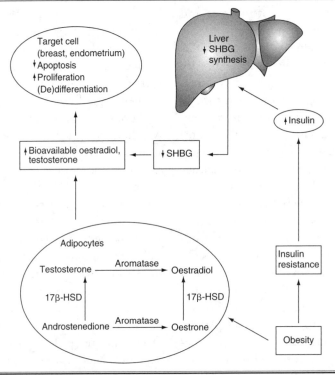

Source: Armant et al., 2005, used with permission.

and increasing cumulative dose. Data is not conclusive, and the benefit to women should always be considered against the risk.[20]

Young women with a family history of colorectal cancer appear to be at increased risk of endometrial cancer, possibly an effect of gene defects, which cause hereditary nonpolyposis colorectal cancer (HNPCC). These women, although a small group, have a significant risk of developing endometrial cancer. Individual risk rises as the woman ages, with age at onset of diagnosis with endometrial cancer occurring 15 years earlier than typically found.[21] Women with a mutation in one of the HNPCC genes develop endometrial cancer at a younger age than the sporadic endometrial cancer cases in the general population.[22]

Prevention/Early Detection

Prevention and detection is aimed at decreasing a woman's exposure to unopposed estrogen.[8] When combination hormone therapy with estrogen and progesterone is used, the incidence of endometrial cancer is decreased. Because estrogen is deposited within fatty tissue, prevention of obesity is key. Women should be encouraged to maintain a low-fat diet, with fresh fruits and vegetables and whole grains and pastas.[7] Women who consistently eat low-fat or vegetarian diets have lower circulating levels of plasma estrone and estradiol.[2] The prevention of obesity will secondarily lead to better blood pressure control and decrease the incidence of hypothyroidism and diabetes.

Prevention of endometrial cancer requires early detection and diagnosis of atypical hyperplasia. Successful eradication of hyperplasia prevents endometrial cancer from developing.[7] Patients with complex and atypical hyperplasia may be treated by hysterectomy or by periodic use of progestins, depending on age and reproductive desire. Twenty-nine percent of women with complex atypical hyperplasia will develop endometrial cancer and 15%–20% of women with atypical hyperplasia will have a coexisting cancer.[6]

Tamoxifen leads to a 2–3-fold increase risk of hyperplasia and the subsequent development of cancer. Women who take tamoxifen should be counseled about the risks of endometrial cancer, and monitored closely for symptoms of endometrial hyperplasia or cancer. Any abnormal vaginal bleeding, discharge, staining, or spotting should be investigated. If atypical endometrial hyperplasia develops, appropriate management should be instituted, and the use of tamoxifen should be reassessed.[20] Screening of women from HNPCC families is recommended to start between ages 25 and 30 years, but optimal methods and benefits have not been determined.[23]

A screening test should be safe, inexpensive, have a high predictive value, and be able to diagnose the disease in a premalignant or early stage.[11] Early, specific, and cost-effective routine screening does not exist for endometrial cancer.

There is no role for it in asymptomatic women at low risk for developing the disease. High-risk populations for whom screening for endometrial cancer is justified include:

- Postmenopausal females on exogenous estrogen therapy without accompanying progesterone therapy
- Women from families with a history of hereditary nonpolyposis colorectal cancer (HNPCC)
- Premenopausal females with anovulatory cycles, such as those with polycystic ovarian disease[24]

The American Cancer Society recommends that women at high risk for endometrial cancer undergo annual screening with endometrial biopsy (EMB) and transvaginal ultrasound starting at age 35 years.[25] The National Cancer Institute (NCI) recommends these same studies be performed at age 25 years for the same population of women.[26] Ultrasonographic measurement of endometrial thickness has been suggested as a screening technique to obtain an image of the endometrial lining and predict the likelihood of disease based on its thickness.

Numerous studies measuring endometrial thickness with the use of transvaginal ultrasonography have indicated that an endometrial thickness of less than 5 mm is rarely associated with carcinoma.[24,27] The choice of initial testing with EMB or ultrasonography depends on the patient's age and preference, disease prevalence, and sensitivity of the ultrasound machine used.[28] Sonohysterography involves placement of fluid within the endometrial cavity to enhance the examination of the endometrial lining. This technique may help differentiate between endometrial cancer and alternative diagnoses, such as polyps, fibroid, and myomas.[14]

Women with significant risk factors should have an endometrial biopsy to screen for cancer. Women with postmenopausal bleeding who are not on hormone replacement therapy (HRT) or have bleeding after being on HRT for longer than 6 months should also undergo screening. Endometrial biopsy and aspiration curettage coupled with endocervical sampling are definitive for the diagnosis if they are positive for cancer. If the endometrial biopsy and curettage are positive, then the advantage exists that the patient will not have to undergo general anesthesia. If a diagnosis is not determined by these methods, then the woman should undergo a dilatation and curettage (D & C) under anesthesia.

Molecular Basis of Disease Carcinogenesis

Endometrial cancer represents one of the few cancers where there is a clear relationship between excessive hormone stimulation and malignant transformation. In incidences associated with estrogen predominance, endometrial cancer develops at the end of a continuum of endometrial hyperplasia and progressive change, each with an increasing malignant potential.[13] Familial cancer syndromes should be considered in women diagnosed with endometrial cancer or multiple primary cancers. This appears to be of more importance in malignancies with a younger onset.[29] The first report of familial endometrial cancer was in conjunction with colorectal cancer.[30]

The majority of familial clustering of endometrial cancers is in association with hereditary nonpolyposis colorectal cancer (HNPCC).[31,32] Germline mutation of one or more of the mismatch repair genes occurs in one or more of four genes: MLH1, MLH3, MSH2, MSH6, and PMS2. Failure of this system leads to the accumulation of single base-pair mismatches, as well as small insertions and deletions in tandem repeats known as microsatellites, which manifest as microsatellite instability (MSI). Endometrial cancer is recognized as the second most common malignancy seen in HNPCC, and in some cases endometrial cancer was seen to develop many years prior to the onset of colon cancer. Women who carry the HPNCC mutation have a lifetime risk reaching 40%–60%, and endometrial cancer occurs in this population at a much younger age.[22,33,34]

Mutations of DNA mismatch repair genes in chromosome 2p (hMSH2) and chromosome 3p (hMLH1) and MSH6 account for 90% of HNPCC cases. This disturbance in DNA mismatch repair leads to genetic instability in somatic cells.[22,35] Mutations and amplifications of oncogenes K-ras, HER2/neu (ERBB2), β_1-catenin (CTNNB1), and E-cadherin (CDH1) or deletions of tumor suppressor genes TP53, p16 (CDKN2A), and pTEN/MMAC1 have been connected with the development of endometrial cancer.[8] Genetic alterations, such as pTEN mutations, microsatellite instability, K-ras mutations, and β-catenin mutations are associated with early stages of endometrial hyperplasia to low-grade endometroid carcinoma.[36] Mutations in the K-ras proto-oncogene have been reported in 10%–46% of endometrial cancer cases. PTEN, found on chromosome 10, expression is altered in endometrial cancer; specifically those of the endometroid type in up to 83% of cases.[4] Overexpression of HER2/neu has been noted in 10%–15% of papillary serous endometrial cancers and is associated with advanced disease and poor prognosis.[37] TP53 mutations have been found in over 90%

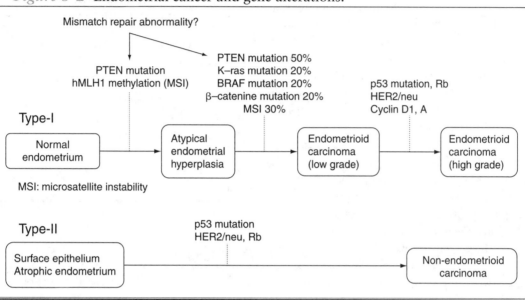

Figure 3-2 Endometrial cancer and gene alterations.

Source: Shiozawa & Konishi, 2006, used with permission.

of serous papillary endometrial cancers, and Type 2 endometrial cancers and are not found in endometroid tumors.[4,36,38] This suggests that different subtypes of endometrial cancers have different genetic pathways behind their pathogenesis[39] (**Figure 3-2**). Relaxin is a naturally occurring hormone that is known to modulate connective tissue remodeling in the uterus and cervix. Relaxin and its receptor, LGR7, are expressed in the majority of EC and EC cell lines. Overexpression of relaxin is associated with aggressive features in EC and is significantly associated with poor clinical outcome.[40]

Histology/Pathology

Endometrial cancer arises from the glandular component of the endometrial mucosa. It is dependent on cyclical changes in estrogen and progesterone. The abnormal imbalance is the most causative factor (**Table 3-1**). Histologically, these tumors are well to moderately differentiated, generally diagnosed at an early stage, and survival is longer. In the majority of cases, these tumors express estrogen and progesterone receptors (ER and PR, respectively), although there is variability in the ratios of the PR isoforms (PRA and PRB).[13]

Type I or adenocarcinoma, endometroid-type is the most common pathology and comprises the majority of cases, though several other histologic subtypes also occur (**Table 3-2**). The majority of endometrial cancers are adenocarcinomas, with endometroid the most common histologic subtype.[41] Risk factors associated with Type I endometrial cancer are associated with risk factors that directly or indirectly influence estrogen levels.[23]

Persistent unopposed estrogenic stimulation leads to endometrial hyperplasia. Endometrial hyperplasia is regarded as a precursor of endometrial carcinoma.[14] Endometrial hyperplasia is classified as simple hyperplasia with or without atypia and complex with or without atypia. Endometrial hyperplasia is overgrowth of the endometrial lining of the uterus as a result of prolific stimulation of the endometrium. This presents clinically as abnormal bleeding. Hyperplasia with atypia is a complex pattern with crowding of the glands. The presence of atypical cells indicates high risk for the progression to cancer. Hyperplasia and endometrial cancer are two different entities, and the distinguishing feature is the presence or absence of cytologic atypia. These two cytologic variants can exist simultaneously. Seventy-five percent of women with atypical hyperplasia have a history of exposure to unopposed estrogen, either exogenous or endogenous. A recent study found that more than 40% of women with atypical hyperplasia developed endometrial cancer, and some of the cancers had invaded the myometrium, some deeply.[42]

Type II endometrial cancers are less common and can appear simultaneously with hyperplasia, but are not clearly related to a transition from atypical hyperplasia. They arise in a background of inert or atrophic endometrium and are associated with more undifferentiated cell types, lower overall survival rates, and a higher risk of metastatic disease at the time of surgical staging.[3,6] Patients with serous (also known as papillary serous) and clear cell carcinomas tend to be older then those with other types and are more likely to have abnormal cervical cytology. The remaining 25% of women develop these types of endometrial cancer and these neoplasms tend to be associated with a more undifferentiated cell type and a poorer prognosis.[12]

Table 3-2 CLASSIFICATION OF ENDOMETRIAL CARCINOMA.

Endometroid adenocarcinoma
Adenocarcinoma with squamous differentiation
Serous adenocarcinoma (papillary serous)
Mucinous adenocarcinoma
Clear cell adenocarcinoma
Squamous cell carcinoma
Mixed müllerian
Undifferentiated
Sarcoma

Assessment

Only 1%–5% of endometrial cancers are diagnosed while the patient is asymptomatic. Diagnosis most often results from the Pap smear showing atypical or malignant endometrial cells or the discovery of cancer in a uterus removed for benign gynecologic indications. Ninety percent of women present with an initial complaint of excessive vaginal bleeding that should be evaluated [6,24] (**Table 3-3**). This usually presents as menometrorrhagia in a perimenopausal woman or menstrual-like bleeding in a woman past menopause. Perimenopausal women relate a history of intermenstrual bleeding, excessive bleeding lasting longer than 7 days, or an interval of less than 21 days between menses. Heavy, prolonged bleeding in patients known to be at risk for anovulatory cycles should have histologic evaluation of the endometrium.

A pregnancy test must be done on all women of childbearing age. Physical examination of the abdomen may reveal ascites, or omental and liver metastases, but is

Table 3-3 Patients in whom a diagnosis of endometrial cancer should be excluded.

1. All patients with postmenopausal bleeding
2. Postmenopausal women with a pyometra
3. Asymptomatic postmenopausal women with endometrial cells on a Pap smear, particularly if it is atypical
4. Perimenopausal women with intermenstrual bleeding or increasingly heavy periods
5. Premenopausal patients with abnormal uterine bleeding, particularly if there is a history of anovulation

Source: Hacker, 2005, used with permission.

usually benign. Retention of blood in the uterine cavity (hematometra) may present as a large midline mass arising from the pelvis. A careful pelvic exam should be performed with inspection and palpation of the vulva, vagina, and cervix to exclude metastatic spread or other causes of abnormal vaginal bleeding. The uterus may or may not be enlarged. A rectovaginal exam should be performed to evaluate the fallopian tubes, ovaries, and cul-de-sac.[24]

Women with endometrial cells on a Pap smear should be evaluated, particularly if atypical cells are present.[24] Fifteen percent of women in the general population with postmenopausal bleeding will develop endometrial cancer. Eighty percent of postmenopausal women will have a complaint of abnormal purulent or blood-tinged vaginal discharge.[12] Some will present with pelvic pain and are found to have hematometra. Premenopausal women usually have complaints of heavy periods and intermittent spotting. Presenting symptoms of advanced disease include pelvic

pressure, ascites, and hemorrhage that are related to uterine enlargement and extrauterine spread of tumor.[6,7]

Diagnosis and Staging

The diagnosis of endometrial cancer involves several steps. A thorough, carefully executed history and physical exam assists in identifying risk factors, including genetically linked cancers, signs, and symptoms. Diagnostic tools used in the diagnosis of endometrial cancer include dilatation and curettage (D & C), endometrial biopsy (EMB), hysteroscopy, and transvaginal sonography (TVS). Endometrial sampling with an EMB and endocervical biopsy should be performed, as well as a hysteroscopy. Hysteroscopy is the direct inspection of the endometrial cavity. The use of hysteroscopy should be used if the diagnosis is not obtainable from usual procedures. This allows the opportunity to obtain a biopsy specimen and remove lesions. An endocervical biopsy is performed to determine cervical involvement.

EMB in combination with hysteroscopy have been found to be a reliable alternative to exam under anesthesia.[43] Because there is a false-negative rate of approximately 10%, a negative EMB in a symptomatic patient must be followed by a D & C under anesthesia.[24] A Pap smear and pelvic exam, along with a rectovaginal exam, assist in determining the extent of disease. The uterus may or may not be enlarged; however, size is not always an indicator of presence or absence of cancer. The Pap smear may be normal.

No diagnostic study has emerged as the standard of care, and multiple modalities are used in the diagnosis/screening of endometrial cancer and include TVS, computed tomography (CT), and/or magnetic resonance imaging (MRI) of the abdomen and pelvis. Imaging is valuable in the pretreatment stage of patients and can assist in two main respects: (1) determining the local extent of the tumor, such as myometrial invasion and cervical involvement, and (2) determining evidence of extrauterine spread, particularly lymph node metastases and, less often, direct spread to the tissues surrounding the uterus. In all cases a chest X-ray (CXR) is mandatory to evaluate the cardiopulmonary status of the patient and identify presence of metastases.

TVS can be used to image endometrial thickness and myometrium and evaluate the uterus for overall size and deformity. TVS is considered to be useful for identifying endometrial malignancies; it is a very sensitive study but not very specific because it has a low positive value and a high false-positive rate. TVS is useful for identification of patients who require further diagnostic evaluation, including EMB.[44] TVS is often the first imaging test undertaken for evaluation of women on tamoxifen therapy and is also helpful in determining which patients should have a biopsy and for use in women on tamoxifen therapy for surveillance.[45] TVS has been studied as an alternative to hysteroscopy, which is an invasive procedure.[43]

More extensive preoperative assessment, such as MRI, CT scan, or barium enema, may be indicated for patients whose disease has features that put them at high risk for metastases (poorly differentiated, papillary serous, clear cell, or sarcomatous histology). MRI may be the most accurate technique for assessing the local extent of disease in terms of myometrial invasion, lymph node, and cervical involvement due to its excellent soft tissue contrast resolution. It has greater sensitivity and accuracy than TVS or abdominal CT. MRI/CT are not sensitive for diagnosing lymph node metastases by size criteria.[44]

Evaluation for metastases is indicated in patients with abnormal liver function tests, an elevated CA 125 value, clinical evidence of metastases, and parametrial or vaginal tumor extension. For locally advanced disease, cystoscopy, proctoscopy, and/or barium enema should be obtained.[6,11]

Surgical staging has been the standard of care since 1988 (Table 3-4). It was found that this was superior to clinical staging in that more patients were found to have disease beyond the uterus. Surgical staging includes an open procedure with removal of the uterus and ovaries, lymph node sampling, and peritoneal cytology. The extent of the surgical procedure is based on the stage of disease, which can only be determined at the time of the operation.

Stage denotes the extent of disease (Figure 3-3). The most important predictor of outcome and survival in women with endometrial cancer is tumor stage.[8,14] Stage I disease is limited to the uterus corpus without involvement of the serosa, with 5-year survival rates of 85%. In stage II, the uterus is involved, and the disease extends to the cervix; survival is 70%. Stage III, survival of 49%, and stage IV, survival of 18%, means the patient has regional or distant metastases; the disease has spread outside the uterus. This may include spread to the adnexa, intraperitoneal spread to other structures, pelvic lymph nodes, aortic lymph nodes, and/or positive peritoneal cytology.

The grade of the tumor signifies how closely the tumor resembles the tissue of origin. In endometrial cancer, the tumor grows in a solid fashion, whereas the normal tissue grows in a glandular fashion. Grade I signifies a tumor that is well differentiated, when 5% or less of the tumor shows a solid growth pattern. Grade II is moderately differentiated, and between 6% and

Figure 3-3 Endometrial cancer staging.

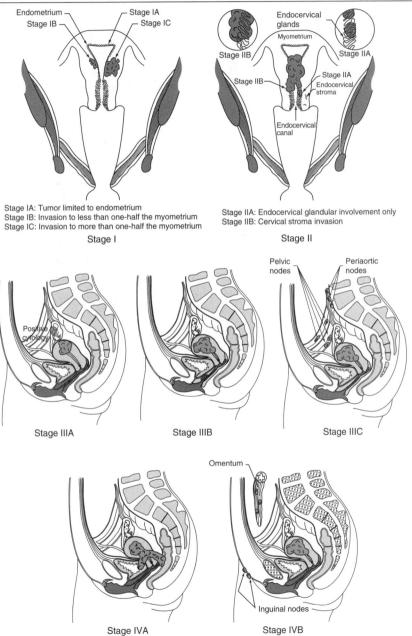

Stage IA: Tumor limited to endometrium
Stage IB: Invasion to less than one-half the myometrium
Stage IC: Invasion to more than one-half the myometrium

Stage I

Stage IIA: Endocervical glandular involvement only
Stage IIB: Cervical stroma invasion

Stage II

Stage IIIA   Stage IIIB   Stage IIIC

Stage IVA   Stage IVB

Source: DiSaia, P.J. & Creasman, W.T. (2007). *Clinical Gynecologic Oncology* 5th ed. St. Louis, MO: Mosby Year Book, Inc., used with permission.

50% of the tumor is growing in a solid fashion. Grade III is poorly differentiated, and more than 50% of the tumor shows a solid growth pattern; a significant nuclear atypia increases the grade of differentiation by one grade.[14,23] Preoperative tumor grade does not predict final histologic results.[46]

The extent of treatment and prognosis are strongly dependent on stage and grade. Prognosis is dependent on:

- Histology/grade
- Tumor stage
- Myometrial invasion
- Extension into cervix
- Peritoneal cytology
- Lymph node metastasis
- Lymphvascular space invasion
- Age

About two-thirds of newly diagnosed women with endometrial cancer have early-stage tumor confined to the uterus with favorable prognostic factors and are typically cured with surgery with or without adjuvant radiation therapy. The remaining one-third of women newly diagnosed with endometrial cancer have more advanced disease (FIGO stage III and IV) tumors and have poor prognostic features. The depth of myometrial invasion, especially invasion of the outer third of the myometrium, cervical involvement, high-grade histologic variants (papillary-serous and clear cell), and aortic node involvement all appear to be important signs of more aggressive disease that is prone to metastasize to distant sites. Positive peritoneal washings at time of surgery is a sign of poor prognosis.[8,12,47]

Metastatic disease on surgical evaluation occurs 6%–10% of the time in those patients with disease clinically confined to the uterus. Lymph node involvement is related to FIGO grade and depth of tumor invasion. Vascular space invasion appears to be an independent risk factor for recurrence and for death from endometrial carcinoma.[24] The presence of deep myometrial invasion is the strongest predictor of lymphatic/hematogenous dissemination in endometrial cancer. Age has been found to be a predictor of survival for endometrial cancer unrelated to surgical stage or grade of adenocarcinoma. As women age over 50 years, factors such as advanced disease at time of diagnosis and deep myometrial invasion cause survival rates to decline.[12,41,48]

Standard therapies include surgery, radiation therapy, chemotherapy, and hormonal therapy. The best outcomes are associated with surgery, or surgery in combination with radiation in women with high-risk features.[8] Women who have endometrial cancer with high-risk features or documented extrauterine disease require adjuvant therapy. Adjuvant therapy should also be considered in those women with grade 1 tumors and additional characteristics such as aneuploidy, p53 overexpression, low ER/PR receptor, and high microvessel density.[36]

Surgical Management/ Advances

Patients with endometrial cancer often have existing comorbidities, often making them at high risk for undergoing surgical procedures. Careful attention and a thorough history and physical will determine the need for preoperative clearance by a medical internist. The exam will also elucidate information that may affect the surgical approach and risks associated with surgery.

In 1988, the International Federation of Gynecology and Obstetrics (FIGO) replaced clinical staging of endometrial cancer, instead favoring surgical staging (**Table 3-4**), including assessment of pelvic and para-aortic lymph nodes for metastases. Approximately 70%–80% of patients with endometrial cancer present with localized disease that potentially can be cured with surgery alone.

The standard surgical procedure for the treatment of endometrial cancer is total abdominal hysterectomy with bilateral salpingo-oophorectomy. This should be accompanied by appropriate staging procedures that include pelvic and para-aortic lymph-adenectomy and peritoneal fluid cytology, especially in patients at risk for metastatic or recurrent disease.[48] Partial omentectomy is performed if the frozen section indicates that there is high-grade tumor invading the myometrium. Aggressive cytoreduction should be performed when extrauterine macroscopic disease is seen. Lymph vascular space invasion (LVSI) leads to an independent and significantly increased risk for pelvic lymph node metastases. The presence of LVSI may indicate the need for lymphadenectomy and subsequent adjuvant therapy.[8,49]

The majority of patients are diagnosed without extrauterine spread, stages I and II, and are medically able to undergo surgery. Radical hysterectomy with pelvic node

Table 3-4 FIGO SURGICAL STAGING FOR ENDOMETRIAL CARCINOMA.

Stage	Grade	Description
IA	1,2,3	Tumor limited to the endometrium
IB	1,2,3	Invasion to less than one-half of the myometrium
IC	1,2,3	Invasion to more than one-half of the myometrium
IIA	1,2,3	Endocervical glandular involvement only
IIB	1,2,3	Cervical stromal involvement
IIIA	1,2,3	Tumor invades serosa, and/or adnexa, and/or positive peritoneal cytology
IIIB	1,2,3	Vaginal metastases
IIIC	1,2,3	Metastases to pelvic and or paraaortic lymph nodes
IVA	1,2,3	Tumor invasion of the bladder and/or bowel mucosa
IVB	1,2,3	Distant metastases including intraabdominal and/or inguinal lymph nodes

Source: FIGO, International Federation of Gynecology and Obstetrics. www.figo.org. International Federation of Gynecology and Obstetrics. Staging classifications and clinical practice guidelines of gynaecologic cancers, 2003. www.figo.org/content/PDF/staging-booklet.pdf, used with permission.

dissection should be considered for women with gross cervical involvement or if MRI indicates cervical involvement.[50] Studies in the advancement in surgical management are attempting to answer if less surgery is better if accompanied by pelvic radiation with or without vaginal brachytherapy in women who are not ideal surgical candidates. [51]

By combining operative laparoscopy with simple vaginal hysterectomy, laparoscopic-assisted surgical staging has been proposed as an alternative to laparotomy for patients with early endometrial cancer. Operative laparoscopy allows for the assessment of the peritoneal cavity, the ability to obtain peritoneal washings, lymph node sampling in indicated cases, and the guaranteed removal of the adnexa. In randomized trials comparing LAVH/BSO with staging and traditional laparotomy with surgical staging, minimally invasive surgery appears to be a reasonable surgical option in 90% of women with early-stage endometrial cancer. Laparoscopy also has an application in the staging of endometrial cancer patients who were incompletely staged initially. Some limitations to this include the surgeon's expertise and the patient's body habitus.[52] Other studies are looking at the benefit of extended surgical staging in stage IV disease. In a review of studies analyzing the benefit of surgical cytoreduction, consistent data was found suggesting that the size of residual disease after surgery has an important impact on the survival of patients with advanced endometrial cancer.[8]

Radiation Therapy/ Advances

In the past, irradiation was often administered in the preoperative setting. At present, irradiation alone is rarely administered; preoperative irradiation is given only in selective cases, with postoperative irradiation administered most commonly.[53] Primary radiation therapy with curative intent is reserved for those women who are medically inoperable and have been clinically staged (**Table 3-5**) through exam under anesthesia, sounding of the uterus, or limited number of other methods such as endocervical curettage, hysteroscopy, cystoscopy, proctoscopy, and radiographic examinations of the lungs and skeleton.[24] Disease-specific survival rates may be 10%–20% lower than similar clinical stage patients who undergo surgery.[3,54] This includes patients with advanced age, severe cardiopulmonary disease or compromise, and those with extreme morbid obesity.

The role of adjuvant radiation for endometrial cancer remains controversial and requires randomized trials to answer the question. Postoperative options include:[24]

- Observation
- Vault brachytherapy
- External pelvic irradiation
- Whole-abdominal irradiation

It has been shown that adjuvant radiotherapy following primary surgery significantly improves pelvic tumor control but has no measurable impact on overall survival in an unselected patient population.[24,55] An analysis of a large number of women with stage IC grade 1 and stage IC grades 3 and 4 supported that adjuvant radiotherapy was significantly associated with improved overall survival and relative survival.[56] Patients who have undergone complete surgical staging receive postoperative adjuvant therapy based on pathologic risk factors identified by examination of the surgical specimen.[53]

Table 3-5 1971 FIGO CLINICAL STAGING FOR ENDOMETRIAL CANCER.

Stage 0	Carcinoma in situ.
Stage I	The carcinoma is confined to the corpus.
Stage IA	The length of the uterine cavity is 8 cm or less.
Stage IB	The length of the uterine cavity is more than 8 cm.

Stage I cases should be subgrouped with regard to the histologic grade of the adenocarcinoma as follows:

Grade 1	Highly differentiated adenomatous carcinoma.
Grade 2	Moderately differentiated adenomatous carcinoma with partly solid areas.
Grade 3	Predominantly solid or entirely undifferentiated carcinoma.
Stage II	The carcinoma has involved the corpus and the cervix but has not extended outside the uterus.
Stage III	The carcinoma has extended outside the uterus but not outside the true pelvis.
Stage IV	The carcinoma has extended outside the true pelvis or has obviously involved the mucosa of the bladder or rectum. A bullous edema as such does not permit a case to be allocated to stage IV.
Stage IVA	Spread of the growth to adjacent organs.
Stage IVB	Spread to distant organs.

Source: FIGO, International Federation of Gynecology and Obstetrics. www.figo.org. International Federation of Gynecology and Obstetrics. Classification and staging of malignant tumors in the female pelvis. *Int J Gynaecol Oncol.* 1971; 9:172, used with permission.

Evidence exists to suggest that in node-negative disease, treatment planning can be more conservative to reduce patient morbidity while maintaining excellent survival.[55] The approaches taken include limiting postoperative radiotherapy to vault brachytherapy or omitting any form of adjuvant radiation.[57] In those patients who are at high risk for relapse after surgery, radiation therapy is used, most often with concurrent chemotherapy as a sensitizing agent to improve locoregional control. Procedures include external beam radiation therapy, brachytherapy, and whole pelvic and whole abdomen radiation therapy. These procedures are shown to have an impact on the local control of disease but not survival.[58]

Vaginal vault brachytherapy used postoperatively has been shown to increase survival and disease-free interval. High-risk histologies, such as papillary serous and clear cell and the presence of lymphvascular space invasion, deep invasion, or grade 3 lesions may warrant adjuvant radiotherapy. Patients with para-aortic and pelvic lymph node involvement should receive radiation therapy to the involved field. Vaginal radiation can be delivered with high-dose-rate (HDR) or low-dose-rate (LDR) equipment. Both techniques have resulted in excellent local control rates and low morbidity. HDR vaginal cuff brachytherapy is one of the most common methods used to deliver postoperative cuff radiation therapy for patients with endometrial cancer. HDR treatments require multiple insertions, generally with one insertion done every week for 3–6 weeks. However, hospitalization is not required, and each insertion takes only a brief amount of time. LDR treatments are delivered once but do require hospitalization for 2–3 days. HDR vaginal brachytherapy in thoroughly staged patients with intermediate-risk endometrial cancer provides excellent overall and disease-free survival with less toxicity and less cost compared with whole-pelvic radiation. Adjuvant whole pelvis radiation therapy is an effective treatment for stage I–III endometrial cancer with high-risk pathologic factors with risk factors for intra-abdominal recurrence, including serous papillary and clear cell variants.[12,59,60]

Intraoperative radiation therapy (IORT) is used as a boost technique in patients who would otherwise require high doses of external radiation therapy. IORT treatment can deliver a single high dose of radiation to a tumor or tumor bed after surgical resection or surgical exposure of high-risk areas. A linear accelerator that produces high-energy electron beams is used to deliver precise, highly concentrated doses of radiation directly to the tumor site while avoiding adjacent normal tissues. A single dose delivered in one treatment during a surgical procedure is equivalent to several weeks of daily radiation treatments. The rationale for this treatment is to increase the therapeutic ratio of local tumor control without significantly increasing the risk of complication.[61]

IORT has been used at various medical centers as a component of aggressive treat-ment approaches for locally advanced primary or recurrent gynecologic cancers, including endometrial cancer.[62] The use of intraoperative radiation therapy in the treatment of endometrial cancer continues to be studied. Current trials are attempting to tailor radiotherapy to the area of highest risk, address the need for pelvic radiotherapy in higher risk patients, and address the distant failure rate seen in high-risk histologies.[63]

Palliative radiation therapy may be used in women with isolated advanced or recurrent disease located in areas not previously irradiated. When palliation is the goal of therapy, it is important to fully evaluate the patient's medical status.[53] In advanced disease, stages III and IV, radiation therapy, chemotherapy, and hormonal therapy are employed.

Chemotherapy/ Hormonal Therapy/ Advances

Surgical management and radiation therapy are not treatment options in young premenopausal women who wish to retain fertility. This includes the 3%–5% of women under the age of 40 when diagnosed with endometrial cancer, most of whom are nulliparous due to infertility issues.[64] Conservative management of endometrial cancer is reserved for candidates who have been carefully selected in regard to grade, receptor status, lymph node status, extrauterine involvement, and imaging to determine depth of invasion.

Fertility conserving approaches deviate from the surgical standard of care. Progestins can induce regression of endometrial cancer and endometrial hyperplasia without atypia.

Therapy with progestins is more effective in young women and in those with well-differentiated tumors. Patient treatment regimens range from 3–6 months and may or may not be combined with a selective estrogen receptor modulator (SERM), and patients are surveilled by EMB or D & C. Following successful treatment, patients should be maintained on an oral contraceptive (OCP) or progestin regimen to prevent recurrent carcinoma. Long-term surveillance should continue every 3–6 months.[64]

Patients who are not interested in or unable to participate in long-term medical care should be offered surgical intervention when fertility is no longer desired or abandoned. In some patients, disease is resistant or refractory to the treatment with progestins. In others, due to side effects, patient compliance is poor. These patients should be offered hysterectomy.[65] Conservative therapy may result in successful pregnancies. Most often, though, this is achieved through assisted reproduction technology.[66] The patient should attempt to become pregnant as soon as complete response is achieved. After childbearing is completed, hysterectomy should be performed.[64]

Systemic therapy is required in cases of initial advanced disease and at the time of relapse. The number of effective chemotherapeutic agents has been found to be limited. Chemotherapy has a role in endometrial cancer in patients with a high risk of relapse, those with stage IIIB or high-grade disease, and those with stage III or IV papillary serous histology.[55,67]

Chemotherapy may be used as a single agent or a multiple agent, or used as combination therapy with radiation. Active agents against endometrial cancer include: doxorubicin, cisplatin, carboplatin, and paclitaxel. In trials enrolling women with advanced or recurrent disease, it is shown that multiagent therapy with a taxane, anthracycline, and platinum regimen is most effective and may increase survival rates from 50%–59%. Studies have also shown that the combination of platinum, doxorubicin, and cyclophosphamide have improved the 5-year survival rate in women with stage I and II disease. The outcome for stage III patients is still unfavorable, depending on the degree of lymph vassular space invasion (LVSI) and deep myometrial invasion. Carboplatin has low toxicity and is active in chemotherapy-naïve advanced endometrial cancer patients. The choice of the initial dose can be determined according to whether the patient has received prior radiotherapy. Taxol is an active agent in the treatment of endometrial cancer in patients who have had previous chemotherapy or advanced disease.[8,47,67,68]

Ongoing studies are determining the use of targeted therapy in the treatment of endometrial cancer. These agents act on a specific population of cells or on a specific molecule of the cell cycle. Targeting the epithelial growth factor receptor (EGFR) pathway would be appropriate on the basis of the biologic characteristic of endometrial cancer or possibly vascular endothelial growth factor (VEGF) on the basis of antiangiogenic effects seen in other malignancies. It is likely these targeted therapies will need to be combined with systemic therapy to assess synergy and to improve outcome.[69]

Endocrine or hormonal therapy is used in endometrial cancer with the aim of prolonging the progression-free interval and time to recurrence in stage I and II lesions after initial surgery and radiation therapy (XRT), and in patients with major comorbidities. This is usually in the form of an oral progestin. Following the theory of estrogen excess as a carcinogenic promoter, progestogens have been used in the treatment of endometrial cancer for their antiestrogenic effects on the endometrium.[69] It has been shown that the increasing of the dose of the medication does not offer a greater response; therefore, higher doses leading to a higher side effect profile are not advocated. The best responders to hormonal therapy are women with well-differentiated lesions and estrogen receptor (ER)/progesterone receptor (PR) positivity.[70] Depo-Provera, Provera, Delalutin, and Megace are the most common progestational agents currently used for women who are estrogen and progesterone receptor positive.[71]

Although regarded as an antiestrogen in breast tissue, tamoxifen is known to have estrogenic or agonist activity at other sites. Tamoxifen blocks the binding of estradiol to the ER of endometrial carcinomas. The benefit of treatment with the drug should outweigh the risk of thromboembolic events and weight gain in women who may already be obese.[72,73]

Advances in the use of hormonal and chemotherapeutic agents, such as Mifeprostine, aromatase inhibitors, and SERMs, have been made. Mifeprostine is an antiprogesterone and noncompeting antiestrogen. It blocks the capacity of the endometrial tissue to grow in response to estrogen. It fights tumors that have progesterone receptors by binding those receptors and also by blocking the growth of new blood vessels that the cancer needs to grow. Aromatase expression is hormonally controlled in adipose cells. Aromatase activity has been reported in endometrial cancer cell lines and endometrial cancer tissues. Disease-free endometrium does not express aromatase. Treatment with aromatase inhibitors decreases cell proliferation in endometrial cancer cells by reducing estrogen production.

SERMs mimic the effect of estrogens in some tissues but act as estrogen antagonists in others. All SERMs act by binding with high affinity to the estrogen receptor and yet produce tissue- and drug-specific responses. SERMs are ER antagonists in the uterus. SERM studies show that the new SERMS are better antagonists in the endometrium; the basic mechanism of action is again binding both ER sites. Each different SERM has a specific affinity for the organ-specific ER alpha and/or ER beta that leads to the unique conformation of the ER-SERM complex. This structure allows coregulatory proteins to induce or stop gene activation.[72,74] Second- and third-generation SERMs, such as raloxifene and arzoxifene, have more selective estrogen antagonism in the uterus. Arzoxifene is more potent than raloxifene by 30–100 times.[75] It may produce clinical responses in both progesterone-sensitive and progesterone-refractory tumors, producing a response of longer duration and increased number of stable disease.[76]

Recurrent Disease/ Nursing Implications

Weight loss, pain, and vaginal bleeding can suggest recurrent disease, which most commonly occurs during the first 3 years following primary treatment.[38] The natural history of endometrial cancers includes extrauterine spread by direct extension to adjacent structures, transtubal passage of exfoliated cells, hematogenous and lymphatic dissemination, or a combination.[24] Deep myometrial invasion, moderately or poorly differentiated tumors, lymphvascular space invasion, node involvement, positive cytology, and cervical involvement are considered to be risk factors for recurrence.[8,77] (See **Figure 3-4**)

Figure 3-4 Metastatic spread of endometrial cancer.

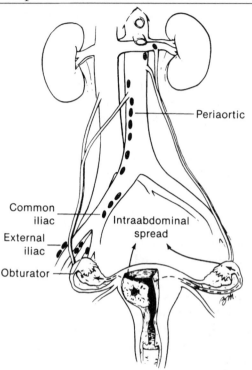

Source: DiSaia, P.J. & Creasman, W.T. (2007). *Clinical Gynecologic Oncology* 5th ed. St. Louis, MO: Mosby Year Book, Inc., used with permission.

Patients with recurrent endometrial cancer must be fully evaluated for sites of recurrent disease. Depending on the site of recurrence and prior therapy, patients may be treated for palliation or for cure.[6] Recurrent endometrial cancer is initially confined to the pelvis in 50% of patients. The major sites of distant metastases are the abdominal cavity, liver, and lungs.[12] Reported median survival times in patients with recurrent disease is rarely more than 1 year.[78] The treatment of recurrent disease is dependent upon the location, extent, and nature of recurrence.

Isolated recurrences, most often seen in the vagina, are still highly curable, especially if confined to the pelvis and treated definitively with surgery or XRT. Patients with recurrent endometrial cancer confined to the pelvis should be treated with external pelvic irradiation and intracavitary or interstitial brachytherapy.[53] Isolated pelvic central recurrence after irradiation is rare. Selected patients in whom it does occur may benefit from pelvic exenteration. Although the long-term survival rate after this procedure is only 20%, it remains the only potentially curative option for the few patients with central recurrence of endometrial cancer who have not responded to standard surgery and radiation therapy. Systemic recurrences may be treated with chemotherapy.[12,41]

Patients with recurrent endometrial carcinoma often receive hormonal therapy with progestins. These agents most often offer only palliation. Toxicity is minimal. Response rates to progestins range from 15%–30%, and therapy can be continued indefinitely. Tamoxifen has been used in the treatment of endometrial cancer both in the salvage setting and as a first-line systemic therapy, though it is not as active as progestins and is of little value as second-line therapy in patients who do not respond to progestins.[12]

For patients whose disease is refractory to hormonal therapy, chemotherapy offers modest efficacy. Active agents include doxorubicin, cisplatin, carboplatin, ifosfamide, and paclitaxel. Combination chemotherapy with cisplatin and doxorubicin results in higher response rates than single-agent doxorubicin chemotherapy. Paclitaxel in combination with cisplatin and doxorubicin chemotherapy improves both response rate and median survival; however, this three-drug combination is associated with increased toxicity. Progression-free survival was limited to 4.8 months.[78]

Topotecan has been shown to have activity in women with advanced or recurrent endometrial cancer that have not received prior cytotoxic therapy; however, more studies are needed to determine the maximum tolerated dose (MTD) and the most efficacious dose in light of the intolerable side effects of hematologic, gastrointestinal, and neurologic toxicities. Support with hematopoietic growth factors is also necessary.[79] Weekly topotecan has also been shown to have efficacy and tolerability in patients that had been previously treated with radiation and chemotherapy.[80]

Follow-Up Care

Surveillance is the observation and follow-up of asymptomatic patients who are clinically free of disease with the aim of diagnosing relapse as soon as possible while disease is still localized and treatable.[81] Most endometrial carcinoma recurrences occur within the first 2 years after therapy.[35] Follow-up for women with endometrial cancer and subsequent therapy is every 2–4 months for 2–3 years depending on the risk recurrence, then every 6 months through the 5th year, and then annually.[81] Several goals for follow-up for women with endometrial cancer are identified: (1) early detection and treatment of recurrent disease, (2) psychologic support of the patient, (3) provision of health maintenance and other screening services, and (4) diagnosis and management of treatment side effects. Patients should be followed by a healthcare professional who is knowledgeable about the natural history of the disease and who is proficient at performing speculum and pelvic exams to diagnose or detect a local (vaginal) recurrence because this type of recurrence is potentially curable.

Exams also should include complete history, pelvic-rectal examination, yearly chest X-ray, and counseling about the signs and symptoms of recurrence and the potential adverse effects of radiotherapy.[82] Women who are young and diagnosed before age 50 years are three times more likely to develop an additional cancer, most often colon cancer. More aggressive colonsocopy-based screening should be encouraged in this group.

Tertiary cancer prevention includes the ongoing surveillance and early detection of secondary primary malignancies and other treatment-related complications in cancer survivors. Survivors are also at risk for psychosocial problems that stem from the effects of the diagnosis and/or treatment. The development of breast cancer and colorectal cancer after endometrial cancer may occur in both long- and short-term survivors of endometrial cancer. Regular mammography and clinical breast exams are indicated in all women who have been treated for endometrial cancer. Women should be counseled about colonoscopy and recommendations based on the magnitude of risk and findings after the first colonoscopy. Anxiety and fear about cancer recurrence in long-term survivors should be addressed. Communication of second cancer risk should focus on screening and prevention to detect cancers early and further increase survival and QOL.[83]

Obesity is a significant risk factor in the development of endometrial cancer and continues to be a health threat to women after treatment. Obese women are likely to also have comorbid conditions that require medical intervention and surveillance. Even in early-stage endometrial cancer, survivors are dying of obesity-driven conditions. Lifestyle and dietary modifications are required to improve overall survival and health outcomes in these women.[84]

Symptom Management/ Advances

Menopause is induced by surgery for endometrial cancer if the woman is not already menopausal preoperatively. The onset of surgical menopause in premenopausal women is abrupt and often dramatic with oophorectomy.

The physical and psychological changes that extend from this precipitous drop in endogenous estrogens and androgens tend to be more dramatic and generally have a significant impact on a woman's quality of life.[85] Whether to offer hormone replacement therapy after surgery for endometrial cancer remains an area of controversy. Women with a history of endometrial cancer have been denied this therapy because adenocarcinoma of the endometrium is considered, and estrogen-dependent neoplasm and the administration of estrogen may stimulate occult disease.[84,86] The postoperative use of supplemental estrogen as treatment for menopausal hot flashes and other symptoms and prophylaxis against osteoporosis and heart disease appear to be safe, although only a small number of patients have been evaluated.[6]

The American College of Obstetricians and Gynecologists Committee Opinion concluded that in women with a history of endometrial cancer, estrogens could be used for the same indications as for any other woman, except the selection of appropriate candidates should be based on prognostic indicators and the risk the patient is willing to assume.[87] A review of estrogen replacement in patients with stage I and II endometrial cancer found no difference in progression-free or overall survival associated with estrogen use. Of note, 53% of patients treated with estrogen received progestin therapy. In addition, patients with estrogen replacement had a lower-stage and lower-grade cancer, and also less depth of invasion, as compared to patients that did not receive estrogen.

In a study initiated in 1997, the GOG followed 1236 patients who had been randomized to placebo versus estrogen replacement therapy. The majority of participants had stage IA or IB disease. Due to the early closure of the study, the group could not conclusively refute or support the safety of exogenous estrogen with regard to risk of endometrial cancer recurrence. The absolute recurrence rate at 35.7 months in the low-risk population was low and did not differ from the placebo group.[86] Treatment with selective serotonin-reuptake inhibitors (SSRIs), the tricyclic antidepressant opipramol, and antiepileptic gabapentin have all shown to reduce the incidence of hot flashes.[88]

Because of the lack of estrogen, the patient may also report decreased vaginal lubrication, vaginal burning and pruritus, and dyspareunia. Nurses can advise on the use of a vaginal moisturizer to restore moisture to vaginal mucosa and water-based lubricants to facilitate sexual relations. The lower acidic environment caused by low levels of estrogen may lead to development of frequent vaginal infections, many times leading to a urinary tract infection. Use of lactobacillus supplements and acidophilus maintains the balance.

Patients may also report joint and back pain as a result of osteoporosis. Calcium with vitamin D supplement and weight-bearing exercise are essential in prevention. Calcium intake for postmenopausal women reaches 1200–1500 mg per day. Vitamin D assists in the absorption of calcium and must be taken with calcium. If taken as a supplement, 400 IU to 800 IU daily is recommended. A minimum of 20 minutes of daily sun exposure also meets the daily recommended intake. Foods that are high in calcium are salmon, dark green vegetables, and dairy products. Prescription medications for prevention and treatment include: bisphosphanates, SERMs, raloxifene, calcitonin, and alendronate and risedronate, both which must be taken on an empty stomach, and the patient should not lie down for half an hour after taking the medication. Women should quit smoking and reduce alcohol consumption.

Exercise also plays an important role after treatment for endometrial cancer. Twenty minutes of exercise 3–4 times weekly is recommended. In a recent study, 70% of subjects did not meet public health exercise guidelines, and as many were overweight or obese. The study of 386 endometrial cancer survivors supported that exercise and body weight had significant, independent, and clinically meaningful associations with QOL.[89] Estrogen therapy, treatment with SERMS, and tamoxifen necessitate the evaluation and monitoring of patients in that they may develop DVT and are ultimately at risk for PE. Another side effect is hot flashes.

Lower extremity lymphedema can be a potentially acute and chronic complication of lymph node dissection, extensive tumor reduction surgery, and radiation. The manifestations range from mild to severe, and it is a life-long condition. Treatment consists of elevation of the lower extremities higher than the heart, compression therapy with either elastic stockings or compression devices, manual massage, exercising, and effective skin care. Women should be encouraged to increase water intake and follow a diet with more fruits and vegetables and less animal fat and dairy. Leg exercises in a pool and swimming have shown results. Obvious avoidance of injury and activities that impede lymphatic flow are stressed. If a change of color of the lower extremity is noted, or if pain increases or fever is present, a physician should be consulted to rule out a blood clot or cellulitis in the lower extremity.

Early and late side effects of radiation therapy include diarrhea, dysuria, and urinary frequency to fistulas, bladder irritation, and vaginal stenosis. Symptom management with appropriate medications should be employed to prevent or stop acute symptoms. Chronic use of a vaginal dilator may be necessary to prevent problems with vaginal shortening and stenosis following brachytherapy and teletherapy. Management of fistulas includes conservative management with TPN, somatostatin, and bowel rest to aggressive surgical procedures.

Patients may also have neurotoxicity issues from the use of platinum and taxanes. Peripheral foot and hand care is important, and the possible deep tendon affect must be addressed to keep the patient mobile and safe. Patients who receive progestins may develop headache, bloating, decreased appetite, premenstrual tension (in those who have not undergone hysterectomy), and vaginal dryness leading to poor patient compliance.

Patients with locally advanced or metastatic endometrial cancer who have symptoms of pain and bleeding may receive external irradiation to the pelvis to relieve these symptoms. Common sites of symptomatic metastasis outside the pelvis that may be treated with radiation therapy are the bone, lung, brain, and lymph nodes.

Conclusion

Endometrial cancer is presently the most common gynecologic malignancy and is expected to remain so for some time, given the rapid aging trends of women and the epidemic of obesity.[76,88] The incidence rates have remained steady since the mid-1980s. The etiology is related directly or indirectly to estrogen stimulation of the endometrial tissue. The standard of care continues to be surgical intervention with or without adjuvant radiation therapy. Those women with high-risk

features and/or advanced/recurrent disease should also receive chemotherapy or hormonal therapy. Most endometrial cancers are diagnosed as stage I disease; however, nearly one in every three women who die of the disease presented with localized disease.[2] More information is needed in the early diagnosis and screening arenas as well as therapeutic options for treatment because the incidence of and death rate from endometrial cancer has not changed significantly in 25 years.[1]

References

1. Jemal A, Siegel R, Ward E, et al. Cancer statistics, 2008. *CA Cancer J Clin.* 2008;58:71–96.

2. Mariani A, Dowdy SC, Keeney GL, Long HJ, Lesnick TG, Podratz, KC. High-risk endometrial cancer subgroups: candidates for target-based adjuvant therapy. *Gynecol Oncol.* 2004;95(1):120–126.

3. Damlo S. ACOG releases guidelines for management of endometrial cancer. *Am Fam Physician.* 2006;74(3):504.

4. Purdie, DM. Epidemiology. In: Luesly DM, Lawton FG, Berchuk A, eds. *Uterine Cancer.* New York, NY: Taylor & Francis; 2006.

5. Maxwell GL, Tian C, Risinger J, et al. Racial disparity in survival among patients with advanced/recurrent endometrial adenocarcinoma: A Gynecologic Oncology Group study. *Cancer.* 2006;107(9): 2197–2205.

6. Barakat RR, Park RC, Grigsby PW, Muss HD, Norris HJ. Corpus: epithelial tumors. In: Hoskins WJ, Perez CA, Young RC, et al., eds. *Principles and Practice of Gynecologic Oncology.* 4th ed. Philadelphia, PA: Lippincott-Raven; 2004.

7. DiSaia PJ, Creasman WT. Adenocarcinoma of the uterus. In: DiSaia PJ, Creasman WT, eds. *Clinical Gynecologic Oncology.* 7th ed. St. Louis, MO: Mosby; 2007.

8. Bakkum-Gamez JN, Gonzales-Bosquet J, Laack NN, Mariani A, Dowdy SC. Current issues in the management of endometrial cancer. *Mayo Clin Proc.* 2008;83(1):97–112.

9. Soliman PT, Oh JC, Schmeler KM, et al. Risk factors for young premenopausal women with endometrial cancer. *Obstet Gynecol.* 2005;105(3):575–580.

10. Yap OWS, Matthews RP. Racial and ethnic disparities in cancers of the uterine corpus. *JAMA.* 2006;98(12):1930–1933.

11. American College of Obstetricians and Gynecologists Committee on Gynecologic Practice. Management of endometrial cancer: committee opinion. Number 65. *Am Fam Physician.* 2006;74(3):504.

12. Barakat RR, Greven K, Markman M, Thigpen JT. Endometrial cancer. In: *Cancer Management: A Multidisciplinary Approach.* 7th ed. Philadelphia, PA: FA Davis Company; 2003.

13. Di Nezza LA, Jobling T, Salamonsen LA. Progestin suppresses matrix metalloproteinase production in endometrial cancer. *Gynecol Oncol.* 2003;89:325–333.

14. Munstedt K, Grant P, Woenckhaus J, Roth G, Tinneberg HR. Cancer of the endometrium: current aspects of diagnostics and treatment. *World J Surg Oncol.* 2004;2(24). www.wjso.com/content/2/1/24.

15. Lachance JA, Everett EN, Greer B, et al. The effect of age on clinical/pathologic features, surgical morbidity, and outcome in patients with endometrial cancer. *Gynecol Oncol.* 2006;101(3):470–475.

16. Chang SC, Lacey Jr JV, Brinton LA, et al. Lifetime weight history and endometrial cancer risk by type of menopausal hormone use in the NIH-AARP diet and health study. *Cancer Epidemiol Biomarkers Prev.* 2007;16(4):723–730.

17. Pavelka JC, Ben-Shachar I, Fowler JM, et al. Morbid obesity and endometrial cancer: surgical, clinical, and pathologic outcomes in surgically managed patients. *Gynecol Oncol.* 2004;95(3):588–592.

18. Trentham-Dietz A, Nichols HB, Hampton JM, Newcomb PA. Weight change and risk of endometrial cancer. *Int J Epidemiol.* 2006;35:151–158.

19. Soliman PT, Wu D, Tortolero-Luna G, et al. Association between adiponenctin, insulin resistance, and endometrial cancer. *Cancer.* 2006;106(11):2376–2381.

20. American College of Obstetricians and Gynecologists Committee on Gynecologic Practice. Tamoxifen and endometrial cancer: committee opinion. *Obstet Gynecol.* 2006;107(5):1475–1477.

21. Robertson G. Screening for endometrial cancer. *Med J Aust.* 2003;178(12): 657–659.

22. Lu KH, Schorge JO, Rodabaugh KJ, et al. Prospective determination of prevalence of lynch syndrome in young women with endometrial cancer. *J Clin Oncol.* 2007;25(33):5158–5164.

23. Goodfellow PJ. Molecular genetics of uterine malignancies. In: Coukas G, Rubin SC, eds. *Cancer of the Uterus.* Monticello, NY: Marcel Dekker; 2005.

24. Hacker NF. Uterine cancer. In: Berek JS, Hacker NF, eds. *Practical Gynecologic Oncology.* 4th ed. Philadelphia, PA: Lippincott, Williams & Wilkins; 2005.

25. American Cancer Society. *Endometrial (uterine cancer).* Atlanta, GA: Author; 2005.

26. National Cancer Institute. (2005). Endometrial cancer (PDQ): screening. Health professional version. http://www.nci.nih.gov/cancertopics/pdq/screening/endometrial/health professional. Accessed June 26, 2008.

27. Saha TK, Amer S, Biss J, et al. The validity of transvaginal ultrasound measurement of endometrial thickness: a comparison of ultrasound measurement with direct anatomical measurement. *BJOG.* 2004;111:1419–1424.

28. Clark TJ, Barton PM, Coomarasamy A, Gupta JK, Khan KS. Investigating postmenopausal bleeding for endometrial cancer: cost-effectiveness of initial diagnostic strategies. *BJOG.* 2006;113:502–510.

29. Soliman PT, Oh JC, Schmeler KM, et al. Risk factors for young premenopausal women with endometrial cancer. *Obstet Gynecol.* 2005;105(3):575–580.

30. Warthin AS. Heredity with reference to carcinoma. *Arch Intern Med.* 1913;12:546–555.

31. Lynch HT, Lanspa SJ, Boman BM, et al. Hereditary non-polyposis colorectal cancer—Lynch syndromes I and II. *Gastroenterol Clin North Am.* 1988;17(4): 679–712.

32. Lynch HT, Smyrk T, Watson P, et al. Genetics, natural history, tumour spectrum, and pathology of hereditary non-polyposis colorectal cancer: an updated review. *Gastroenterol.* 1993;104(5):1535–1549.

33. Black D, Soslow RA, Levine DA, et al. Clinicopathologic significance of defective DNA mismatch repair in endometrial cancer. *J Clin Oncol.* 2006;24(11):1745–1753.

34. Schmeler KM, Lynch HT, Chem LM, et al. Prophylactic surgery to reduce the risk of gynecologic cancers in the Lynch syndrome. *N Engl J Med.* 2006;354:261–269.

35. Hernandez E, Houck KL. Endometrial carcinoma. In: Bieber EJ, Sanfilippo JS, Horowitz IR, eds. *Clinical Gynecology.* Philadelphia, PA: Churchill Livingstone, Elsevier; 2006.

36. Shiozawa T, Konishi I. Early endometrial carcinoma: clinicopathology, hormonal aspects, molecular

genetics, diagnosis, and treatment. *Int J Clin Oncol.* 2006;11:13–21.

37. Maxwell GI, Rosinger JI, Barrett C, Berchuk A. Molecular genetics of endometrial cancer. In: Luesly DM, Lawton FG, Berchuk A, eds. *Uterine Cancer.* New York, NY: Taylor & Francis; 2006.

38. Armant F, Moerman P, Neven P, Timmerman D, Van Limbergen E, Vergote I. Endometrial cancer. *Lancet.* 2005;366:491–503.

39. Lalloo F, Evans G. Molecular genetics and endometrial cancer. *Best Pract Res Clin Obstet Gynaecol.* 2001;15(3):355–363.

40. Kamat AA, Feng, Shu, et al. The role of relaxin in endometrial cancer. *Cancer Biol Ther.* 2006;5(1):71–77.

41. ACOG Practice Bulletin. Management of endometrial cancer. *Obstet Gynecol.* 2005;106(2):413–425.

42. Trimble CL, Kauderer J, Zaino R, et al. Concurrent endometrial carcinoma in women with a biopsy diagnosis of atypical endometrial hyperplasia. *Cancer.* 2006;106:812–819.

43. Bettochi S, Nappi L, Ceci O, Pontrelli G, Pinto L, Selvaggi L. Hysteroscopy and menopause: past and future. *Curr Opin Obstet Gynecol.* 2005;17:366–375.

44. Barwick TD, Rockall AG, Barton DP, Sohaib SA. Imaging of endometrial adenocarcinoma. *Clin Radiol.* 2006;61(7):545–555.

45. Fong K, Causer P, Atri M, Kung R. Transvaginal US and hysterosonography in postmenopausal women with breast cancer receiving tamoxifen: correlation with hysteroscopy and pathologic study. *Radiographics.* 2003;23(1):137–150.

46. Frumovitz M, Singh DK, Meyer L, et al. Predictors of final histology in patients with endometrial cancer. *Gynecol Oncol.* 2004;95(3):463–468.

47. Sarosky JI. Endometrial cancer. *Obstet Gynecol.* 2008;11(2):436–447.

48. Chu, CS. The surgical management of early endometrial cancer. In: Coukas G, Rubin SC, eds. *Cancer of the Uterus.* Monticello, NY: Marcel Dekker; 2005.

49. Mariani A, Webb MJ, Keeney GL, Aletti G, Podratz KC. Endometrial cancer: predictors of peritoneal failure. *Gynecol Oncol.* 2003;89:236–242.

50. Cohn DE, Woeste EM, Cacchio S, et al. Clinical and pathologic correlates in surgical stage II endometrial carcinoma. *Obstet Gynecol.* 2007;109(5): 1062–1067.

51. von Gruenigen VE, Gil KM, Frasure HE, Jenison EL, Hopkins MP. The impact of obesity and age on quality of life in gynecologic surgery. *Am J Obstet Gynecol.* 2005;193:1369–1375.

52. Schlaerth AC, Abu-Rustum NR. Role of minimally invasive surgery in gynecologic cancers. *Oncologist.* 2006;11(8):895–901.

53. Grigsby PW. Radiation treatment for early stage endometrial cancer and uterine sarcoma. In: Coukas G, Rubin SC, eds. *Cancer of the Uterus.* Monticello, NY: Marcel Dekker; 2005.

54. Viani GA, Patia BF, Pillizon AC, et al. High-risk surgical stage 1 endometrial cancer: analysis of treatment outcome. *Radiat Oncol.* 2006;1:24. www.ro-journal. com/content/1/1/24.

55. Ramondetta LM, Burke TW, Broaddus R, Jhingran A. Treatment of endometrial cancer. In: Eifel PJ, Gershenson DM, Kavanagh JJ, Silva EG, eds. *Gynecologic Cancer.* New York, NY: Springer; 2006.

56. Lee CM, Szabo A, Shrieve DC, Madonald OK, Gaffney DK. Frequency and effect of adjuvant radiation therapy among women with stage I endometrial adenocarcinoma. *JAMA.* 2006;295(4):389–395.

57. Rittenberg PVC, Lotocki RJ, Heywood MS, Jones KD, Krepart GV. High-risk surgical stage I endometrial cancer: outcomes with vault brachytherapy alone. *Gynecol Oncol.* 2003;89:288–294.

58. Tangjitgamol S, Manusirivithaya S, Lertbutsayanukul C. Adjuvant therapy for early-stage endometrial cancer: a review. *Int J Gynecol Cancer.* 2007;17:949–956.

59. Deeks E. Local therapy in endometrial cancer: evidence based review. *Curr Opin Oncol.* 2007;19:512–515.

60. Grigsby PW. Radiation treatment for early stage endometrial cancer and uterine sarcoma. In: Coukas G, Rubin SC, eds. *Cancer of the Uterus.* Monticello, NY: Marcel Dekker; 2005.

61. Domanovic M, Ouzidane M, Ellis R, Kinsella T, Beddar A. Using intraoperative radiation therapy—a case study. *AORN.* 2003;77(2):412, 414–417.

62. Dowdy SC, Mariani A, Cliby WA, et al. Radical pelvic resection and intraoperative radiation therapy for recurrent endometrial cancer: technique and analysis of outcomes. *Gynecol Oncol.* 2006;101:280–286.

63. Shaeffer DT, Randall ME. Adjuvant radiotherapy in endometrial carcinoma. *Oncologist.* 2005;10:623–631.

64. Frumovitz M, Gershenson DM. Fertility-sparing therapy for young women with endometrial cancer. *Expert Rev Anticancer Ther.* 2006;6(1):27–32.

65. Bowen G, Randall T. Conservative treatment of endometrial hyperplasia and early endometrial cancer.

In: Coukas G, Rubin SC, eds. *Cancer of the Uterus*. Monticello, NY: Marcel Dekker; 2005.

66. Ramirez PT, Frumovitz M, Bodurka DC, Sun CC, Levenback C. Hormonal therapy for the management of grade 1 endometrial adenocarcinoma: a literature review. *Gynecol Oncol*. 2004;95(1):133–138.

67. Lincoln S, Blessing JA, Lee RB, Rocereto TF. Activity of paclitaxel as second-line chemotherapy in endometrial cancer: a Gynecologic Oncology Group study. *Gynecol Oncol*. 2003;88:277–281.

68. van Wijk FH, Lhomme C, Bolis G, et al. Phase II study of carboplatin in patients with advanced or recurrent endometrial cancer. A trial of the EORTC Gynaecologic Cancer Group. *Eur J Cancer*. 2003;39:78–85.

69. Kieser K, Oza AM. What's new in systemic therapy for endometrial cancer. *Cur Opin Oncol*. 2005;17:500–504.

70. DeCruze SB, Green JA. Hormone therapy in advanced and recurrent endometrial cancer: a systematic review. *Int J Gynecol Cancer*. 2007;17:964–978.

71. Langhorne M, Fulton J, Otto S. Gynecologic cancers. In: *Oncology Nursing*. 5th ed. St. Louis, MO: Mosby; 2005.

72. Leslie KK, Walter SA, Torkko K, Stephens JK, Thompson C, Singh M. Effect of tamoxifen on endometrial histology, hormone receptors and cervical cytology: a prospective study with follow-up. *Appl Immunohistochem Mol Morphol*. 2007;15(3):284–293.

73. Ring A, Dowsett M. Mechanisms of tamoxifen resistance. *Endocr Relat Cancer*. 2004;11(4):643–658.

74. Shang Y. Molecular mechanisms of oestrogen and SERMs in endometrial carcinogenesis. *Nat Rev Cancer*. 2006;6:360–368.

75. Slomovitz BM, Lu KH. Systemic therapies for endometrial carcinoma. In: Coukas G, Rubin SC, eds. *Cancer of the Uterus*. Monticello, NY: Marcel Dekker; 2005.

76. Burke TW, Walker CL. Arzoxifene as therapy for endometrial cancer. *Gynecol Oncol*. 2003;90:S40–S46.

77. Straughan JM, Huh WK, Orr JW, et al. Stage IC adenocarcinoma of the endometrium: survival comparisons of surgically staged patients with and without adjuvant radiation therapy. *Gynecol Oncol*. 2003;89:295–300.

78. Carey MS, Gawlik C, Fung-Kee-Fung M, Chambers A, Oliver T. Systematic review of systemic therapy for advanced or recurrent endometrial cancer. *Gynecol Oncol*. 2006;101:158–167.

79. Wadler S, Levy DE, Lincoln ST, Soori GS, Schink JC, Goldberg G. Topotecan is an active agent in the first-line treatment of metastatic or recurrent endometrial carcinoma: Eastern Cooperative Group study E3E93. *J Clin Oncol*. 2003;21(11):2110–2114.

80. Traina TA, Sabbatini P, Aghajanian C, Dupont J. Weekly topotecan for recurrent endometrial cancer: a case series and review of the literature. *Gynecol Oncol*. 2004;95(1):235–241.

81. Landoni F, Maggioni A, Crippa G. Molecular genetics of endometrial cancer. In: Luesly DM, Lawton FG, Berchuk A, eds. *Uterine Cancer*. New York, NY: Taylor & Francis; 2006.

82. Fung-Kee-Fung M, Dodge J, Elit L, Lukka H, Chambers A, Oliver T. Follow-up after primary therapy for endometrial caner: a systematic review. *Gynecol Oncol*. 2006;101(3):520–529.

83. Mahon S. Tertiary prevention: implications for improving the quality of life of long-term survivors of cancer. *Semin Oncol Nurs*. 2005;21(4):260–270.

84. Fader AN, Gibbons HE, vonGruenigen VE. Helping endometrial cancer. *Contemp OB/GYN*. 2007;Nov:54–60.

85. Chung-Park M. Anxiety attacks following surgical menopause. *Nurse Pract*. 2006;31(5):44–49.

86. Barakat RR, Bundy BN, Spirtos NM, Mannel RS. Randomized double-blind trial of estrogen replacement therapy versus placebo in stage I and II endometrial cancer: a Gynecologic Oncology Group study. *J Clin Oncol*. 2006;24(4):587–592.

87. American College of Obstetricians and Gynecologists Committee on Gynecologic Practice. Hormone replacement therapy in women treated for endometrial cancer. Committee opinion. 2000;May:Number 234.

88. Mueck AO, Seeger H. Hormone therapy after endometrial cancer. *Endocr Relat Cancer*. 2004;11:305–314.

89. Courneya KS, Karvinen KH, Campbell KL, et al. Associations among exercise, body weight, and quality of life in a population-based sample of endometrial cancer survivors. *Gynecol Oncol*. 2005;97:422–430.

Chapter 4

Epithelial Ovarian Cancer—The Disease and Survivorship

Sheryl Redlin Frazier, RN, BSN, OCN®

Ovarian cancer ranks eighth in new cancer cases among women, comprising about 3% of all women's cancers, but it ranks as the fifth leading cause of cancer death in women.[1] Ovarian cancer is the most lethal of all the gynecologic malignancies. In 2008, the American Cancer Society estimates that 21,650 women will be diagnosed with ovarian cancer and 15,520 women will die of cancer of the ovary.[1] There was a modest but statistically significant decline in incidence between 1975 and 2003.[2] However, the most significant problems of early diagnosis, curative therapies, and symptom management persist as challenges for women who have been or will be diagnosed with ovarian cancer and the people who care for them.

Epidemiology and Risk Factors

The exact molecular cause of ovarian cancer is not yet clearly understood, although a number of epidemiological studies have been conducted. Presumptions and evidence indicate a pathway that includes incessant and uninterrupted ovulation in an environment conducive to tumorigenicity to be contributory.[3] Epidemiological data indicates familial incidence and aging are two of the strongest risk factors and has also yielded data that indicates certain protective benefits that can reduce risk.

Incidence

Cancers of the ovary can occur virtually at any time during the lifetime of a female. Germ cell tumors are more likely to occur in adolescent and young women;[4] however, the age range can be from infants to the elderly, with the prevalence beginning around 8 years of age with a mean of 19 years of age. There has been no increase in germ cell tumor incidence in the United States over the past 30 years.[5] Stromal tumors may occur at any age and are characterized by hormonal secretions.[6] Epithelial tumors most commonly occur later in life, typically in postmenopausal women, with only 10%–15% occurring prior to menopause.[7] Surveillance, epidemiology, and end results (SEER) data from 2000–2003 shows an overall median age at diagnosis of epithelial tumors to be 64 years of age.[8]

wanes in the postmenopausal time when the risk for ovarian carcinogenesis increases.[20] Childbearing and breastfeeding offer protective benefits by reducing the number of ovulations in a lifetime, thereby reducing the number of times the ovarian capsule is interrupted, damaged, and repaired.[7] If a woman has had two children and has taken oral contraceptives for 5 years or more, her risk is reduced by 70%.[7] Surgical interventions that reduce risk include tubal ligation and oopherectomy with or without hysterectomy, and it seems these interventions are helpful for high-risk women as well.[21] The implication for the high-risk group would be to utilize oral contraceptives, complete childbearing, and undergo oopherectomy with or without hysterectomy, although even after a total hysterectomy there persists a risk of developing peritoneal cancer[7,21] (see **Table 4-1**).

Screening

Ovarian cancer strikes approximately 1 in 70 women and does not command the attention of the public and national resources like breast cancer, which, in turn, impacts funding and strategies for treatment and prevention. Nevertheless, 23% of the National Cancer Institute's 2005 annual budget for ovarian cancer was dedicated to early detection, diagnosis, and prognosis research.[22] Routine screening is not recommended for the general population because of the lack of efficient and cost-effective tests currently available. The CA 125, a tumor marker that is useful in women who have been diagnosed with ovarian cancer, is not specific enough to use alone in screening efforts. In early results from the Prostate, Lung, Colorectal, and Ovarian Cancer Screening Trial (PLCO), the CA 125 and transvaginal ultrasound continue to prove to be poor predictors of disease in the general population.[23] The CA 125 is less than 60% effective in detecting the cancer in early stage disease.[24] Efforts continue to be focused on cancer screening strategies that demonstrate an improvement over the currently best available methods for high risk groups: biannual bimanual rectovaginal pelvic examination, transvaginal color Doppler imaging, and the CA 125, or what is referred to as multimodal screening.[14] Future screening strategies include the development of tumor markers of greater specificity than the CA 125 and the field of proteomics.[14] Recently, a group of researchers developed a biomarker blood test that has a sensitivity of 95.3% and a specificity of 99.4% in the detection of ovarian cancer.[24] Further testing will answer whether

Table 4-1 Risk factors and risk reduction strategies.

Risk Factors	Prevention/Risk Reduction Strategies
Age	Parity, breastfeeding
Heredity	Oral contraceptives
Nulliparity/infertility	Tubal ligation, oopherectomy
Personal cancer history	Regular healthcare provider visits

this new test will be the answer to screening or early detection for the disease;[25] however, at the moment, without the necessary tools for adequate screening, it remains the work of advocacy groups and healthcare providers to persist in inspiring the case for early detection. Survivors report having seen as many as three or more providers before getting to a definitive diagnosis of ovarian cancer.[26]

Biology and Carcinogenesis

Transformation to ovarian neoplasm requires a cascade of genetic events that include activation of oncogenes, such as K-ras, that is overexpressed in 30% of tumors and HER2/neu overexpression in up to 30%.[27] Other growth factors involved are interleukin-6 (IL-6), epidermal growth factor (EGF), and transforming growth factor (TGF).[27] As previously discussed, the role of tumor suppressor genes is predominant as evidenced by mutations found in the BRCA1 gene in 30% of hereditary cases and 10% of sporadic cases.[27] The p53 gene, which functions in regulation of cell proliferation and apoptosis, is found mutated in 30% of cases and overexpressed in 50% of cases.[27] The significance of these abnormalities are important in the development and utilization of novel agents for therapeutic management of ovarian cancer.

Pathology

There are three basic categories for malignant ovarian tumor types: tumors that arise from the germ cell layer, stromal tissue, or the epithelial layer of the ovary.[28] Epithelial cancers of the ovary are the most common, comprising approximately 90% of all ovarian tumors.[18] Epithelial ovarian tumors can be further categorized as benign, tumors of low malignant potential (sometimes called borderline tumors), and malignant.[28] The less common nonepithelial types of ovarian cancer, germ cell and stromal tumors, occur much less frequently and comprise approximately 10% of malignant ovarian tumors.[29] The tumors of low malignant potential comprise about 15% of the epithelial histology, are usually diagnosed in an early stage, rarely undergo malignant transformation, and have an excellent prognosis.[30] In addition to other very rare types of nonepithelial ovarian cancer, the ovaries can be the sites of metastasis from other organs, such as the breast and gastrointestinal tract, and from melanoma.[6]

In addition to cancers that arise specifically from the ovaries, fallopian tube cancers and primary peritoneal cancers occur infrequently but are no less problematic. Primary peritoneal cancers arise from the lining of the peritoneum, which is comprised of the same embryologic tissue as the ovaries.[31] Fallopian tube cancer arises in the fallopian tube, is found arising simultaneously from both tubes approximately 30% of the time, and behaves in a similar fashion as ovarian and primary peritoneal cancers.[18]

Diagnosis and Staging

Early diagnosis of ovarian cancer remains one of the most difficult and confounding problems facing women and their healthcare providers. Although many of the symptoms are common, they are not specific and infrequently yield the opportunity for early detection. Clinicians who are alert to the common complaints and utilize appropriate diagnostic testing sometimes are able to make a diagnosis early, but those instances are rare. The most common scenario is late diagnosis and advanced stage disease. Ovarian cancer is a surgically staged disease involving a highly technical and precise staging procedure and tumor debulking best performed by a gynecologic oncologist.

Anatomy and Pattern of Spread

The ovaries are two small, pinkish gray organs that lie adjacent, in a slightly posterior and caudal position, to the fallopian tubes and lateral to the uterus.[18] The size of the ovaries increases gradually from infancy as the female matures to their maximum size achieved in the premenopausal state, and then begins to decrease in size through perimenopause until, when in postmenopause, the ovaries are so small as to not be palpable on pelvic examination.[18] Considering the location of the ovaries, it is easy to visualize the manner in which tumor excrescences on the ovary would communicate with other organs of the pelvis and, as such, transcoelomic migration is one of the three commonly recognized ways the tumor metastasizes.[32] Unfortunately, the efficiency of the fluid in the peritoneum, mobilized by peristalsis, diaphragmatic fluctuation, and generalized body movement, disperses the malignant cells throughout the abdominal cavity.[32] The other mechanisms of spread are hematologic and lymphatic.[11]

Diagnosis

Women who are diagnosed with ovarian cancer typically have a constellation of symptoms that are characterized by abdominal complaints that confound the women who are experiencing the problems and the providers they see. The characteristics of the abdominal complaints are ones that many women experience on a monthly basis throughout their lives and often don't acknowledge the problems as serious. This ambiguity of symptoms led to the label of "Ovarian Cancer: A Silent Killer." However, advocacy groups and ovarian cancer survivors vehemently oppose this suggestion that this cancer is "silent." In a novel study involving the readership of *Conversations!*, a newsletter authored by Cindy Melancon, a nurse and ovarian cancer survivor, researchers found 71% of those responding had stage III/IV disease, 77% had complaints of abdominal symptoms, 70% had gastrointestinal symptoms, 58% had pain, 50% had constitutional symptoms, 34% had urinary symptoms, and 26% had pelvic symptoms prior to their definitive diagnoses.[26] Sadly, but replicated many times over, the women surveyed were often told there was nothing wrong (13%); that their symptoms were related to depression (6%) or stress (12%); their symptoms were related to gastrointestinal problems, such as IBS, constipation, or gastritis (30%); or their symptoms were related to other various diagnoses (47%).[26] Of the survey responders, only 20% were told they might have ovarian cancer.[26]

After taking a thorough clinical history, paying particular attention to symptoms, the physical assessment should include a bimanual rectovaginal exam. The rectovaginal exam is necessary to palpate the ovaries, which in a postmenopausal woman as a result of aging will shrink from a premenopausal size of 3.5 × 2.0 × 1.5 cm to a nonpalpable size.[18] If the ovaries are palpable in this circumstance, the examiner should have a degree of suspicion that leads to further testing and assessment. In addition to the tests previously mentioned as multimodal screening tools, an abdominal/pelvic CT scan would be the next best choice for diagnostic purposes. It is important to emphasize the need for the pelvic view of the CT scan to locate disease in the pelvis that an abdominal scan alone would miss. Other tests include an evaluation of the bowel with a barium enema or colonoscopy, chest X-ray, mammogram, and MRI or PET scan.[18] When the index of suspicion indicates the possibility of ovarian cancer, a referral to a gynecologic oncologist is essential.

In 1985, gynecologic oncologists found that nearly half of women with early ovarian cancer were inadequately staged at their original surgeries, were actually upstaged at the second surgery, and showed a survival advantage for women with ovarian cancer when they received adequate debulking surgeries performed by gynecologic oncology surgeons.[33] Today that data can still be replicated as evidenced by a recent study showing improved outcomes when women are operated on by a gynecologic oncologist over a general gynecologist, and a superior outcome is shown over surgeries performed by general surgeons.[34] Surgical skills in debulking tumors and surgeon specialty are especially important in terms of the survival advantages of early stage disease and in the application of treatment of the appropriate stage of disease for intraperitoneal chemotherapy.[34]

Surgery

The surgical procedure involves a vertical incision, usually made from a point above the umbilicus to the symphysis pubis, which provides for adequate visualization, inspection, and palpation of all abdominal surfaces. The goal of this surgery is to adequately stage the disease, remove as much of the bulky tumor as possible, and leave behind as little as possible.[18] Ascitic fluid is obtained, or if there is none present, washings of the cavity are performed, and

this sample is sent for cytologic examination. All surfaces are examined, including the liver and diaphragm, and a complete hysterectomy is performed including removal of the uterus, fallopian tubes, and ovaries. In circumstances such as a low malignant potential tumor or stage I disease, fertility-sparing surgery can be performed with adequate staging[18] (see **Table 4-2**). It is important to establish the extent of disease, particularly for early stages, because it has been estimated that as many as 30% will have metastatic disease in lymph nodes or the upper abdomen, and treatment decisions are based on staging.[7] To further emphasize the importance of proper staging and tumor debulking, recent findings suggest that younger women diagnosed with ovarian cancer have longer survival rates than women over age 60 years.[35] The value of adequate cytoreduction on survival has been proven in several trials.[11]

The role of laparoscopy in ovarian cancer is to minimize morbidity, but it has limitations in visualization, and with the discovery of adhesions, the surgery would be inadequate.[18] However, with the recent development of intraperitoneal treatment recommendations, laparoscopy is being used for placement and removal of intraperitoneal catheters with increasing frequency.

Chemotherapy

On January 4, 2006, the National Cancer Institute issued a clinical announcement for the preferred method of treatment for optimally debulked (less than one centimeter in size) stage III disease.[36] The treatment involves intraperitoneal chemotherapy, which, although it is a treatment modality that has been used for several years, had not been widely

Table 4-2 AJCC STAGING OF CANCER OF THE OVARY.

American Joint Committee on Cancer (AJCC) Staging—Ovary				
Primary Tumor (T): Corresponds with staging criteria of the Federation Internationale de Gynecologie et d'Obstetrique (FIGO)				
Regional Lymph Nodes (N):				NX – Regional lymph nodes cannot be assessed N0 – No regional lymph node metastasis N1 – Regional lymph node metastasis
Distant Metastasis (M):				MX – Distant metastasis cannot be assessed M0 – No distant metastasis M1 – Distant metastasis (excludes peritoneal metastasis)
Stage I	T1	N0	M0	Tumor limited to ovaries (one or both).
Stage IA	T1a	N0	M0	Tumor limited to one ovary; capsule intact, no tumor on ovarian surface. No malignant cells in ascites or peritoneal washings.*
Stage IB	T1b	N0	M0	Tumor limited to both ovaries; capsules intact, no tumor on ovarian surface. No malignant cells in ascites or peritoneal washings.*
Stage IC	T1c	N0	M0	Tumor limited to one or both ovaries with any of the following: capsule ruptured, tumor on ovarian surface, malignant cells in ascites or peritoneal washings.
Stage II	T2	N0	M0	Tumor involves one or both ovaries with pelvic extensions.
Stage IIA	T2a	N0	M0	Extension and/or implants on uterus and/or tube(s). No malignant cells in ascites or peritoneal washings.
Stage IIB	T2b	N0	M0	Extension to other pelvic tissues. No malignant cells in ascites or peritoneal washings.
Stage IIC	T2c	N0	M0	Pelvic extension (2a or 2b) with malignant cells in ascites or peritoneal washings.
Stage III	T3	N0 or N1	M0	Tumor involves one or both ovaries with microscopically confirmed peritoneal metastasis outside the pelvis and/or regional lymph node metastasis; includes liver capsule metastasis.
Stage IIIA	T3a	N0	M0	Microscopic peritoneal metastasis beyond pelvis.
Stage IIIB	T3b	N0	M0	Macroscopic peritoneal metastasis beyond pelvis 2 cm or less in greatest dimension.
Stage IIIC	T3c	N0 or N1	M0	Peritoneal metastasis beyond pelvis more than 2 cm in greatest dimension and/or regional lymph node metastasis.
Stage IV	Any T	Any N	M1	Distant metastasis (excludes peritoneal metastasis); includes liver parenchymal metastasis and pleural effusion evidenced by positive cytology.

*The presence of malignant cells in ascites or washings affects staging.

accepted as a standard. The recommendation was the result of data gathered from trials that showed a significant improvement in survival of women with advanced disease.[36] The treatment involves intravenous paclitaxel over 24 hours on day 1, intraperitoneal cisplatin on day 2, followed by intraperitoneal paclitaxel on day 8, and the cycle was repeated on day 22.[37] Although this regimen was intensive, and many subjects were unable to complete the treatment as described by the trial, when compared to the standard treatment group, there was significant improvement in progression-free and overall survival.[37]

For other stages of disease, treatment with intravenous paclitaxel (or docetaxel) and carboplatin (or cisplatin) have proven to be the superior regimen and remain the standard of care outside the application of clinical trials.[7] In early stages, it is possible to treat stage I, grade 1 patients with surgery alone, and for early stage, high-risk patients, three to six cycles of intravenous paclitaxel and a platinum compound is sufficient.[7]

There is a subset of women who present in advanced disease states, such as advanced age with comorbidities such as deep vein thromboses, malnutrition, and pulmonary compromise from pleural effusion(s), who are in such challenged states of health (poor performance status) that they are deemed to be poor surgical candidates.[11] There have been studies conducted to address the group of patients who are poor surgical candidates as previously mentioned or were suboptimally debulked. The findings have supported using neoadjuvant chemotherapy, three cycles of paclitaxel and platinum, followed by interval cytoreduction, followed by additional cycles of the same chemotherapeutic regimen, that have excellent responses.[11] These studies

have shown feasibility, some improvement in quality of life, and a slight improvement in survival providing providers with a reasonable alternative to the standard of care.[11]

Radiation

In the United States, the use of radiotherapy is primarily for targeting small tumors, controlling pain, and usually in the salvage setting.[7] There may be a role for radioimmunotherapy in intraperitoneal treatment of ovarian cancer. A number of trials investigating radiolabeled monoclonal antibodies are underway; however, there is no data available at this time.

Hormonal Therapy

The use of hormonal therapy is typically reserved for recurrent disease during treatment holidays or when more aggressive chemotherapy regimens are not tolerable. Tamoxifen and megace are the more frequently used agents.[7]

Biotherapy/Immunotherapy/ Targeted Therapy

The field of biologic therapy is the most promising area of research for all cancer patients, including ovarian cancer. Several different agents are being explored in the clinical trial setting, such as monoclonal antibodies, angiogenesis inhibitors, anti-VEGF, and tyrosine kinase inhibitors.[38] One monoclonal antibody that acts on the HER2/neu receptor sites is trastuzumab (Herceptin(R)), but HER2/neu is expressed in only 15%–30% of ovarian cancers, making this a treatment that is unlikely to be mainstreamed.[7] These targeted therapies have proven to successfully treat a number of other diseases, and there is great hope that due to the biologic nature of epithelial ovarian cancer, some of these agents will also be effective. Vaccines are another immunotherapy that are being closely analyzed for therapeutic purposes. MAb-B43.13 or oregovomab (OvaRex) is one such agent that has shown some exciting activity.[7]

Survival and Recurrent Disease

In spite of the best available therapies, ovarian cancer continues to be a difficult cancer to diagnose in its early stages, when the chance of cure and long-term survival is at the maximum opportunity. Although there have been some modest improvements in 5-year survival over the past 20 years with the addition of more active agents, the fact remains that 75% of women who are diagnosed with epithelial ovarian cancer will eventually succumb to the disease[11] (see **Table 4-3**). When the disease recurs, there is no current therapy available that will provide cure. Management of the recurrent disease state occupies much of the care given by gynecologic oncology healthcare providers.

In the setting of recurrent disease, several treatment modalities are possible. Surgical intervention, radiation, clinical trial investigation, chemotherapy, and supportive care are all elements of recurrent disease management. In particular, and in the absence of a clinical trial, chemotherapy is the most

frequently used therapeutic. There are a number of agents that are approved for use in recurrent disease, and there are concepts of "chronic disease," platinum sensitivity, and sequencing that are applied to the individualized treatment plan.[39] The value of platinum-based therapy in response rates has been well established and continues to be a predictor of disease response.[11] If the disease is "platinum resistant," meaning it does not respond to platinum-containing therapy, then the likelihood of disease response to other therapies is very low[39] (see **Table 4-4**). The importance of managing, in concert with the patient, the type and timing of chemotherapy becomes a delicate balancing act between securing stable disease, minimizing toxicities associated with treatment, and prolonging quality of life.[40] Many women with recurrent disease will receive four to five or more different regimens of treatment before dying.[39]

Nursing Implications

Nurses play an immensely important role in the entire disease trajectory of ovarian cancer including in screening and prevention. Nurses and nurse practitioners who see clients in the

Table 4-3 SURVIVAL RATES BY STAGE OF DISEASE.

Stage of Disease	Survival Rates (Relative 5-year)
Stage I	84.7%–92.7%
Stage II	64.4%–78.6%
Stage III	31.5%–50.8%
Stage IV	17.5%

Source: ACS, 2006, "How is ovarian cancer staged?"

Table 4-4 Agents used in recurrent disease.

Drug	Response Rate (%)	
	Platinum-Resistant	Platinum-Sensitive
Docetaxel		
Doxil		
Etoposide		
Gemcitabine		
Paclitaxel	10%–25%	20%–55%
Platinum		
Topotecan		
Vinorelbine		
Hexamethamelamine – 20% (Active in platinum resistant and sensitive)		

Source: Adapted from Coleman & Monk, 2006, Table 4, Response rates for platinum-resistant and platinum-sensitive disease.

community should be educated to perform in-depth clinical history and assessment, being careful to inquire and listen to clues for family history of cancer and to symptoms that might indicate ovarian cancer. Where there are indications of a familial cancer trend, the nurse should recommend a referral to a genetic counselor for pedigree assessment, evaluation, and counseling. For general care, recommendations should include oral contraceptive counseling, avoidance of talcum powder or talc-containing products, exercise, and a low-fat diet, achieving and maintaining a BMI less than 25. Women who are considered to be high risk should be referred to a gynecologic oncologist for recommendations for follow-up, interventions after childbearing years, and genetic counseling.

Gynecologic oncology nurses are a subspecialty of oncology nursing and are particularly trained in advocating for and care of the ovarian cancer patient. Their focus is on optimum disease and symptom management. In the face of long-term chronic disease, the nurse is uniquely positioned to take on the role of advocate for support of women living with ovarian cancer in the aspects of body-image changes, performance of activities of daily living with fatigue and neuropathies, psychological distress and social isolation, and the ongoing threat of recurrence and mortality.[41] These issues are a small representation of the many faced by women who live with ovarian cancer and their families. The future will continue to challenge nurses to find evidence through research to provide better care and support for ovarian cancer survivors.

Chapter 5

Nonepithelial Ovarian Malignancies

Margaret M. Fields, MSN, ANP-BC, AOCNP®

Nonepithelial ovarian malignancies are much less common than those that arise from the outer covering, or epithelium, of the ovary. Nonepithelial malignancies account for only about 10% of all ovarian malignancies. There are two broad categories of nonepithelial tumors: germ cell tumors and sex cord stromal tumors.[1] We will look at these categories individually, as well as several subgroups in detail within each category.

Pathogenesis

The ovary is comprised of germ cells, stromal cells, and mesenchymal tissue. At fertilization, the sex of the embryo is determined; however, the characteristics of being male or female do not develop until the seventh week. Initially, the urinary system and the genital system are closely related both anatomically and embryologically. Both develop from the same mesodermal ridge.[2] The primitive germ cells are originally formed in the wall of the yolk sac and migrate to the gonadal ridge, where they cause the gonad to develop into either an ovary or testis. If the germ cells do not reach the gonadal ridge, it results in a lack of gonadal development.[3]

After the germ cells reach the gonadal ridge, the coelomic epithelium begins to rapidly proliferate. Some of these cells penetrate the stroma and develop into the primitive sex cords. This connection between the surface epithelium and the sex cords produces a gonad that is able to be identified as male or female. Prior to this time (at about the seventh week), this tissue is referred to as the indifferent gonad.[2] Dysgerminomas and seminomas are felt to arise from cells at this level of development.[3]

In the ovary, the primitive sex cords are broken into cell clusters, which contain groups of primitive germ cells. Later these sex cords disappear and are replaced by the vascular stroma, which forms the ovarian medulla. The surface epithelium continues to proliferate and forms a second set of cords, the cortical cords, which penetrate the mesenchyme but remain close to the surface. At the fourth month, the sex cords split into isolated cell clusters, which surround one or more of the primitive germ cells. The germ cells develop into oogonia, which will become the primary oocytes. The surrounding epithelial cells form the follicular cells.[2] See **Figure 5-1** for an overview of the sites of origin of ovarian malignancies.

Figure 5-1 Origins of ovarian tumors.

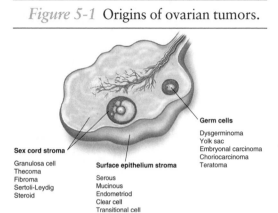

Germ cells
Dysgerminoma
Yolk sac
Embryonal carcinoma
Choriocarcinoma
Teratoma

Sex cord stroma
Granulosa cell
Thecoma
Fibroma
Sertoli-Leydig
Steroid

Surface epithelium stroma
Serous
Mucinous
Endometriod
Clear cell
Transitional cell

Ovarian Germ Cell Tumors

Ovarian germ cell tumors arise from the primordial germ cell of the ovary. Germ cell tumors account for 3%–5% of all malignant ovarian neoplasms in western countries. They are more common in Asian and black populations, where they represent up to 15% of ovarian malignancies.[4] Ovarian germ cell tumors tend to arise in the first two decades of life. In this age group, almost 70% of ovarian tumors are of germ cell origin, and up to 30% of these are malignant. The incidence of germ cell tumors is rare after the third decade, but they have been reported in women up to 70 years of age.[5] Due to the young age of the majority of these patients, preservation of fertility is an important consideration. This is often achieved due to advances in surgical staging and chemotherapy regimens.

Germ cell tumors of the ovary, which tend to grow rapidly, are unlike epithelial ovarian neoplasms in that they are often diagnosed while still confined to one ovary (stage IA). The majority of patients will present with abdominal pain related to capsular distention, hemorrhage, or ovarian torsion and an abdominal mass. Due to the rapid rate of growth of germ cell tumors, the mass is frequently quite large, often exceeding 20 cm. The median size of the mass at presentation is 16 cm.[6]

Surgery

The goal of surgical staging in germ cell tumors is the same as in epithelial tumors, that is, to remove as much of the disease as is technically possible. Superior response rates to chemotherapy, as well as improved rates of remaining disease free, have been demonstrated in optimally debulked patients. However, due to the highly chemosensitive nature of germ cell tumors, a mix of surgical aggressiveness as well as caution is indicated. Because these are very often young patients, preservation of fertility is an important consideration. Care should be taken to avoid unnecessary biopsy of a normal-appearing contralateral ovary that could compromise fertility due to peritoneal adhesions or ovarian failure. An exception is in the case of dysgerminoma, where 10% of normal-appearing ovaries will have occult metastasis and biopsy may be indicated.

Often a complete staging surgery will involve unilateral salpingo-oophorectomy with pelvic washings, pelvic and para-aortic lymph node sampling, and random staging biopsies of high-risk areas such as the omentum, bilateral paracolic gutters, cul-de-sac, lateral pelvic walls, vesicouterine reflection, subdiaphragmatic areas, and any adhesions.[7]

Chemotherapy

Before the advent of adjuvant chemotherapy for nondysgerminomatous ovarian germ cell malignancies, a high percentage of patients with completely resected, early stage disease relapsed and died.[8] Improvements in survival in germ cell malignancies over the past several decades can be directly attributed to advances in chemotherapeutic regimens. Prior to the development of cisplatin and the regimens we use today, survival rates were less than 50%. Now at least 90% of early stage patients, and as many as 75% to 80% of patients with advanced disease, will be long-term survivors.[6] Due to the rarity of ovarian germ cell tumors, many of these advances have resulted from studies of germ cell tumors of the testis.[9]

The first regimen used in the treatment of germ cell malignancies was vincristine, dactinomycin, and cyclophosphamide (VAC). The number of long-term survivors using this regimen was under 50%.[7] The success of platinum-based regimens in testicular cancer led to the development of the PVB combination. This regimen combined cisplatin, vinblastine, and bleomycin and resulted in a 53% long-term survival rate. When used for salvage therapy, the 4-year overall survival rate was 70%.[7] Later, when etoposide was substituted for vinblastine, long-term survival rates rose to 95% to 100% for early stage disease, with 75% to 80% survival in advanced disease.[6,7] Not only was this regimen more efficacious, it also was better tolerated with less neurotoxicity and less constipation. BEP is the standard regimen used in ovarian germ cell malignancies both for adjuvant therapy and for treatment of disease. It is important that full doses be given on schedule to avoid compromising the curative potential of chemotherapy due to development of drug resistance.[10]

Carboplatin, rather than cisplatin, is routinely used in treatment of epithelial ovarian malignancies with no decrease in efficacy.

However, in testicular germ cell malignancies, these agents are not interchangeable. There is a decrease in efficacy when carboplatin is substituted. There aren't sufficient data in the ovarian germ cell malignancy population to answer this question definitively. The data that does exist comes primarily from children with ovarian germ cell malignancies and seems to suggest the carboplatin is an acceptable substitute. Mann et al. in the United Kingdom treated 137 children with carboplatin, etoposide, and bleomycin and achieved a 5-year survival rate of 91%.[11] Similar results were obtained by Stern et al. in a smaller study with 23 children treated with carboplatin, etoposide, and bleomycin. The 5-year survival rate was 87% in this group.[12] Because no data are available in the adult population regarding the efficacy of this substitution, the treatment guidelines recommend BEP.

The salvage regimens used for recurrent or persistent ovarian germ cell malignancies are derived from protocols established in the setting of recurrent or persistent testicular germ cell tumors. Patients are generally rechallenged on BEP chemotherapy if recurrence is several months after the completion of treatment. For patients with platinum-sensitive disease, treatment regimens generally include ifosfamide and cisplatin. Examples are VIP (etoposide, ifosfamide, and cisplatin), VeIP (vinblastine, ifosfamide, and cisplatin), or TIP (paclitaxel, ifosfamide, and cisplatin). See **Table 5-1** for schedule and dosing information.[13-15] Results are poor for patients with platinum refractory disease. New salvage regimens of gemcitabine and paclitaxel with or without cisplatin or epirubicin and cisplatin are being tried with some success.[16-18]

40%–50% of malignant nonepithelial ovarian neoplasms. It is the histologic equivalent of the seminoma of the testis, the most common germ cell tumor in men. Of the germ cell tumors, dysgerminoma is the one most likely to occur bilaterally. Ten percent of women will have gross disease of the other ovary, while an additional 10% will have microscopic disease of the other ovary.[4] Because this is a disease of young women, 20%–30% of the ovarian malignancies diagnosed during pregnancy are dysgerminomas.[20]

Approximately 5% of dysgerminomas are found in females with phenotypically abnormal gonads. These will generally be very young, premenarcheal girls. In the setting of a premenarcheal female with a pelvic mass, the karyotype should be assessed preoperatively because the removal of the other ovary is indicated if phenotypic abnormality is found.[1]

Seventy-five percent of women will be diagnosed with stage I disease. Of these, 85%–90% will have disease confined to one ovary (stage IA). For patients treated with unilateral salpingo-oophorectomy and staging, there is a 5%–10% risk of developing disease in the remaining ovary in the next 2 years.[21]

In the 25% of patients with spread of disease, the route is most often lymphatic. Hematologic spread also occurs with metastasis to the lung, liver, and brain. This generally reflects long-standing or recurrent disease. Surgery with staging is the primary treatment.[21]

Cure rates for stage IA disease are greater than 95%. Dysgerminomas are very chemosensitive. Even in the face of advanced disease, 5-year survival rates are 85%–90% with the use of BEP combination chemotherapy. In completely resected disease, adjuvant chemotherapy in the form of three to six cycles of BEP

is generally the recommendation for stage IB or greater.[6] Due to the high salvage rate of recurrent disease (greater than 90%), some clinicians advocate adjuvant chemotherapy only for stage II or greater. Patients with stage I disease treated with surgery alone have a 15%–25% risk of recurrence, and virtually all of these patients will be salvaged.[4] Dysgerminoma is radiosensitive as well. However, this option is generally reserved for recurrent disease already treated with chemotherapy, due to the impact on future fertility.[19]

The highest risk for recurrent disease is within the first 2 years. Of the patients who recur, 90% will do so within this time frame. Careful monitoring is indicated with serum tumor markers and frequent examinations, including CT scan of the chest, abdomen, and pelvis every 3 months for the first 2 years, then every 6 months for 3 years. Late recurrence occurs in dysgerminoma; therefore, annual surveillance is indicated for 10 years.[22] The most common sites of recurrence are the peritoneal cavity and the retroperitoneal lymph nodes. Recurrent disease is treated with BEP combination chemotherapy or radiation therapy.[7]

Pure dysgerminomas do not produce alpha fetoprotein. However, in dysgerminomas with mixed embryonal components, this may be a useful marker. In general, the markers used for monitoring disease status are placental alkaline phosphatase and lactate dehydrogenase (LDH).[4]

Immature Teratoma

The pure immature teratoma accounts for less than 1% of all ovarian malignancies and for 15%–20% of germ cell malignancies. This tumor generally occurs in the first 2 decades of life; it is rare in postmenopausal women. It is the only form of ovarian germ cell tumor that is histologically graded. The grade is a measure of the number of immature neural elements present per low power field (LPF). Grade 1 (well differentiated) has less than one immature neural element per LPF, grade 2 (moderately differentiated) has one to three, and grade 3 (poorly differentiated) has more than three of these elements per LPF. This is the most important prognostic factor, with grade 1 having an 82% overall survival for all stages, grade 2 having a 62% overall survival for all stages, and grade 3 having a 30% overall survival for all stages.[1]

Surgical staging with unilateral oophorectomy is the recommended initial approach for women who desire future fertility. Contralateral ovarian involvement is rare, so wedge biopsy or resection of a normal-appearing ovary is not necessary. The contralateral ovary may contain a mature teratoma in 10% of cases.[4] The most common sites of disease spread are the peritoneum and, to a lesser extent, the retroperitoneal lymph nodes. Hematologic dissemination to organ sites of liver, lung, and brain are uncommon and often present only in recurrent or grade 3 disease.[21] Due to the less favorable prognosis for grade 2 and grade 3 disease, it is recommended for adjuvant chemotherapy to be given to all patients except those with stage IA grade 1 disease.[4] The recommended regimen is BEP combination chemotherapy for four to six cycles. It is vital that patients be treated with full doses on time to avoid chemo resistance.[10]

The presence of yolk sac features is an indicator of more aggressive disease. Extra ovarian spread is likely with an overall worse outcome. Tumors with yolk sac foci may have elevated alpha fetoprotein or LDH levels. In general, immature teratomas do not have the ability to secrete hormones and tumor markers, and hormonal abnormalities are usually not present.[6]

Immature teratomas that were not completely resected at initial staging may benefit from second look surgery if they have persistent masses present after chemotherapy. Occasionally these are found after resection to be mature teratomas that do not require further chemotherapy after resection.[21]

The highest rates of recurrence occur in the first 2 years; therefore, careful monitoring is indicated with serum tumor markers (if initially elevated) and frequent examinations, including CT scan of the chest, abdomen, and pelvis every 3 months for the first 2 years, then every 6 months for 3 years. Recurrent disease is treated with chemotherapy.[21]

Endodermal Sinus (Yolk Sac) Tumors

Endodermal sinus (yolk sac) tumors are the second most common form of ovarian germ cell tumor, accounting for approximately 20% of ovarian germ cell malignancies.[23] These tumors occur in young girls, with the median age at presentation being 18 years. One-third of patients will be premenarcheal at presentation. Endodermal sinus tumors secrete alpha fetoprotein (AFP) and are characterized histologically by the presence of Schiller-Duval bodies.[24]

Endodermal sinus tumors do not affect the contralateral ovary. They have a tendency toward distant hematogenous spread to the lungs, or they may be metastatic to the peritoneum with surface disease on the other ovary. Any gross disease should be removed in the initial surgery; however, aggressive staging is not necessary because all patients will require chemotherapy. Most patients will have early stage disease: 71% stage I, 6% stage II, and 23% stage III.[23] Prior to the routine use of chemotherapy for all patients, the 2-year survival rate for this disease was 25%. With the introduction of BEP chemotherapy for all patients, long-term cure rates for stage I disease are greater than 90%, and for stage III disease the cure rate is 60%–80%.[20] It is important to start chemotherapy as soon as possible after surgery, generally in 7–10 days, because some of these patients will recur rapidly. The optimal number of cycles of chemotherapy has yet to be determined. The general consensus is to give three cycles in stage I and completely resected disease, and to give two cycles past normalization of AFP in patients with residual disease after surgery.[21]

There are no data to support second look laparotomy after chemotherapy. In general, it is felt to be unnecessary. Patients with normal AFP levels are placed on surveillance, and patients with elevated levels are presumed to have persistent disease, and alternative chemotherapy regimens are indicated.[1]

As with the other ovarian germ cell malignancies, the highest rates of recurrence occur in the first 2 years after treatment. Close surveillance with monitoring of serum AFP, physical examination, and appropriate radiologic imaging (CT of chest, abdomen, and pelvis) is indicated. Recurrent disease is treated with chemotherapy.[21]

Embryonal Carcinoma and Ovarian Choriocarcinoma

Embryonal carcinoma and ovarian choriocarcinoma are very rare tumors that are generally diagnosed in women younger than age 20 years. The premenarcheal patient will often exhibit signs of precocious puberty. Embryonal carcinomas secrete AFP and HCG, while choriocarcinomas display HCG elevations. Ovarian choriocarcinoma, like that arising from the placenta, tends to have early hematogenous spread to distant organs. However, unlike placental choriocarcinoma, the ovarian type is not chemosensitive and is generally fatal.[4]

Classes of Ovarian Sex Cord Stromal Tumors

Ovarian sex cord stromal tumors are a heterogeneous group of rare tumors that develop from the cells that surround the oocytes. They include the cells that originate from the sex cords (the granulosa cells and the Sertoli cells, as well as the cells that originate from the mesenchyme), the theca cells, Leydig cells, and fibroblasts. Ovarian sex cord stromal tumors constitute 5%–8% of ovarian neoplasms.[25]

Most ovarian sex cord stromal tumors produce steroid hormones. Therefore, patients will often present with symptoms of estrogen excess (precocious puberty in premenarcheal patients, abnormal uterine bleeding in perimenopausal women, or postmenopausal bleeding in the postmenopausal patient) or with symptoms of androgen excess (virilization such as hirsutism, voice deepening, clitoral enlargement, breast atrophy, oligomenorrhea, or acne).[25]

An additional presenting symptom may be abdominal or pelvic pain related to a large mass. Although most ovarian sex cord stromal tumors are diagnosed at stage I, the presenting mass is often quite large. The median size of granulosa cell tumors is 12 cm, thecomas can be up to 40 cm in size, and Sertoli-Leydig tumors have an average size of 16 cm at presentation.[26]

In general, these tumors are of low malignant potential with a favorable long-term prognosis. The peak incidence is in the perimenopausal years, with the average age at diagnosis being 52 years. The exceptions to this are juvenile granulosa cell tumors, in which approximately one-half of the patients are below the age of 10 years at diagnosis; and Sertoli-Leydig tumors, which generally present at a younger age, with the majority being diagnosed in the second and third decade.[4]

Surgery

Surgery is utilized for diagnosis and treatment. Frequently, the affected population may be young and desirous of maintaining fertility. Because the majority of these tumors are diagnosed at stage IA, they rarely affect the contralateral ovary, and because several (i.e., thecoma, fibroma) are benign, a bilateral salpingo-oophorectomy is not required. Unilateral oophorectomy with staging to include pelvic and para-aortic lymph node sampling as well as directed biopsies (if the tumor is malignant) is recommended. If the patient has completed childbearing and is not desirous of future fertility, a bilateral salpingo-oophorectomy with hysterectomy is advised.[27] If no hysterectomy is to be performed, it is necessary to include a dilatation and curettage of the uterus during the surgery because there is about a 25%–50% incidence of endometrial hyperplasia and a 5%–10% incidence of endometrial carcinoma in those tumors with excess estrogen production.[28] In patients with sex cord tumors with annular tubules (SCTAT), there is a 35% incidence of Peutz-Jeghers syndrome. In this population, careful attention must also be paid to the cervix because 15% of these women will develop adenoma malignum of the cervix, a highly aggressive malignancy.[4]

Surgical resection is also indicated in the setting of localized disease recurrence because this may provide long-term disease control.[29]

Chemotherapy

There are no data to support the use of adjuvant treatment in stage I disease with either chemotherapy or radiotherapy in ovarian sex cord stromal tumors. Because stage I is the most common stage at diagnosis, the numbers of patients with advanced disease are very small and often not a homogenous population. This makes accrual to clinical trials to demonstrate the benefits of chemotherapy and radiotherapy treatment difficult.[4]

Early chemotherapy regimens included dactinomycin, 5-fluorouracil, and cyclophosphamide and had response rates of 23%. Later trials with BEP (bleomycin, etoposide, and cisplatin) chemotherapy regimens increased the response rate to 82%. Later trials with BEP in poor prognosis stromal tumors achieved a 37% pathologic complete response on second look.[4] At this time, the most commonly used regimen for advanced and recurrent disease is BEP.[28] Alternative regimens that have been tried include etoposide plus cisplatin (EP), cyclophosphamide, doxorubicin, plus cisplatin (CAP) or cisplatin as a single agent.[30]

For children with advanced stage juvenile granulosa cell tumors, adjuvant chemotherapy appears to confer benefits that contribute to long-lasting remissions. Therefore, the recommendation is for adjuvant therapy for those with stage IC disease with a high mitotic index (greater than 20 mitoses per 10 high power field) and for anyone with advanced disease.[25,31] However, due to differences in biology, which results in a lower mitotic rate and a risk of late recurrences, it is difficult to extrapolate these results to adult type granulosa cell tumors. Retrospective review of the literature reveals some studies that show a benefit to adjuvant chemotherapy in advanced adult granulosa cell malignancies,[31] while others show no improvement in survival.[32-34]

Radiotherapy

Granulosa cell tumors are known to be radiosensitive, and there have been documented responses in patients with gross residual disease after resection and in patients with recurrent disease. In one series of 34 patients, there was a 43% complete clinical response among the 14 patients who had measurable disease at the start of therapy.[35]

The optimal approach for patients with advanced or recurrent ovarian sex cord stromal tumors has yet to be determined. The decision of whether to offer adjuvant therapy in the setting of completely resected advanced disease or to observe closely must be made at the discretion of the clinician without the benefit of definitive data.

There are several subgroups of ovarian sex cord stromal tumors. They include granulosa cell (adult and juvenile), thecoma, fibroma, Sertoli, Leydig stromal cell, gynandroblastoma, and sex cord tumor with annular tubules (SCTAT). We will look at these individually, due to differences in treatment and prognosis. For an overview of the subclasses of ovarian sex cord stromal tumors, tumor markers expressed, treatment, and unique features, refer to **Table 5-3**.

Granulosa Cell Tumors (Adult)

The most common type of sex cord stromal tumor is the adult type granulosa cell tumor. It comprises 70% of ovarian sex cord stromal tumors; however, this translates to only 5% of all ovarian malignancies. Ninety-five percent of granulosa cell tumors are of the adult type. These tumors occur most often in middle-aged and older women, and present as a large unilateral pelvic mass. Additional symptoms often relate to the excess estrogen production of this type of tumor and include menometrorrhagia or postmenopausal bleeding.[9]

The histologic presentation consists of round pale cells with scant cytoplasm and a "coffee bean" grooved nuclei. These cells tend to be arranged in clusters around a central cavity. These typical arrangements are termed "Cal-Exner bodies."[27] The cells are generally well differentiated with few mitoses. Approximately 70% of adult granulosa cell tumors will contain theca cells, which produce estrogen and are responsible for the endocrine symptomatology associated with adult granulosa cell tumors.[27]

The most important indicator of prognosis is stage at presentation. These tumors are often referred to as low-grade malignancies due to their tendency to remain localized and to demonstrate indolent growth. The majority of women, 80-90%, will present with stage I disease. Five-year survival rates for stage I disease are 90%. Only 10% of patients will recur. Patients with extra ovarian spread have a less favorable prognosis, with 5-year survival rates of 33%–53% and recurrence rates of 30%. Other factors that may contribute to prognosis include tumor size, rupture, mitotic activity, and nuclear atypia.[9]

Due to the excess estrogen production associated with granulosa cell tumors, there is a strong association with endometrial hyperplasia and adenocarcinoma. Preoperative workup should include an endometrial biopsy to determine whether either of these conditions is present.[28]

The hormonal activity of adult granulosa cell tumors allows for the use of several tumor

Table 5-3 OVERVIEW OF THE SUBCLASSES OF OVARIAN SEX CORD STROMAL
TUMORS, TUMOR MARKERS EXPRESSED, TREATMENT, AND UNIQUE FEATURES.

Types	Tumor Marker	TX	Unique Feature
Adult granulosa cell	Inhibin A, inhibin B, estradiol	USO with staging and D & C of the uterus or TAH/ BSO with staging; no consensus regarding adjuvant chemotherapy	Generally considered a tumor of low malignant potential; can have late recurrences; is radiosensitive
Juvenile granulosa cell	Inhibin or estradiol	Staging surgery with BEP adjuvant chemotherapy if stage IC with high mititotic index or stages II–IV	Stage at diagnosis is the most important prognostic factor; 97% occur in pts. <30; known for early relapse
Thecoma	Estradiol	USO with D & C or TAH/BSO	Benign tumors occur primarily in sixth or seventh decade; associated with excess estrogen production
Fibroma	Hormonally inert	Surgical resection	Benign tumors with 10%–15% incidence of ascites (called Meigs syndrome)
Sertoli cell	Estradiol	USO with staging and D & C of the uterus or TAH/BSO with staging	Rare tumors of low malignant potential; 2/3 produce excess estrogen; average age at diagnosis is 27 years
Sertoli-Leydig	Testosterone	USO with staging: BEP chemotherapy for adjuvant tx if poorly differentiated tumor or presence of heterologous elements	Average age at diagnosis is 25 years; behavior (benign→malignant) is dependent on level of cellular differentiation

(continues)

Table 5-3 OVERVIEW OF THE SUBCLASSES OF OVARIAN SEX CORD STROMAL TUMORS, TUMOR MARKERS EXPRESSED, TREATMENT, AND UNIQUE FEATURES *continued.*

Types	Tumor Marker	TX	Unique Feature
Gynandroblastoma	Estradiol or testosterone	USO with D & C if excess estrogen is present	Must contain at least 10% of both granulosa cell and tubules of Sertoli cells; a tumor of low malignant potential
Ovarian sex cord tumor with annular tubules (SCTAT)	Estradiol	USO if associated with PJS; non-PJS SCTATs require staging; BEP chemo if advanced disease	30% of SCTAT are associated with PJS; of PJS associated SCTAT, there is a 15% incidence of adenoma malignum of the cervix; PJS assoc. SCTATs are benign tumors

markers in diagnostic evaluation and the monitoring for recurrent disease. The most useful markers are inhibin A and inhibin B.[36,37] One of the first markers identified in the serum of granulosa cell tumor patients was estradiol. It is generally a less sensitive marker than inhibin. Additionally, approximately 30% of granulosa cell tumors do not produce estradiol, which may be related to a lack of theca cells.[28,30]

Surgical staging is essential in the treatment of adult granulosa cell tumor. If the patient is a young woman and wishes to maintain her fertility, unilateral salpingo-oophorectomy with pelvic and para-aortic lymph node sampling and staging biopsies, along with dilatation and curettage of the endometrial lining, is appropriate. In the setting of the postmenopausal woman, a total abdominal hysterectomy, bilateral salpingo-oophorectomy, pelvic and para-aortic lymph node sampling, and staging biopsies is the standard.[28,30]

The question of the value of adjuvant chemotherapy in this malignancy remains unanswered. At present, patients with stage IA or IB disease are not offered adjuvant therapy. There is mixed opinion on whether or not to treat women with high-risk resected disease (stages IC through IV). Schumer et al. recommend postoperative adjuvant platinum-based therapy but offer no specific recommendation as to regimen or number of cycles.[28] Dorigo and Berek offer chemotherapy only to women with residual disease. Women with completely resected disease are followed closely for recurrence.[30]

Adult granulosa cell tumors (AGCT) can recur very late after diagnosis. The median time to recurrence is 4 to 6 years; however, recurrences have been documented as long as 40 years after initial treatment.[26,28] Therefore, prolonged surveillance with physical examination and serum inhibin levels with or without estradiol is indicated. Routine radiographic imaging studies are not recommended and are generally reserved for evaluation of new symptoms or elevations in tumor markers.[29]

Most often, the site of disease recurrence is the pelvis or upper abdomen, and surgery is the preferred intervention because complete resection of localized disease may provide long-term control.[38] In instances of diffuse or unresectable disease, the treatment options include chemotherapy, most often with BEP, or radiotherapy.[38,33] Both have been used successfully, but unfortunately many patients do not achieve durable remissions, and over 70% of women who recur will die of their disease.[27] Another reasonable option, given that most of these tumors express hormone receptors, is that of hormonal therapy. An advantage of this approach is that hormone therapy is generally well tolerated. Responses to medroxyprogesterone, as well as to leuprolide, have been documented.[39]

Granulosa Cell Tumor (Juvenile)

Ovarian neoplasms in children and adolescents are quite rare, and the majority of those that occur will be germ cell tumors. Ovarian sex cord stromal tumors make up 5%–7% of ovarian neoplasms. The preponderance of these tumors when they do occur in the young or adolescent population are juvenile granulosa cell tumors (JGCT). Only 3% percent of JGCTs occur after the third decade, with more than 30% occurring prior to age 10 years.[40]

The primary presenting symptoms are abdominal pain due to increasing abdominal girth and a large pelvic mass. Ascites is present in 10%–36% of cases. Additional presenting signs are precocious puberty, most commonly

with isosexual features and occasionally with virilization.[40]

In 95% of the cases JGCT will be unilateral, and nearly 90% will be stage IA. The most important prognostic factor is stage at presentation, with stage IA or IB achieving 97% survival. Survival rates drop dramatically as stage increases, with stages II–IV achieving only 23% survival. JGCT is different from AGCT in several respects. While AGCT tends to have long latency periods with median time to relapse of 4 to 6 years, JGCT is aggressive, with time to relapse and death of limited duration. Virtually no patients recur after 3 years from diagnosis.[27] Secondly, while the benefit of adjuvant therapy in advanced stages of AGCT is unclear, there is documented benefit to adjuvant treatment in JGCT, which appears to contribute to long-lasting remissions. Therefore, the recommendation is for adjuvant therapy for those with stage IC disease with a high mitotic index (greater than 20 mitoses per 10 high power field) and for anyone with advanced disease.[31,38]

Surveillance of JGCTs can be of limited duration due to the lack or late recurrences in this malignancy. Tumor markers of inhibin and estradiol have been reported in the literature in association with JGCT. Patients with advanced stage disease will require very close surveillance in the first 3 years due to the speed of recurrence.[27]

Thecoma

Thecomas account for about 1% of ovarian neoplasms. They occur primarily in the sixth and seventh decade.[41] Thecomas are benign tumors. In a review of the literature, there have been reports of metastatic or so-called malignant thecomas. Upon review, Waxman et al. felt that these tumors were misnamed and were in fact more likely low-grade stromal sarcomas or fibrosarcomas rather than thecomas.[42]

Thecomas vary in size, with ranges from 1 cm to 40 cm in diameter. Ascites is an occasional component. Thecomas are among the most hormonally active of the sex cord stromal tumors, and 60% of the time present with symptoms of abnormal vaginal bleeding as a result of excess estrogen.[41] Due to the excess estrogen, thecomas are associated with endometrial hyperplasia and adenocarcinoma in 25% and 15% of patients, respectively.[30]

The recommended intervention is total abdominal hysterectomy with bilateral salpingo-oophorectomy in the perimenopausal and postmenopausal patient. Unilateral salpingo-oophorectomy with endometrial sampling may be substituted in younger women for whom fertility or avoidance of exogenous estrogen replacement is desired.[30]

Fibroma/Fibrosarcoma

The most common ovarian sex cord stromal tumor is the fibroma. They tend to be unilateral and to occur in postmenopausal women. These tumors are hormonally inert. Fibromas are benign tumors of varying size. When these tumors become large (greater than 10 cm), there is a 10%–15% incidence of ascites as fluid escapes from the surfaces of the tumor. There is also a 1% incidence of hydrothorax in addition to the ascites. The association of ovarian fibroma with ascites and hydrothorax is termed Meigs syndrome.[43]

In contrast to fibromas, fibrosarcomas are rare malignant sarcomas whose aggressiveness directly relates to number of mitoses and the degree of atypia.[30]

Sertoli Cell

Sertoli cell tumors are extremely rare, accounting for less than 5% of all Sertoli-Leydig cell tumors. Two-thirds of these tumors are noted to produce estrogen and be associated with symptoms of precocious puberty or abnormal vaginal bleeding. The average age at diagnosis is 27 years, with an average tumor size of 9 cm. Sertoli cell tumors are occasionally associated with excess rennin production, resulting in refractory hypertension and hyperkalemia.[27] These are lesions of low malignant potential, and all reported cases have been stage I. Generally, these tumors have fairly mild cytologic features and rarely demonstrate moderate nuclear atypia.[27]

Sertoli-Leydig

Sertoli-Leydig is a very rare malignancy that accounts for less than 0.2% of all ovarian tumors. The majority of these tumors occur in the second and third decade, with 75% occurring in women less than age 40 years. The mean age at diagnosis is 25 years. Most of these tumors are unilateral and large, with an average size of 16 cm in diameter. Presenting symptoms generally include pelvic mass and pain. These tumors contain testicular structures that produce androgens and can cause virilization. However, not all Sertoli-Leydig tumors are functionally active; frank virilization is present in 35% of patients, with another 10%–15% with clinical signs of androgen excess.[27]

Sertoli-Leydig cell tumors may display benign or malignant behavior depending on their degree of differentiation. Some tumors may contain other tissue types, such as mucinous epithelium cartilage and skeletal muscle. The presence of nonepithelial tissues is linked with a poorer prognosis.[44] The majority of Sertoli-Leydig cell tumors, 97%, will be stage IA at diagnosis, and fewer than 20% will display malignant behavior. The overall 5-year survival rate is 70%–90%. In a series of 207 patients, all well-differentiated tumors behaved in a benign manner, while malignant behavior occurred in 11% of intermediate grade and 59% of poorly differentiated tumors. Nineteen percent of tumors with heterologous elements displayed malignant behavior. Those tumors that display malignant behavior tend to recur early, with only 6%-7% of recurrences occurring after 5 years.[44]

Metastatic disease is treated with platinum-based chemotherapy. Adjuvant therapy is often used for those patients with poorly differentiated tumors or those with heterologous elements. The most commonly used regimen is BEP combination chemotherapy. Additionally used regimens include cyclophosphamide; doxorubicin plus cisplatin (CAP); carboplatin and epirubicin plus etoposide; or cisplatin and vinblastine plus bleomycin.[30,44]

Gynandroblastoma

Gynandroblastoma is a very rare tumor, if strict criteria are followed, because it must contain an intermingling of both granulosa cells and tubules of Sertoli cells, with at least 10% of the minor element being present. The range of ages at presentation is 16–65 years, with an average age of 29.5 years. Because both granulosa and Sertoli cells are present, symptoms of either excess estrogen or androgen may appear. These are considered to be tumors of low malignant potential. Treatment consists of unilateral oophorectomy.[30]

Unclassified Sex Cord Stromal Tumors

Unclassified sex cord stromal tumors account for less than 10% of sex cord stromal tumors. They are characterized by tumors in which the predominant pattern of ovarian or testicular differentiation is unable to be discerned.[21]

Ovarian Sex Cord Tumor with Annular Tubules (SCTAT)

Ovarian sex cord tumors with annular tubules (SCTAT) are a unique type of sex cord tumor that is thought to represent an intermediate between Sertoli cell and granulosa cell tumors. They are characterized by simple and complex ring-shaped tubules.[45]

Many of the clinical signs are related to excess estrogen production and include abnormal vaginal bleeding or precocious puberty in children. Because SCTATs possess characteristics of both Sertoli cells and granulosa cells, tumor markers that are produced by either cell type may be present.[30]

One-third of SCTATs are associated with Peutz-Jeghers syndrome (PJS). In this setting, the tumor is generally small (less than 3 cm), multifocal, bilateral, and asymptomatic.[46] All SCTATs associated with PJS are benign; therefore, unilateral oophorectomy is curative. It is important to note that SCTATs associated with PJS have a 15% incidence of malignant adenoma of the cervix.[46] This is often demonstrated by multicystic cervical mass on imaging studies. Cervical cytology and colposcopy can be normal in the presence of this malignancy. Any lesions should be evaluated with excisional biopsy.[30,46]

Non-PJS associated SCTATs are almost always large, unilateral, and uncalcified. The affected population is also younger: mid- to late 20s. These women have a 20% incidence of metastatic disease at presentation; therefore, surgical staging is essential. Patients who present with metastatic disease may respond to chemotherapy.[30,45]

Long-Term/Late Effects

Due to the young age at which patients with germ cell and sex cord stromal ovarian malignancies are diagnosed, as well as improvements in long-term survival, attention has turned to the potential late- or long-term effects of treatment. Advances in our knowledge of the natural history of these disease processes, as well as advances in surgical techniques, have made preservation of fertility, for those patients who wish to do so, an attainable goal.[1,4-7,22] Although many women will experience ovarian dysfunction during platinum-based chemotherapy, most (up to 68% in one series) will recover normal ovarian function, and the majority will be able to conceive and have healthy children.[6]

Much of the data regarding long-term toxicities associated with platinum-based chemotherapy comes from research in men with testicular cancer. Among the reported long-term effects are renal and gonadal dysfunction, neurotoxicity, and cardiovascular toxicity.[1] The most serious long-term risk of BEP chemotherapy is risk of secondary malignancies, particularly acute leukemia related to etoposide administration. The level of risk is directly related to the total cumulative dose. In patients receiving less than 2000 mg/m^2, the incidence of leukemia is 0.4%–0.5%. This is approximately a 30-fold increase over the risk

of the general population. However, this risk increases to 5%, or a 336-fold increase, in the likelihood of developing leukemia when the dose exceeds 2000mg/m^2. Patients who receive a typical three- or four-cycle course of BEP will receive less than 2000mg/m^2. Despite the increased risk of developing a secondary malignancy with etoposide, it is felt that the benefit exceeds the risk because one case of treatment-induced leukemia would be expected for every 20 additionally cured patients who receive BEP as compared to PVB.[1]

Finally, bleomycin-induced pulmonary fibrosis is a potential long-term effect of BEP chemotherapy. Although rare, it must not be overlooked, particularly if general anesthesia is needed.[22]

Symptom Management and Nursing Issues

Because young women are a high-risk population for chemotherapy-induced nausea and vomiting and cisplatin is highly emetogenic, it is important to ensure adequate antiemetic prophylaxis. A $5HT_3$ antagonist plus or minus a substance P inhibitor, with dexamethasone for premedication, should be used with continuation of antiemetic medication on a scheduled basis for 2 to 3 days following treatment.[47,48]

Supportive nursing care is essential throughout all phases of treatment for the woman with nonepithelial ovarian cancer. These are often young patients and require extensive teaching and emotional support. Information is crucial to helping the patient and her family to understand the disease process and its treatment.

Patients with nonepithelial ovarian tumors will undergo at least one surgical procedure at diagnosis and staging. It is very important to make sure that the patient has a clear understanding of what the surgical procedure will involve, including what tissues will be removed and the effect, if any, on her future fertility. Additionally, teaching should include expected postoperative recovery information.[49]

For those patients who require further treatment with chemotherapy, it is necessary to instruct them on the expected side effects (nausea, hair loss, myelosuppression, etc.), as well as the necessary precautions (risk of infection, importance of hand washing, etc).

Finally, the importance of follow-up care and surveillance for disease recurrence must be communicated to the patient. It is essential to provide a supportive environment that allows the patient to feel free to ask questions and express concerns or fears.

References

1. Berek JS, Non epithelial ovarian and fallopian tube cancers. In: Berek JS, Hacker NF, eds. *Practical Gynecologic Oncology*, 4th ed. Philadelphia, PA: Lippincott, Williams & Wilkins; 2005.

2. Tanagho EA, Heip, N.T. Embryology of the urinary system. In: Tanagho EA, McAninch JW, Smith DR, eds. *Smith's General Urology*, 17th ed. New York, NY: McGraw Hill; 2008.

3. DeUgarte CM, Bast JD. Embryology of the urogenital system and congenital anomalies of the female genital tract. In: DeCherney AH, ed. *Current Diagnosis and Treatment: Obstetrics and Gynecology*, 7th ed. New York, NY: McGraw Hill; 2007.

4. Lu KH, Gershenson DM, Poynor EA, Sabbatini PJ. Germ cell and ovarian sex cord stromal tumors. In: Barakat RR, Bevers MW, Gershenson DM, Hoskins WJ, eds. *Handbook of Gynecologic Oncology*, 2nd ed. London: Martin-Dunitz Ltd; 2002.

5. Pectasides E, Pectasides D, Kassanos D. Germ cell tumors of the ovary. *Cancer Treat Rev.* In press.

6. Gershenson DM. Management of ovarian germ cell tumors. *J Clin Oncol.* 2007;25(20):2938–2943.

7. Guillem V, Poveda A. Germ cell tumours of the ovary. *Clin Transl Oncol.* 2007;4:237–243.

8. Lai CH, Chang TC, Hsueh S, et al. Outcome and prognostic factors in ovarian germ cell malignancies. *Gynecol Oncol.* 2005;96:784.

9. Feldman, DR, Bosl GJ, Sheinfeld J, Motzer RJ. Medical treatment of advanced testicular cancer. *JAMA.* 2008;299(6):672–684.

10. Hussain SA, Ma YT, Cullen MH. Management of metastatic germ cell tumors. *Expert Rev Anticancer Ther.* 2008;(5):771–784.

11. Mann JR, Raafat F, Robinson D, et al. The United Kingdom Children's Cancer Study Group's second germ cell tumor study: carboplatin, etoposide, and bleomycin are effective treatment for children with malignant extracranial germ cell tumors, with acceptable toxicity. *J Clin Oncol.* 2000;18:3809.

12. Stern JW, Bunin N. Prospective study of carboplatin based chemotherapy for pediatric germ cell tumors. *Med Pediatr Oncol.* 2002;39:163.

13. Sonpavde G, Hutson TE, Roth BJ. Management of recurrent testicular germ cell tumors. *Oncol.* 2007;(1):51–61.

14. Kondagunta GV, Bacik J, Donadio A, et al. Combination of paclitaxel, ifosfamide, and cisplatin is an effective second line therapy for patients with relapsed testicular germ cell tumors. *J Clin Oncol.* 2005;23:6549.

15. Mead GM, Cullen MH, Huddart R, et al. A phase II trail of TIP (paclitaxel, ifosfamide and cisplatin) given as second line (post BEP) salvage chemotherapy for patients with metastatic germ cell cancer: a medical research council trial. *Br J Cancer.* 2005; 93:178.

16. Hinton S, Catalano P, Einhorn LH, et al. Phase II study of paclitaxel plus gemcitabine in refractory germ cell tumors (E9897): a trial of the Eastern Cooperative Oncology Group. *J Clin Oncol.* 2002;20:1859.

17. Pizzocaro F, Nicolai N, Salvioni R, Gianni L. Paclitaxel, cisplatin, gemcitabine (TPG) third line therapy in metastatic germ cell tumors (GCT)

of the testis [abstract]. *Proc Am Soc Clin Oncol.* 2001;20:194a.

18. Bedano PM, Brames MJ, Williams SW, Einhorn LH. A phase II study of cisplatin plus epirubicin in refractory germ cell tumors. *J Clin Oncol.* 2005;23:384s.

19. Tewari KS, DiSaia PJ. Radiation therapy for gynecologic cancer. *J Obstet Gyanecol Res.* 2002(3);123–140.

20. Berek JS. Germ cell malignancies. In: Berek JS, Adashi EY, Hillard PA, eds. *Novak's Gynecology,* 13th ed. Philadelphia, PA: Lippincott, Williams & Wilkins; 2002.

21. Chalas E, Valea FA, Mann WJ. Treatment of malignant germ cell tumors of the ovary. In: Rose BD, ed. *UpToDate.* Waltham, MA: Author; 2006.

22. Dorigo O, Berek J. Overview of ovarian germ tumors. In: Rose BD, ed. *UpToDate.* Waltham, MA: Author; 2006.

23· Dallenbach P, Bonnefoi H, Pelte MF, Vlastos G. Yolk sac tumors of the ovary: an update. *Eur J Surg Oncol.* 2006;10:1063–1075.

24. Williams SD, Gershenson DM, Horowitz CJ, Silva E. Ovarian germ cell tumors. In: Hoskins WJ, Perez CA, Young RC, eds. *Principles and Practice of Gynecologic Oncology,* 3rd ed. Philadelphia, PA: Lippincott, Williams &Wilkins; 2000.

25. Columbo N, Parma G, Zanagnolo V, Insingna A. Management of ovarian stromal cell tumors. *J Clin Oncol.* 2007;25(20):2944–2951.

26. Pectasides D, Pectasides E, Psyrri A. Granulosa cell tumor of the ovary. *Cancer Treat Rev.* 2008;34(1): 1–12.

27. Hartman LC, Young RH, Podratz KC. Ovarian sex cord stromal tumors. In: Hoskins WJ, Perez CA, Young RC, eds. *Principles and Practice of Gynecologic Oncology,* 3rd ed. Philadelphia, PA: Lippincott, Williams &Wilkins.

28. Schumer ST, Cannistra GA. Granulosa cell tumor of the ovary. *J Clin Oncol.* 2003;21:1180.

29. Sehouli F, Drescher RS, Mustea A, et al. Granulosa cell tumor of the ovary: 10 years follow up data of 65 patients. *Anticancer Res.* 2004;24:1223.

30. Dorigo O, Berek J. Sex cord stromal tumors of the ovary. In: Rose BD, ed. *UpToDate.* Waltham, MA: Author; 2006.

31. Schneider DT, Calaminus G, Wessalowski R, et al. Ovarian sex cord stromal tumors in children and adolescents. *J Clin Oncol.* 2003;21:2357.

32. Al-Badawi IA, Brasher PM, Ghatage P, et al. Postoperative chemotherapy in advanced ovarian granulosa cell tumors. *Int J Gynecol Cancer.* 2002;12:119.

33. Chan JK, Zhang M, Kaleb V, et al. Prognostic factors responsible for survival in sex cord stromal tumors of the ovary: a multivariate analysis. *Gynecol Oncol.* 2005;96:204.

34. Zanzgnolo V, Pasinetti B, Sartori E. Clinical review of 63 cases of sex cord stromal tumors. *Eur J Gynaecol Oncol.* 2004;25:431.

35. Wolf JK, Mullen J, Eifel PJ, et al. Radiation treatment of advanced or recurrent granulosa cell tumor of the ovary. *Gynecol Oncol.* 1999;73:35.

36. Pectasides D, Papaxoinis G, Fountzilas G, et al. Adult granulosa cell tumors of the ovary: a clinicopathologic study of 34 patients by the Hellenic Cooperative Oncology Group. *Anticancer Res.* 2008;28(2B): 1421–1427.

37. Farinola MA, Gown AM, Judson K, et al. Estrogen receptor alpha and progesterone receptor expression in ovarian adult granulosa cell tumors and Sertoli-Leydig cell tumors. *Int J Gynecol Path.* 2007;26(4):375–382.

38. Uygun K, Aydiner A, Saip P, et al. Clinical parameters and treatment results in recurrent granulosa cell tumor of the ovary. *Gynecol Oncol.* 2003;88:400.

39. Ameryckx L, Fatemi HM, De Sutter P, Amy JJ. GnRH antagonist in the adjuvant treatment of a recurrent ovarian granulosa cell tumor: a case report. *Gynecol Oncol.* 2005;99:764.

40. Gittleman AM, Price AP, Coren C, Akhtar M, Donovan V, Katz DS. Juvenile granulosa cell tumor. *Clin Imaging.* 2003;27(4):221–224.

41. Nocito AL, Sarancone S, Bacchi C, Tellez T. Ovarian thecoma: clinicopathological analysis of 50 cases. *Ann Diagn Pathol.* 2008;12(1):12–16.

42. Waxman M, Vuletin JC, Urcuyo R, Belling CG. Ovarian low grade stromal sarcoma with thecomatous features: a critical reappraisal of the so-called "malignant thecoma." *Cancer.* 1979;44:2206.

43. Ishiko O, Yoshida H, Sumi T, et al. Vascular endothelial growth factor levels in pleural and peritoneal fluid in Meigs' syndrome. *Eur J Obstet Gynecol Reprod Biol.* 2001;98:129.

44. Tandon R, Goel P, Saha PK, Takkar N, Punia RP. A rare ovarian tumor—Sertoli-Leydig cell tumor with heterologous element. *MedGenMed.* 2007;9(4):44.

45. Roth LM. Recent advances in the pathology and classification of ovarian sex cord-stromal tumors. *Int J Gynecol Pathol.* 2006;25(3):199–215.

46. Lembo AJ. Peutz-Jeghers syndrome. In: Rose BD, ed. *UpToDate.* Waltham, MA: Author; 2008.

47. Alexander J. Symptom management. In: Gullatte MM, ed. *Clinical Guide to Antineoplastic Therapy.* Pittsburgh, PA: Oncology Nursing Society; 2001.

48. Fieler VK. Aprepitant approved for treatment of nausea and vomiting. *Oncol Nurs Forum.* 2003;30:699.

49. Winkelman LA, Birk CL. Nonepithelial cancers of the ovary. In: Moore GJ, ed. *Women and Cancer: A Gynecologic Oncology Nursing Perspective,* 2nd ed. Boston, MA: Jones and Bartlett; 2000.

Chapter 6

Preinvasive Cervical Cancer

Margaret Fischer, RN, MSN, ANP-BC

Introduction

The diagnosis and management of preinvasive diseases of the cervix has changed greatly over the past 50 years. With the development of the Pap smear and the colposcope, the cervix can be directly visualized, examined, and tested. Pathology techniques have allowed us to differentiate between normal cervical cells, squamous intraepithelial lesions (SIL), and cancer. A clear progression from normal cervical cells to cancer has been identified. Liquid-based cervical cytology smears provide more accurate results by removing blood and mucous, which can obscure the cells. The process also arranges the cells in a single layer so that they can be seen clearly. The discovery of the influence of human *Papillomavirus* (HPV) on the development of cervical cancer opened up multiple possibilities for screening, treatment, and prevention of cervical cancer. The development of the Loop Electrosurgical Excision Procedure (LEEP) and various other surgical techniques has given us effective tools for evaluating and treating SIL. Ideally, screening and treatment would prevent the progression of normal cells to SIL and cervical cancer. Presently, scientists are looking at molecular biology to give us more answers to explain what factors initiate the progression to cancer and how to reverse that change.

Epidemiology/Risk Factors

The presence of oncogenic HPV types has been proven to be the greatest risk factor for developing preinvasive and invasive disease of the cervix. HPV was noted in greater than 85% of cervical cancers.[1] Although many women have HPV, only a few will progress to cervical cancer. It has been proposed that other factors in the presence of oncogenic HPV may stimulate the development of SIL and cancer. Some "plausible cofactors in cervical and lower genital tract carcinogenesis include the use of tobacco products, infection by other microbial agents, specific vitamin deficiencies, hormonal influences, and immunosuppression."[2] There are probably other factors that affect development of preinvasive cervical cancer that have yet to be established. Additional risk behaviors that increase potential for exposure to HPV include multiple sexual partners, early age of first intercourse, and unprotected sexual contact.

Human *Papillomavirus* (HPV)

Human *Papillomavirus* is a virus that is implicated in the pathogenesis of warts or papillomas. There are over 100 different types of HPV, of which approximately 40 are known to be sexually transmitted.[3] HPV has a propensity for the transformation zone of the cervix, where cells are continually changing. HPV has to be integrated into the cervical epithelial cells before changes that lead to SIL or cervical cancer can occur. When the virus has been integrated into the cell, it affects the tumor suppressor proteins, such as P53, which allows cells to grow uncontrolled. The CDC identifies HPV 16, 18, 31, 33, and 35 as the strains that are oncogenic in the anogenital region and are highly associated with cervical cancer in the United States.[4] Williamson et al. (2005) also identified HPV 39, 45, 51, 52, 58, 68, 73, and 82 as high-risk when they looked at HPV types across nine different countries.[5]

HPV 16 is associated with the majority of high-grade squamous intraepithelial lesions (HSIL) and invasive squamous cancers.[2] HPV 18 is more commonly associated with adenocarcinomas of the cervix, which are seen in a younger population and tend to be more aggressive tumors.[2] According to CDC estimates, up to 50% of sexually active men and women will develop HPV at some point in their lifetime.[3] Research has demonstrated that 90% of those infections will become undetectable within 2 years due to a natural regression of the HPV infection. The CDC estimates that approximately 20 million people currently have a genital HPV infection that can be transmitted.[3]

Prevention

Until recently, there was no way to prevent the transmission of HPV except for abstinence. For those who choose to be sexually active, "condoms may lower the risk of HPV, if used all the time and the right way. Condoms may also lower the risk of developing HPV-related diseases, such as genital warts and cervical cancer."[3] For SIL and cervical cancer to develop, the high-risk HPV needs to persist for a prolonged period of time. If the HPV can be treated and eradicated before any changes can occur, there is the potential to prevent development of cervical cancer.

Two vaccines for HPV have been developed: Gardasil (Silgard) by Merck and Cervarix by Smith Kline.[6] To date, only Gardasil is approved by the FDA for use in the United States. Gardasil is approved for the prevention of HPV 6, 11, 16, and 18, which most commonly cause cervical cancer and genital warts. It is recommended to be administered to young women between the ages of 9 through 26. It is given as a series of three injections; the second and third doses should be administered 2 and 6 months after the first dose.[7] Cevarix specifically targets HPV 16 and 18.

Prior to having a vaccine to prevent transmission of HPV, screening was focused on detecting high-grade lesions and treating them before they had the chance to convert to cervical cancer.

Histology/Pathology

Before we can understand the changes, which are occurring at the cellular level, we need to have an understanding of what the normal cervix is. **Figure 6-1** is a picture of a normal cervix. The cervix is round, approximately 2.5 cm in size.

Figure 6-1 A normal cervix.

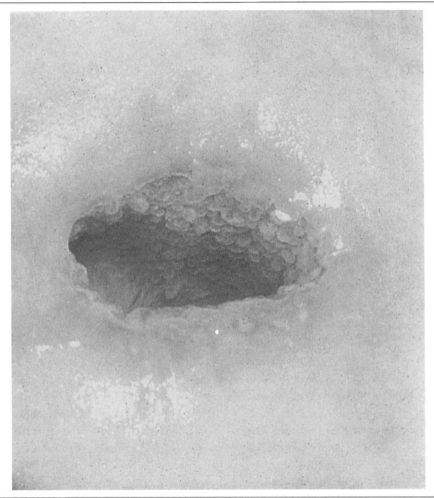

Normally the cervical opening is either round, as in nulliparous women, or can look like a slit in multiparous women. The cervix is smooth and pink. On examining the cervix under the microscope, there are three layers.[8] **Figure 6-2** is a microscopic view of a normal cervix.

The basal layer is a single layer of cells that binds the epithelium to the basement membrane. The next layer, composed of a few layers of cells, is the parabasal layer. Cell proliferation occurs here, so mitosis is commonly seen. The cells in the parabasal area have darkened round nuclei with very little cytoplasm. As the cells get further from the parabasal layer they flatten out, and fewer nuclei are noted.

Figure 6-2 A microscopic view of a normal cervix.

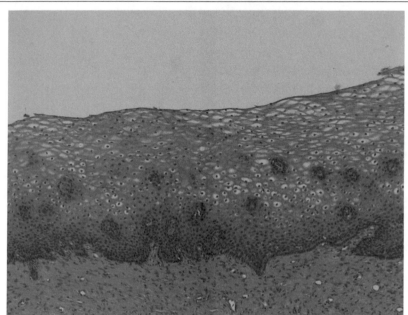

When SIL is found on colposcopy, a biopsy is performed. **Figure 6-3** is what is seen on colposcopy when SIL is found. Microscopically when a woman develops SIL, undifferentiated basaloid cells replace the epithelium. Where the cells normally had become flattened, there are multiple nuclei, sometimes atypically shaped with mitosis. The grading of the SIL is determined by how much of the epithelial layer is involved. **Figure 6-4** is a microscopic view of cervical HSIL.

Assessment/Screening

The ideal screening tool should be able to detect preinvasive disease or early invasive disease while it can be easily cured and while it is also cost effective and easily tolerated by patients. The gold standard for many years was the Papanicolaou (Pap) smear in addition to visual examination of the cervix. A scraping of cells was taken from the cervix and transformation zone and smeared on a glass slide. The smear was then sprayed with a fixative. Today that same technique is used in many places. Though this may sound rather simple, there are many opportunities in the process for error: improper labeling or handling of the slide, improper technique for obtaining the sample, improper interpretation of the results or loss of the specimen, and so on. Numerous efforts have been made to improve this process and decrease errors.

Out of these efforts came the development of liquid-based Pap smears. The sampling of cells is placed in solution, and then the cells can be separated from the mucous and blood and placed as a single layer of cells on a slide to be

Figure 6-3 Colposcopy view when SIL is found.

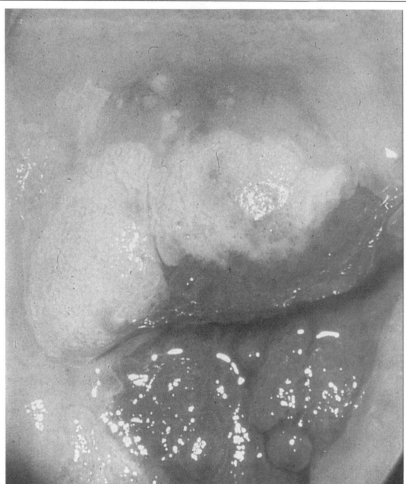

read. The benefits of the new technique are that there is an increased detection of SIL and that it detects significantly more cases of HSIL than conventional cytology.[8] There is more accurate diagnosis of glandular disease as well.[9]

Guidelines from the American Society of Cytopathology recommend the use of plastic spatulas when using glass slides because there are more cells lost when wooden spatulas or cotton swabs are used.[10] The cytobrush, plastic spatula, or broom-type device can be utilized with the liquid-based solutions.

A Pap smear, whether standard or liquid-based, is interpreted utilizing the Bethesda System. The Bethesda System identifies the specimen type and specimen adequacy, identifies

Figure 6-4 A microscopic view of cervical HSIL.

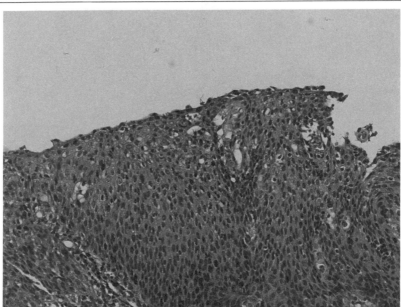

whether ancillary testing or automated review were performed, and gives an interpretation of the results. In 2001, the system was revised to decrease areas of confusion and to incorporate new technology. HPV testing was noted to be a clinically valid tool to determine the risk of developing SIL or invasive cancer.[11] The American Society of Cytopathology additionally emphasized that the Pap smear is a screening tool and does not replace diagnostic tools. **Table 6-1** is a listing of the 2001 Bethesda System.[12]

According to Bethesda guidelines, the interpretation of a Pap smear can be either "negative for intraepithelial lesion or malignancy" or "epithelial cell abnormalities." Included within the "negative for intraepithelial lesion or malignancy" are a variety of infectious organisms, reactive changes, or atrophy. The epithelial cell abnormalities are divided into either squamous cell or glandular cell abnormalities.

Squamous cell abnormalities include: atypical squamous cells of undetermined significance (ASC-US), atypical squamous cells cannot exclude HSIL (ASC-H), low-grade squamous intraepithelial lesion (LSIL), high-grade squamous intraepithelial lesion (HSIL), and squamous cell carcinoma. Glandular cell abnormalities include: atypical glandular cells (AGC) from endocervix, endometrial, or an unspecified area; AGC favor neoplastic; adenocarcinoma in situ (AIS); and adenocarcinoma.

Historically ASCUS, the old Bethesda terminology, included anything that didn't fit into either the normal or the SIL category. The interpretation of ASCUS on a Pap smear

Table 6-1 THE 2001 BETHESDA SYSTEM.

- **Specimen Type**

  Indicate conventional smear (Pap smear) versus liquid-based preparation versus other

- **Specimen Adequacy**

  - Satisfactory for evaluation
    (describe presence or absence of endocervical/transformation zone component and any other quality indicators, e.g., partially obscuring blood, inflammation, etc.)

  - Unsatisfactory for evaluation (specify reason)

    - Specimen rejected/not processed (specify reason)

    - Specimen processed and examined, but unsatisfactory for evaluation of epithelial abnormality because of (specify reason)

- **Interpretation/Result**

  - **Negative for Intraepithelial Lesion or Malignancy**
    (when there is no cellular evidence of neoplasia, state this in the General Categorization above and/or in the Interpretation/Result section of the report, whether or not there are organisms or other nonneoplastic findings)

    - **Organisms**

      - *Trichomonas vaginalis*

      - Fungal organisms morphologically consistent with *Candida* spp

      - Shift in flora suggestive of bacterial vaginosis

      - Bacteria morphologically consistent with *Actinomyces* spp

      - Cellular changes consistent with herpes simplex virus

    - **Other nonneoplastic findings (optional to report; list not inclusive)**

      - Reactive cellular changes associated with:

        - Inflammation (includes typical repair)

        - Radiation

        - Intrauterine contraceptive device (IUD)

        - Glandular cells status posthysterectomy

        - Atrophy

  - **Other**

    - Endometrial cells (in a woman >= 40 years of age)
      (Specify if 'negative for squamous intraepithelial lesion')

(continues)

Table 6-1 THE 2001 BETHESDA SYSTEM *continued.*

- Epithelial Cell Abnormalities
  - Squamous cell
    - Atypical squamous cells
      - Of undetermined significance (ASC-US)
      - Cannot exclude HSIL (ASC-H)
    - Low-grade squamous intraepithelial lesion (LSIL)
      Encompassing: HPV/mild dysplasia/CIN 1
    - High-grade squamous intraepithelial lesion (HSIL)
      Encompassing: moderate and severe dysplasia, CIS; CIN 2 and CIN 3
      - With features suspicious for invasion (if invasion is suspected)
    - Squamous cell carcinoma
  - Glandular cell
    - Atypical
      - Endocervical cells, NOS or specify in comments
      - Endometrial cells, NOS or specify in comments
      - Glandular cells, NOS or specify in comments
    - Atypical
      - Endocervical cells, favor neoplastic
      - Glandular cells, favor neoplastic
    - Endocervical adenocarcinoma in situ
    - Adenocarcinoma
      - Endocervical
      - Endometrial
      - Extrauterine
      - Not otherwise specified (NOS)
  - Other Malignant Neoplasms (specify)
- Ancillary Testing
- Automated Review
- Educational Notes and Suggestions (optional)

left healthcare providers uncertain as to how to proceed. Was the cervix safe to just watch when there could be SIL that was just unidentified? How much testing and what procedures should the patient be subjected to in order to prove a normal Pap smear? It was also problematic when the pathologist identified the sample as satisfactory *but* not optimum due to such problems as inflammation. Frequently, results were confusing. Erring on the side of safety, the Pap smear was repeated, as well as colposcopy and even biopsies, leading to much overtreatment.

The revised Bethesda System aimed to decrease the confusion. Samples are now listed as either satisfactory or unsatisfactory, removing the confusion of whether the sample was adequate or not. The results that previously were called ASCUS are now better defined. If reactive changes or inflammation is present, those results are now read as normal. ASC-US includes those results that probably are associated with SIL; however, obvious SIL is not seen. ASC-H is an intermediate level between ASCUS and SIL where it is thought that there is a higher possibility of SIL being present. The term "benign cellular changes" has been eliminated. The updated Bethesda System allows for better interpretation of the Pap smear.

There still remains a continued controversy over how often and who to screen. The American Cancer Society (ACS) and the US Preventive Services Task Force (USPSTF) recommend beginning screening 3 years after onset of sexual activity or 21 years of age, whichever is earlier.[13] ACS & USPSTF suggest that waiting 3 years will avoid overtreatment as the young woman is exposed to HPV and then has time to clear the virus. The ACS and American College of Obstetricians and Gynecologists (ACOG) suggest that after the woman has three normal

Pap smears, screening can be decreased to every 2-3 years unless the woman has risk factors that would make her more likely to develop SIL or cervical cancer.[13] USPSTF recommends screening every 3 years.[13] ACS suggests stopping screening after the age of 65 or 70 years if the woman has previously had normal Pap smears. Elderly women who have not had a Pap smear recently or who have a history of "cervical cancer, DES exposure before birth, HIV infection, or a weakened immune system should continue to have screening as long as they are in good health."[14]

Women who have had previous exposure to diethylstilbestrol (DES) or who have previously had cervical cancer are recommended to continue annual screening. They also suggest that there is no need to do screening in women who have had a hysterectomy for benign conditions.[14]

Women who are infected with HIV have an increased progression of both preinvasive and invasive cervical neoplasia.[15] The only significant predictor of developing an incident high-risk HPV infection was low CD4 count, defined as a CD4 count below 200 and a high viral load.[16] The US Public Health Service Infectious Disease Society of America recommends screening twice in the first year and then yearly thereafter if the Pap smear for the HIV-infected woman has been normal.[17] HPV testing can be helpful in determining if high-risk HPV is present, which would put the woman at risk. It makes sense then that if antiretroviral therapy can improve CD4 counts, it may decrease the risk of HSIL and cervical cancer in women who are HIV seropositive.

Presently, HPV testing is not being used as a routine screening tool to replace the Pap smear. Many times, it is utilized as a secondary test with abnormal Pap smears to determine the woman's risk. Reflex HPV testing can be ordered, which will automatically be run if an abnormal Pap smear is diagnosed.

Diagnosis

If ASC-US is noted on a Pap smear, additional testing is suggested with the goal to determine if SIL is actually present. The 2001 Consensus Guidelines recommend using a program of two repeat cytology tests, immediate colposcopy, or DNA testing for high-risk types of HPV for women with ASC-US.[8] Initially, the Pap smear may be repeated. The repeat Pap smear cannot be performed for at least 6–8 weeks from the previous Pap smear so that any inflammation from performing the previous test has resolved. With patients who are postmenopausal and atrophy is suspected, the patient can be treated with a course of intravaginal estrogen before the Pap smear is repeated.

When the Pap smear is repeated, a liquid-based solution can be utilized with reflex HPV testing so that HPV testing will automatically be performed if ASC-US or LSIL is identified. HPV testing can be helpful in trying to triage women with ASCUS Pap smears.[8] Women whose Pap was interpreted as ASCUS and had high-risk HPV, as well as abnormally high DNA content, are at an elevated risk of developing cervical cancer.[18] Patients with repeat biopsies that were ASCUS or who were found to have high-risk HPV were then screened for SIL using colposcopy and biopsy.

Women whose Pap was interpreted as ASC-H should be referred immediately for colposcopy.[8] Twenty-four percent to 94% of women with Pap smears of ASC-H will have CIN 2 or 3 identified on sampling.[8]

For women with a Pap smear interpreted as AGUS or AGC, immediate colposcopy

is recommended. "Atypical glandular cell cytology confers a risk (38%) of either preinvasive disease or carcinoma, with the risk of carcinoma increasing significantly for women aged older than 40."[19]

Usually women with SIL will be referred for colposcopy. The exception to this is with adolescents who have ASC-US or LSIL. Adolescents with either ASC-US or LSIL should be followed by Pap smears since many of these abnormalities regress over time.[20] In addition, adolescents who have not been immunized with the HPV vaccine should be immunized to prevent exposure to other strains of HPV.[21] All other women will be referred for colposcopy. When a Pap smear indicates that SIL or invasive cancer is present, a colposcopy and biopsy is usually recommended.

Colposcopy is the examination of the cervix and vagina using a magnified light source. Normal saline is initially applied to remove mucous and debris. Hyperkeratosis, which is a thickening of the epithelial layer or atypical blood vessels, should be able to be visualized at this point. Three to five percent acetic acid solution is then applied with a waiting time of 30 seconds for the reaction to occur. Acetowhite epithelium or abnormal vascular patterns are indicative of SIL or cancer. If the patient is not allergic to iodine, Lugol iodine one-quarter strength may be applied. The normal squamous epithelium will stain mahogany brown. Metaplastic tissue or neoplastic epithelium will appear mustard yellow.[2]

When the abnormal tissue is identified, a biopsy is performed. A colposcopy is considered to be adequate if the entire lesion and transformation zone can be visualized. If the lesion cannot be totally visualized or appears to extend up the canal, an endocervical biopsy can be performed to rule out disease in the cervical canal. If abnormal endometrial cells are noted or a source of the abnormality cannot be identified, an endometrial biopsy may be helpful to diagnosing abnormalities within the endometrial cavity.

For women who are pregnant, a colposcopy and biopsy can be performed. Endocervical curettage is avoided during pregnancy. As long as invasive cancer is not present, the woman will be monitored throughout her pregnancy and then be retested approximately 6 weeks postpartum.[22]

Treatment

If an infectious organism is identified on Pap smear, the infection can be treated. Fungal organisms can either be treated with Monistat, Terazol, Diflucan, or one of the other antifungal agents. Bacterial vaginosis can be treated with MetroGel. Treatment of a suspected infection may also treat unexplained inflammation.

When HSIL or LSIL with high-risk HPV is identified, the affected tissue is usually removed. The specific procedure that will be performed will depend on whether the entire lesion can be visualized.

If the whole lesion cannot be visualized, a cone biopsy will be performed to determine if the disease extends up into the canal. The cone biopsy can be both diagnostic as well as therapeutic. A cold knife conization or cone biopsy is a surgical excision of the affected area. A cone-shaped specimen is removed from the cervix, making sure that adequate margins are obtained around the lesion. Bleeding is minimized by injecting the cervix with a vasospastic agent prior to the procedure and then by cauterizing the surgical bed afterward. Because the specimen itself is not cauterized, the entire specimen can be evaluated by the pathologist. If the entire SIL lesion is removed with adequate normal tissue margins, the patient will not require additional surgical treatment unless the disease recurs.

Other options for treatment, where the entire lesion can be seen, include: cryotherapy, laser ablation, loop excision of the transformation zone (LLETZ), or LEEP. Cryotherapy uses liquid nitrogen to freeze the affected area. The freezing causes tissue necrosis. This is used primarily on small lesions. Laser ablation is similar to cryotherapy except that instead of using cold, the lesion is lasered, which burns the tissue. It has a similar affect on the tissue. The treated layers slough off, as with a burn. The LLETZ and LEEP utilize an electrocautery loop that can be directed to remove a specific sample of tissue. **Figure 6-5** shows how a LEEP is performed.

With HSIL there is a risk of recurrence of the SIL after a cone biopsy. Almog et al. suggested checking an HPV viral load after cone biopsy to try to determine which women were at risk for developing a recurrence of SIL.[23] Some women may be offered a hysterectomy as definitive treatment for the SIL if it continues to persist or recurs. Research is being conducted to evaluate the use of HPV vaccines to treat SIL or prevent recurrence of SIL after treatment.

Nursing Implications

Nurses have varied roles in the care of women with SIL. Some may be responsible for ensuring that patients have appropriate screening and follow-up. The American Society for Colposcopy and Cervical Pathology (ASCCP) states that a good follow-up system ensures that: (1) the patient is notified of abnormal Pap results, (2) the recall system ensures that the patient returns for follow-up, and (3) guidelines exist so that uniform teaching and advisement are given.[24]

Figure 6-5 How a LEEP is performed.

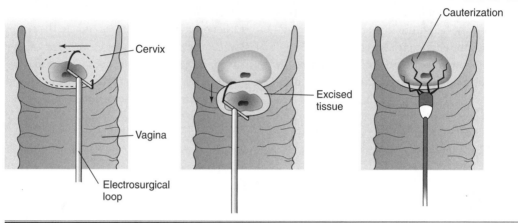

Nurses are well aware of the difficulties that many women have in getting access to care. Undeveloped countries have many issues regarding providing availability of screening tests or treatment for these women; however, even in our own country there are many women who go for 15–20 years without a Pap smear and then are found to have cervical cancer. Nurses can be instrumental in community education by instructing women in the need for Pap smears as well as helping women find access to care.

Many times the nurse is the one who explains to the patient what a Pap smear is, how is it performed, what the results mean, what a colposcopy is, and what to expect. A resource that can be useful in explaining to patients about abnormal Pap smears is *Abnormal Pap Smears: What Every Woman Needs to Know*.[25] There are also many other resources available from the American Cancer Society (ACS), the American College of Obstetricians and Gynecologists (ACOG), and the National Cancer Institute (NCI).

Nurse practitioners may be involved with screening, diagnosing, treating, and follow-up of abnormal Pap smears. For nurse practitioners in the medical field or family practice, it is important to ensure that women get regular Pap smears. Many women do not see a gynecologist regularly after childbearing age. It is the nurse or nurse practitioner in family practice that has the opportunity to ensure that women continue to have adequate follow-up. It is women who have not had regular Pap smears who are probably at the highest risk of developing cervical cancer.

Many nurses who work in physician's offices, clinics, or hospitals may be involved with caring for the women who are having treatment for SIL or cervical cancer. Education is very important for these women. The initial role of education is to allay fears and to help the woman understand what SIL is and what the procedure is that will be done. The woman is given postoperative or postprocedure instructions to minimize pain and risk of bleeding or infection.

Many women will require some type of pain medication to control their discomfort. The woman is instructed that she cannot put anything into the vagina or have intercourse for

4 weeks after a cone biopsy or LEEP to prevent infection. The woman generally will have a watery discharge after the procedure for a few weeks. Approximately 10–14 days after a cone biopsy or LEEP procedure, the woman is at risk for having heavy vaginal bleeding. Women are instructed to contact their care provider if they have any problems with bleeding. It is important that follow-up care is provided because many women will have a recurrence of SIL.

Nurses have multiple opportunities for involvement in ongoing clinical trials that look at vaccines to prevent or treat HPV and cervical cancer. They may collect data or recruit women or men to participate in the clinical trials. They may administer the vaccines and monitor the women afterward for side effects or response to the treatment.

Now that the first HPV vaccines are available, nurses will be instrumental in vaccination programs. Because the focus is for young women and teenagers, it will require education not only of the young woman but potentially also her parents.

Conclusion

Cervical cancer is a preventable disease. Regular screening can detect preinvasive disease, which can be treated before it progresses to invasive cancer. There are still women, however, who are not getting regular Pap smears or do not have access to care. In many areas, either access to care needs to be improved or women need to be instructed to obtain the preventative care that they require to remain healthy.

Even though we know a great deal more than we did 50 years ago about HPV and its effect on cervical tissue, there is still a great deal of work needed to understand the stimulants that initiate the progression to cancer and how we can halt that process.

We now have vaccines available to prevent HPV and its effects. Much education needs to be done to ensure that all young women and children are vaccinated. Clinical trials continue to look at the use of HPV vaccines to assist in the treatment of cervical cancer. In addition, clinical trials are being done to test the efficacy of vaccines in young men. Continued studies are needed to determine the length of immunity, which is provided with immunization. Globally, studies need to be done to test the prominent HPV strains in different regions so effective vaccines can be determined for those areas. This has the greatest potential to decrease the incidence of cervical cancer in indigent areas where Pap smears are not routinely performed due to lack of resources. Cervical cancer can be prevented.

Suggested Readings

Harper DM, Franco EL, Wheeler C, et al. Efficacy of bivalent L1 virus-like particle vaccine in prevention of infection with human papillomavirus types 16 and 18 in young women: a randomized controlled trial. *Lancet.* 2004;364:1757–1765.

Villa LL, Costa RLR, Petta CA, Andrade RP. Prophylactic quadrivalent human papillomavirus (types 6, 11, 16, and 18) L1 virus-like particle vaccine in young women: a randomized double-blind placebo controlled multicentre phase II efficacy trial. *Lancet Oncology.* 2005;6:271–278.

References

1. Creasman, WT. Preinvasive disease of cervix. In: DiSaia, PJ, Creasman, WT, eds. *Clinical Gynecologic Oncology.* Philadelphia, PA: Mosby Elsevier; 2007:1–36.

2. Campion, M. preinvasive disease. In: Berek, JS, Hacker, NF, eds, *Practical Gynecologic Oncology.* New York, NY: Lippincott Williams & Wilkens; 2005:265–336.

3. Centers for Disease Control and Prevention, Division of Sexually Transmitted Diseases Prevention. STD Facts—human papillomavirus (HPV). http://www.cdc.gov/std/HPV/STDFact-HPV.htm. Published 2008. Accessed July 7, 2008.

4. Centers for Disease Control and Prevention, Division of Sexually Transmitted Diseases Prevention. Sexually transmitted diseases treatment guidelines 2006. http://www.cdc.gov/std/treatment/2006/hpv.htm. Published 2006. Accessed July 7, 2008.

5. Williamson AL, Passmore JA, Rybicki EP. Strategies for the prevention of cervical cancer by human papillomavirus vaccination. *Best Pract Res Clin Obstet Gynaecol.* 2005;19(4):531–544.

6. Schmiedeskamp MR, Kockler DR. Human papillomavirus vaccines. *Ann Pharmocother.* 2006;40: 1344–1352.

7. Merck & Co. Gardasil (quadrivalent human papillomavirus [types 6, 11, 16, 18] recombinant vaccine). http://www.merck.com/product/usa/pi_circulars/g/gardasil/gardasil_pi.pdf. Published 2007. Accessed July 7, 2008.

8. Wright TC Jr. Pathogenesis and diagnosis of preinvasive lesions of the lower genital tract. In: Hoskins WJ, Perez CA, Young RC, Barakat RR, Markman M, Randall ME, eds. *Principles and Practice of Gynecologic Oncology.* New York, NY: Lippincott Williams & Wilkins; 2005:627–664.

9. Sharpless KE, Schnatz PF, Mandaulli S, Greene JF, Sorosky JI. Dysplasia associated with atypical glandular cells on cervical cytology. *Obstet Gynecol.* 2005; 105(3):494–500.

10. American Society of Cytopathology. Cervical Cytology Practice Guideline. http://www.cytopathology.org/website/article.asp?id=384 Published 2000. Accessed July 24, 2008.

11. American Society of Cytopathology. ASC Statement on New Technologies in Cervical Cytology Screening. http://www.cytopatholgy.org/website/article.asp?id=10 Published 2008. Accessed July 24, 2008.

12. NIH News Release. Bethesda 2001: a revised system for reporting pap test results aims to improve cervical cancer screening. http://bethesda2001.cancer.gov/terminology.pdf. Published April 23, 2002. Accessed July 7, 2008.

13. Twombly R. Guidelines recommend less frequent screening interval for cervical cancer. *J Natl Cancer Inst.* 2003;95(6):424–425.

14. American Cancer Society. American Cancer Society Guidelines for the Early Detection of Cancer. http://www.cancer.org/docroot/PED/content/PED_2_3X_ACS_Cancer_Detection_Guidelines_36.asp?sitearea=PED Published 2008. Accessed July 24, 2008.

15. Centers for Disease Control. Epidemiologic Notes and Reports Risk for Cervical Disease in HIV-Infected Women-New York City. Http://www.cdc.gov/mmwR/preview/00001844.htm Published 1990. Accessed July 25, 2008.

16. Denny L, Boa R, Williamson AJ, et al. Human Papillomavirus Infection and Cervical disease in Human Immunodeficiency Virus-1-Infected Women. *Obstet & Gynecol.* 2008;111(6):1380–1387.

17. Harris TG, Burk RD, Palefsky JM, et al. Human Papilloma test results associated with HIV serostatus, CD4 cell counts, and incidence of cervical squamous intraepithelial lesions. *JAMA.* 2005;293(12): 1471–1476.

18. Bollmann R, Mehes G, Torka R, Speich N, Schmitt C, Bollmann M. Determination of features indicating progression in atypical squamous cells with undetermined significance. *Cancer Cytopath.* 2003;99(2):113–117.

19. DeSimone CP, Tovar NM, Dietrich CS, et al. Rate of pathology from atypical glandular cell Pap tests classified by the Bethesda 2001 nomenclature. *Obstet Gynecol.* 2006;107(6):1285–1291.

20. Moscicki AB. Conservative management of adolescents with abnormal cytology and histology. *J Natl Compr Netw.* 2008;61(1):101–106.

21. CDC Media Relations. CDC's advisory committee recommends human papillomavirus virus vaccination. http://www.cdc.gov/od/oc/media/pressrel/r060629.htm. Published October 30, 2006. Accessed July 7, 2008.

22. Hunter MI, Monk BJ, Tewari KS. Cervical neoplasia in pregnancy. Part 1:screening and management of preinvasive disease. *Am Jrnl Obstet Gynecol.* 2008; 199(1):3–9.

23. Almog B, Gamzu R, Kupermine MJ, et al. Human papilloma virus testing in patient follow-up post cone biopsy due to high-grade cervical intraepithelial neoplasia. *Gyn Oncol.* 2003; 88:345–350.

24. Cox, JT. ASCCP practice guidelines: the follow-up system for abnormal cervical cytological findings. *J Lower Genital Tract Dis.* 1997;1(3):167–170.

25. Rushing L, Joste N. *Abnormal Pap Smears: What Every Woman Needs to Know.* NewYork, NY: Prometheus Books, 2008.

Chapter 7

Invasive Cervical Cancer

Connie L. Birk,
RN, BSN, OCN®

Introduction

The advent of regular Pap smear screening and recent advances in screening with liquid-based Pap cytology has resulted in a steady decline in the annual death rate from cervical cancer in the United States.[1] According to the American Cancer Society, approximately 11,070 women will be diagnosed with cervical cancer in the United States in 2008, with a predicted death rate of 3870 women.[1] Globally, cervical cancer affects over 500,000 women and is the second most common cause of cancer-related mortality in developing countries, with approximately 234,000 deaths annually.[2] Although cervical cancer is highly curable in early stages, this disease continues to be a worldwide problem due to inadequate or lack of regular screening and access to health care in many developing nations.

Epidemiology and Risk Factors

The majority of data in the epidemiology of cervical cancer relates to squamous cancers of the cervix, which account for the majority of all cervical cancer cases.[3] Several risk factors that predispose a woman to be at a higher risk of developing cervical cancer have been delineated. One of the most consistent and statistically significant risk factors is a woman's age at first intercourse. Several studies have shown that if a woman has sexual intercourse prior to the age of 17 years, the relative risk to develop an invasive cervical cancer can be significantly higher.[4,5] A similar risk is the time between menarche and first intercourse. If a woman has sexual intercourse less than 1 year postmenarche, her relative risk is 26 times greater to develop an invasive cancer.[6] In addition, women who have had multiple sexual partners or whose male partner has had multiple partners are at higher risk.[7]

Socioeconomic status can also contribute to the risk of developing cervical cancer. For example, women with a lower socioeconomic status, who are of Hispanic, Latin American, or African American descent, and particularly those who live in rural areas have a higher incidence of invasive cervical cancer.[8–10] Furthermore, uninsured women or those with limited access to health care are also at higher risk not just of developing invasive cervical cancer but also of having a statistically significant survival disadvantage.[9,11] As research has demonstrated, if a woman cannot or elects not to participate in regular cervical cancer screening, she is at increased risk of developing this disease. Cervical cancer prevention efforts must ensure that particularly low-income women have access to preventive services, including education, screening, and human *Papillomavirus* (HPV) vaccines, or existing disparities in cervical cancer may increase.[12]

HPV can also predispose a woman to develop invasive cervical cancer. More than 100 distinct types of HPV have been identified, but particularly HPV 16 and 18 have been found in actual cervical tumors. HPV 16, together with HPV 18, accounts for approximately 70% of all cervical cancers.[2] HPV 16 is more commonly found in the squamous cancers.[13,14] HPV 18 is the most common subtype in cervical adenocarcinoma, but additional subtypes, such as HPV 33, 45, and 56, have also been associated with an increased incidence of invasive cervical cancer.

The role of cigarette smoking and tobacco use as a cofactor in developing invasive cervical cancer has long been established. Numerous studies have demonstrated the ability to identify nicotine and the other specific carcinogens, such as cotinine and benzo[a]pyrene (BaP), in the actual cervical mucus and genital tract of women.[15,16] The process of cervical carcinogenesis is proposed to be a result of the exposure of cervical cells to high concentrations of cigarette smoke carcinogens, which will induce DNA-altering changes to the basement membrane of the cervix and will allow an invasive cervical cancer to develop. Coupled with high-risk HPV DNA such as HPV 16 and HPV 18, a woman can greatly increase

her risk of developing cervical cancer if she continues cigarette smoking.[17] Some studies also report that exposure to passive smoking may increase the risk of developing cervical neoplasia.[16,18] In addition, recent studies have indicated that smoking can predict a worse overall survival in locally advanced cervical cancer patients undergoing chemotherapy and radiation.[19]

The link between oral contraceptive use and the risk of invasive cervical cancer is not completely understood, but there appears to be an increased incidence of cervical cancer in women who use oral contraceptives longer than 10 years.[20]

Immunosuppression is also a known risk factor, particularly in the development of preinvasive and invasive disease of the cervix. The Centers for Disease Control and Prevention (CDC) has designated cervical cancer as an AIDS-related illness. Women who are infected with the human immunodeficiency virus (HIV) are at a much higher risk of developing higher grade squamous intraepithelial lesions (SIL) of the cervix and invasive cervical cancer compared to the normal population.[21] These lesions tend to be more aggressive and behave in unpredicted patterns. Women who are on immunosuppressive medications, such as transplant patients, are also at an increased risk.

Finally, the male partner may also play a role in the increased risk of cervical cancer in a female partner. Women whose husbands were previously married to a woman with cervical cancer or whose husband had penile cancer appear to have a higher incidence of invasive cervical cancer. In addition, one study has shown that husbands of women with invasive cervical cancer are more likely to have had multiple sexual partners and sexually transmitted diseases.[22]

Prevention and Early Detection

Similar to most cancers, the ability to have a large-scale, cost-effective, and specific screening tool is essential to early detection of invasive cervical cancer. Since the development of the Pap smear over 60 years ago, the cancer-related mortality of cervical cancer has steadily declined in the United States.[23] Newer liquid-based cytology has become more prevalent with its ability to conduct HPV subtyping and detect more cervical dysplasia or precancerous lesions of the cervix.[24] Cells from the cervix and endocervix are placed in a liquid medium and transported to the cytology lab. The lab then processes the liquid by using a one-layer technique on a slide, avoiding any air drying, which has long been criticized in distorting cervical cells with the traditional Pap smear. The FDA recently approved the digene High-Risk HPV hc2 DNA test manufactured by QIAGEN to assist in cervical cancer screening. This test allows cervical cytology to undergo DNA HPV subtyping to determine if a woman has high-risk HPV and allows for closer identification of those high-risk individuals for screening. There are other similar liquid-based technologies on the market, and although they are more expensive than the standard Pap smear, the liquid-based technology can provide HPV subtyping, which otherwise cannot be done on the standard Pap smear. It is important to note that cervical cancer screening and detection only is successful if women undergo the screening process and continue screening throughout their lives. The World Health Organization (WHO) has designated HPV as a "necessary cause of cervical cancer"[25] and those women who continue to have limited access to care and screening will unfortunately still be at risk for developing invasive cervical cancer.

In 2002, an initial clinical trial of a prophylactic vaccine against HPV 16 was reported with promising results.[26] This vaccine was established to affect the L1 HPV capsid protein, which is thought to allow HPV to actually enter the individual cells of the cervix. In a randomized double-blind study of 2392 women, significant reduction in the incidence of HPV-16 infection and preinvasive disease (cervical intraepithelial neoplasia) was found. The placebo group contained all nine cases of cervical intraepithelial neoplasia, while no cases of cervical intraepithelial neoplasia were found in the vaccine group. In addition, a multinational, multicenter study of a recombinant virus vaccine that expresses HPV 16, HPV 18, E6, and E7 genes with modifications was recently reported.[26] The E6 and E7 proteins are HPV proteins, which have oncogenic potential and can cause tumor progression.[27] This recombinant vaccine was given to 29 patients with stage Ib and IIa invasive cervical cancer. The first vaccine was given 2 weeks prior to the radical hysterectomy, followed by a second administration given 4 to 8 weeks after surgery. At least 60% of the patients tested exhibited evidence of vaccination by serological testing. Kaufman et al. also report that 39 patients with high-grade CIN 2 and 3 received two doses of the HPV 16 L1E7 viruslike particle vaccine. Thirty-nine percent of the patients who received the phase 1 vaccine showed improvement from a CIN 3 lesion to a lesion of CIN 1 or normal with minor adverse events related just to the administration of the vaccine.[27] Long-term and sustained efficacy of the several vaccines has been demonstrated 5 years post vaccination.[28–30]

In 2006, the US Food and Drug Administration (FDA) approved the first vaccine for prevention of cervical cancer implicated by HPV subtypes 16 and 18. This quadrivalent vaccine is also for the prevention of HPV subtypes 6 and 11, which are associated with the majority of genital warts.[31] Gardasil (Merck) is a vaccine comprised of viruslike particles (VLP) intended to be prophylactic in individuals who are not yet exposed to HPV. It is not indicated for those affected by other high-risk subtypes, such as HPV 33 and 45. Vaccination is recommended for girls and women between the ages of 9 and 26 years of age. Gardasil should be given intramuscularly at day 1, month 2, and month 6. Each dose is approximately $150 and may be covered by insurance. Screening for precancerous lesions and disease cannot be eliminated because the vaccine is not designed to protect against other HPV subtypes. Issues regarding cervical cancer screening in an era with HPV vaccination must be addressed, such as high-frequency screening and higher cost of cytology, which may not be needed in a vaccinated population.[32] Pharmacoeconomic analyses indicate that a combination of cytology and HPV testing every 3 years in women over 30 years old is comparable in sensitivity to annual liquid-based cytology and is more cost effective.[23] Recent studies have demonstrated continued prevention of persistent HPV infections for over 4.5 years after initial vaccination.[33] In follow-up to its 2004 trial, Harper et al. demonstrated vaccine efficacy of 100% against cervical intraepithelial neoplasia (CIN) lesions. In addition, cross protection was defined against HPV subtypes 31 and 45.

Mao et al. identified 100% vaccine efficacy in that there were no cases of HPV 16 infection in the vaccinated group 3.5 years after vaccination, while the placebo group had 111 cases of persistent HPV 16 infection. Current trials are again investigating other vaccine combinations to hopefully be effective against other subtypes of high-risk HPV.

Cervarix, a bivalent vaccine, is currently under development for launch in 2008–2009 in the United States. It has already been released in Australia and the Philippines in 2007. This vaccine, effective against HPV 16 and 18 subtypes, has also shown some cross effectiveness against HPV strains 31 and 45.[34,35] Research is continuing with developing targeted vaccines using DNA, viruslike particles (VLP), recombinant viral vectors or peptides, and oral vaccines to hopefully vaccinate women against HPV 16 and thus decrease the incidence of invasive cervical cancer. Studies will continue to delineate the role of vaccination against HPV subtypes and the modification of cervical cancer screening recommendations over time.

The American Cancer Society, with support from the Society of Gynecologic Oncologists (SGO), Gynecologic Cancer Foundation (GCF), and other groups, revised its guidelines for cervical cancer screening in 2002. With consideration of newer screening and diagnostic technologies, such as the liquid-based cytology and HPV subtyping, the guidelines changed in four major areas. The initiation of screening should begin approximately 3 years after a woman begins having vaginal intercourse, but no later than 21 years of age. Screening should be done annually with a standard Pap test or may be extended every 2 years using liquid-based cytology. Women who have had three consecutive normal Pap tests and are at least 30 years old can continue screening every 2 to 3 years but are recommended to see a healthcare provider yearly for regular health checkups and other disease prevention. Finally, women who are 70 years of age and older who have had three or more normal Pap tests and have had no abnormal results in the last 10 years may choose to stop cervical cancer screening.

Additional areas of prevention include smoking cessation programs due to tobacco being a cofactor in the development of pre-invasive and invasive disease of the cervix. The education of young women regarding the risks of vaginal intercourse prior to the age of 17 years, using barrier contraception to limit contact with the immature cells in the cervical transformation zone, and limiting sexual partners may also decrease the incidence. In addition, the Breast and Cervical Cancer Mortality Prevention Act of 1990 mandated a nationwide program to help in the establishment of efficient and effective screening through the National Breast and Cervical Cancer Early Detection Program (NBCCEDP) linked to the Centers for Disease Control and Prevention (CDC). Data continues to be analyzed in determining participation in cervical cancer screening and determining what factors are still limiting women to receive screening and early detection.

Carcinogenesis

Throughout the last decade, a significant amount of research has been devoted to documenting the role of the human *Papillomavirus* (HPV) in the initiation of carcinogenesis of invasive cervical cancer. The HPV DNA appears to be integrated into the host genome with a predilection of two oncogenic proteins E6 and E7. These proteins may affect the transformation of cells by interfering with the tumor suppressor genes p53 and Rb. The E6 protein of certain high-risk HPV types binds to p53, causing the protein to basically disintegrate, while E7 binds to the Rb protein, causing its inactivation. It is theorized that with the inactivation of p53 and Rb, cells can proliferate more quickly, potentially causing malignant or genetic alterations with each cell line.[27] Only a small percentage of women infected by HPV develop invasive cervical cancer, so HPV alone cannot cause the malignant changes.[36]

Carcinogenesis most likely arises in the transformation zone of the cervix, the area of the cervix that was originally covered by columnar epithelium, which is transformed into squamous epithelium via metaplasia. This carcinogenic process usually takes many years and is due to DNA changes to the immature metaplastic epithelium through carcinogens (e.g., nicotine). It is further theorized that viral persistence with oncogenic HPV subtypes, as well as persistently infected cervical epithelium, will cause a progression to precancerous and cancerous lesions in the cervix. These processes may induce a much quicker transformation of precancerous lesion to invasive cancers than previously reported.[3]

Cervical cancer usually will progress either by direct extension in any direction or by lymphatic invasion. The tumor can be exophytic, or growing out toward the vagina, causing infiltrating tumor in the upper vagina (**Figure 7-1**). Cervical tumors can also be endophytic and invade the uterus if the tumors are located higher up in the endocervical canal. Through lymphatic invasion, the cancer will spread initially to the cardinal ligaments from the drainage of the cervical tissue. Cervical cancer will continue its pattern of growth, affecting either the anterior or posterior parametrium before spreading into any nodal metastasis. Pelvic and parametrial nodes are first breached, followed by the common iliac, the aortic, and finally the supraclavicular nodes in advanced stages.[37] If the tumor continues to grow, the bladder may be infiltrated with tumor because the base of the bladder rests on the upper cervix. When a tumor invades or extends into the uterosacral ligaments, the tumor can spread to the rectum and sacral lymph nodes. In advanced stages, the hematogenous spread of a tumor via the venous plexus and paracervical veins can cause lung, liver, and sacral bone involvement. Tumors of the cervix can spread intraperitoneally if the tumor grows through the posterior cervix or through the uterus. This will result in presentation of abdominal ascites in advanced disease.

Figure 7-1 Invasive cervical cancer.

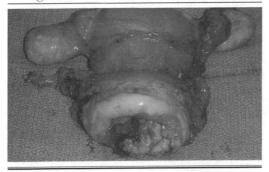

Histology and Pathology

The primary histology of all invasive cervical cancers is squamous carcinoma. These cancers generally arise in the squamocolumnar region of the cervix due to preexisting dysplastic cells or lesions. While 80% to 90% of cervical cancers are squamous in origin, the remainder arise

in the lining of the endocervical canal, causing invasive adenocarcinoma. Adenocarcinomas have been associated with more aggressive tumors in women under the age of 35 years, and some studies have found that survival is worse when corrected for age variations.[38] Additional cell types include poor prognostic tumors, such as the clear cell, adenosquamous, sarcoma, adenoid cystic, undifferentiated, and melanoma cancers.

Squamous carcinomas of the cervix can be further subdivided into large-cell nonkeratinizing, large-cell keratinizing, and small-cell tumors. These tumors can also be graded based on how closely the tumor resembles cervical cells under the microscope. Grade 1 tumors are classified as well differentiated, grade 2 tumors are moderately differentiated, and grade 3 tumors are poorly differentiated and associated with a worse prognosis. Historically, the large-cell nonkeratinizing squamous cancers have the most favorable prognosis and occur most frequently. The presence of keratin within the cells is thought to provide some protection. Several studies have shown a greatly reduced survival rate for small-cell tumors in comparison to both the large-cell keratinizing and nonkeratinizing tumors.[38]

Another critical issue is whether there is lymph vascular space invasion (LVSI) in the tumor. This feature appears to increase the incidence of lymph node metastasis in women if LVSI is present. Particularly in recent years, further studies have attempted to delineate between actual blood vessel involvement and tumors that just invade the lymphatic space. In addition, many studies have demonstrated both a higher risk of recurrence as well as decreased survival.[39,40] The determination of LVSI in pathology has always been subjective, and continued research in this area is needed to further clarify the predicted risk of lymph node involvement when LVSI is present.

The depth of stromal invasion in cervical tumors has long been a predictor of both lymph node metastasis and prognosis. Tumors that invade 5 millimeters or less tend to have a better prognosis than tumors that are more invasive. Both LVSI and lymph node involvement are related to depth of invasion of the primary tumor. LVSI and lymph node metastasis occur more frequently the greater the depth of the invasion by the cervical tumor. LVSI and depth of invasion have been researched extensively to help assist in predicting disease-free survival (DFS) and overall survival (OS) in cervical cancer patients.[41,42]

Tumor size and volume have been critical in determining risk for nodal metastasis, survival, and rates of recurrence, particularly in stage I tumors. Lesions that are less than 4 cm in size have historically been associated with longer disease-free survival than lesions greater than 4 cm in size. Not surprisingly, the larger the tumor, the greater the chance of LVSI and nodal metastasis within the pelvic lymph nodes. Additionally, the tumor volume measured in cubic millimeters also predicts an increased risk for lymph node metastasis and a decreased survival.[43] Sentinel lymph node (SLN) identification and lymphatic mapping have been used to help identify lymph node metastases in early cervical cancer.[44]

Research has shown that these multiple variables, such as tumor size, volume, LVSI, depth of invasion, lymph node involvement, and grade of tumor, can all impact survival.

Assessment

The majority of cervical cancer is detected in the early stages by Pap smear screening during routine examination. It has been estimated that only 20% of women with an invasive cancer are asymptomatic at time of diagnosis. Most women experience some type of irregular or abnormal bleeding prompting medical evaluation. This bleeding is usually reported by the patient and can include postcoital bleeding, intermenstrual bleeding, extremely heavy menstrual periods, or even postmenopausal bleeding. Unfortunately, practitioners can treat patients for menstrual disorders without even a pelvic exam or relying on a Pap smear for diagnosis, even if an abnormality can be seen on cervical exam.

A second common presenting symptom is some type of vaginal discharge. This discharge is not necessarily foul in odor, and it can vary in consistency from watery, purulent, or mucoid. Cervical adenocarcinomas tend to produce a mucinlike discharge, which is sometimes overlooked because many young women will complain of a discharge when there is a cervical or vaginal infection. Any woman with a persistent vaginal discharge, particularly after treatment with local antifungals, should be evaluated by a medical professional to preclude an occult cervical cancer and to assess any abnormal discharge.

Many women who are diagnosed with cervical carcinoma will have a normal physical examination. In fact, the cervix may look normal to physical inspection if the cancer is small or if the cancer arises from within the endocervical canal. If a woman has glandular atypia on a routine Pap screening, an endocervical curettage or scraping is warranted to assess the lining of the endocervical canal and to verify that an early adenocarcinoma has not manifested itself within the canal.

Late symptoms of cervical cancer are a result of advanced disease. Women can present with ascites due to intraperitoneal spread of tumor. Edema in the lower extremities can occur due to venous obstruction by tumor or lymphatic involvement in the pelvis preventing lymphatic return. Sciatic pain is common in late stages as involvement of the sacral nerve plexus or sciatic nerve roots by tumor affect the leg, back, or tailbone. Pelvic pain, urinary frequency, and rectal symptoms, such as frequency or urgency, can indicate involvement by tumor. Some women with advanced-stage disease present with ureteral obstruction or renal failure due to the obstruction of ureters by tumor. It is also not uncommon for women with advanced disease to have vaginal hemorrhaging due to development of blood vessels in the primary tumor, which can result in severe cases of anemia. A woman can also present with an enlarged supraclavicular node, usually on the left side in advanced disease. The thoracic duct enters the subclavian vein at that site, and malignant cells from the lymphatic system in the pelvis will migrate to that area. Practitioners must be aware of these symptoms to assess the patient and make steps toward the diagnosis and clinical staging of invasive cervical cancer.

Diagnosis and Staging

A speculum examination is necessary to physically inspect the cervix, particularly if a woman is having abnormal bleeding or persistent discharge. If the patient has an abnormal-appearing cervix, a cervical biopsy is obtained in addition to the standard Pap smear screening. The cervical biopsy should always be taken in the center of the lesion to avoid an inadequate specimen or a missed diagnosis. Equally important is the evaluation of the endocervical canal by endocervical curettage (ECC), even if the cervix appears

normal. If the biopsy reveals carcinoma in situ or cervical intraepithelial neoplasia 3 (CIN 3), further evaluation by a cervical cone biopsy may be required to verify there is not an early invasive cancer or to determine the depth of invasion of a cervical tumor prior to additional surgery if indicated.

As cervical cancer is staged clinically, it is critical that the practitioner perform a rectovaginal examination to assess the true extent of the cancer. It is not uncommon for cancers arising within the endocervix to progress and grow posteriorly, which can only be assessed by rectal exam. It is important to verify if the tumor is mobile or fixed to the pelvic side wall and to determine the actual size of the tumor by palpation or physical inspection. In addition to the physical exam, imaging studies may be necessary to make treatment decisions. Primarily, the chest X-ray and CT scan of the abdomen and pelvis are indicated to verify the presence of any metastatic disease, particularly in advanced stage diagnosis. Magnetic resonance imaging (MRI) can also be utilized, depending on the preference of gynecologic oncologist.[45]

Additionally, laboratory testing may be necessary in advanced disease because there is a higher likelihood of abnormal results. Treatment decisions may be based upon the presence of anemia, elevated serum creatinine, and blood urea nitrogen or other electrolyte abnormalities that are prevalent in renal obstruction or failure. Bone involvement can cause hypercalcemia, although this is rare.

The International Federation of Gynecology and Obstetrics (FIGO) modified its clinical staging in 1995 to further subdivide stage Ib cervical cancer into Ib1 for lesions that are equal to or less than 4 cm in size and Ib2 for cervical tumors greater than 4 cm in size. Because of the importance of tumor size in the prognosis of survival, the occurrence of lymph node metastasis, and recurrence rates, particularly in stage I disease, this delineation was accomplished. **Table 7-1** lists the FIGO stages of cervical cancer.

Again, the FIGO staging is a clinical staging with surgery being utilized to make any further treatment decisions. There have been advocates of surgical staging in conjunction with the clinical staging, for example, in the removal of bulky tumor in lymph nodes prior to initiation of radiation in a radiation field and sampling of both pelvic nodes and para-aortic nodes in poorly differentiated tumors.[46] Clinical staging will help to determine those patients who will require surgery or radiation, radiation followed by surgery, or radiation and/or chemotherapy. Surgery is almost always the treatment of choice in stage I tumors of the cervix, while a combination of radiation and chemotherapy can be utilized in stage III and IV tumors. It is noteworthy that women who present with stage IVb cervical cancer are candidates for local control of disease with radiation to decrease the risk of excessive bleeding and subsequent systemic chemotherapy.

Table 7-1 FIGO STAGING OF CERVICAL CANCER.

Stage 0	Carcinoma in situ; intraepithelial carcinoma
Stage I, Ia, Ia1, Ia2	Carcinoma strictly confined to the cervix. Ia lesions show invasive microscopic disease and invasion limited to measured stromal invasion with a maximum depth of 5 mm and no wider than 7.0 mm. Ia1 lesions with stromal invasion not greater than 3.0 mm deep and not greater than 7.0 mm wide. Ia2 lesions with stromal invasion 3.0-5.0 mm deep and not greater than 7.0 mm wide.
Stage Ib, Ib1 Ib2	Clinical lesions confined to the cervix or preclinical lesions greater than Stage Ia. Stage Ib1 demonstrates lesions not greater than 4 cm in size. Ib2 lesions are greater than 4 cm in size.
Stage II, IIa, IIb	Carcinoma extends beyond the cervix but has not extended onto the pelvic side wall or involves the upper two-thirds of the vagina. IIa lesions have no parametrial involvement, while IIb shows obvious parametrial involvement.
Stage III, IIIa, IIIb	Carcinoma has extended onto the pelvic wall; on rectal examination there is no cancer-free space between the tumor and the pelvic wall; the tumor involves the lower third of the vagina; all cases with a hydroureter or nonfunctioning kidney should be included. IIIa lesions have no extension onto the pelvic wall but involve the lower third of the vagina. IIIb lesions extend to the pelvic wall and/or hydronephrosis or nonfunctioning kidney.
Stage IV, IVa, IVb	Carcinoma has extended beyond the true pelvis or has clinically involved the mucosa of the bladder or rectum. IVa lesions have spread to adjacent organs. IVb lesions have spread to distant organs.

Source: Adapted from Morrow CP, Curtin JP. *Synopsis of Gynecologic Oncology*. 5th ed. New York, NY: Churchill Livingstone; 1998.

The treatment of microinvasive cervical carcinoma is one of the most discussed and debated fields of gynecologic oncology. This debate particularly is centered on fertility-sparing options for women diagnosed with microinvasive disease who wish to retain their fertility status. The tumors that fall within this category are no greater than 3 mm of stromal invasion, without lymphovascular involvement (LVSI), and clear cervical cone biopsy margins. Several studies have indicated that cervical cone biopsy alone may be an option to preserve fertility.[47] The patient must agree to undergo close surveillance cancer screening at regular intervals. This consists of Pap smear screening every 3 months for 2 years and every 6 months thereafter. In addition, an endocervical curettage (ECC) is usually done at least every 3 to 6 months to assess the lining of the endocervical canal. Despite adherence to screening, there is a potential for tumor recurrence with cervical cone biopsy alone. Consequently, some women elect to have one child, followed by a vaginal hysterectomy when childbearing is complete.

An additional topic of debate is the role of radical trachelectomy in women who wish to preserve fertility. This procedure involves a vaginal approach with a laparoscopic lymph node dissection. There has been recent discussion regarding the role of neoadjuvant chemotherapy followed by fertility-preserving surgery in selected patients.[48] Pelvic lymph node dissection must be done first to exclude the presence of lymph node involvement. If there is involvement, the procedure is stopped. If there is no lymph node involvement, the cervix is removed just below the isthmus so that sufficient cervical tissue is remaining to perform a cervical cerclage and prevent cervical incompetence during future pregnancy. Several studies have

demonstrated successful live births following radical trachelectomy, although there is a higher incidence of premature delivery. Shepherd et al. followed a series of 123 women, reporting 55 pregnancies in 26 women and 28 live births in 19 women, with a 5-year cumulative pregnancy rate of 52.8% among women who were trying to conceive.[49] All women underwent cesarean section, with some instances of local recurrence following radical trachelectomy.[50,51]

For women with stage Ia and Ia1 cervical carcinoma who have completed childbearing, a vaginal hysterectomy is an option, provided there is less than 3 mm of stromal invasion and no LVSI in the pathology according to the cervical cone biopsy. Reported incidences of tumor recurrence in this population of women have been negligible. One area of controversy within the Ia and Ia1 lesions is related to the microinvasive adenocarcinoma of the cervix. The FIGO staging of cervical cancer has been based on squamous carcinoma data, and historically the debate within this venue is that adenocarcinomas of the cervix have been treated more radically with surgery because these tumors are typically more aggressive. The risk of a cervical cone biopsy in this particular subset of patients is that the glandular cells can be multifocal, and thus tumor detection can be compromised with a cone biopsy.[37] Therefore, some gynecologic oncologists will perform a simple vaginal hysterectomy if the depth of invasion is less than 3 mm with no LVSI. For stages Ia1 or Ia2, the surgery may vary from a modified radical hysterectomy with pelvic lymphadenectomy (lymph node dissection) or radical hysterectomy with pelvic lymphadenectomy.

Radical hysterectomy with pelvic lymphadenectomy is one of the most common options of treatment for early stage cervical squamous carcinoma. A radical hysterectomy involves the removal of the cervix, uterus, and portions of the upper vagina, cardinal and ureterosacral ligaments, and bladder and rectal pillars. This surgery may be modified based on each patient's extent of disease. The removal of the ovaries is usually recommended in postmenopausal women. For young women who wish to preserve ovarian function, an ovarian transposition can be performed in which the ovaries are moved out of the central pelvis to avoid the field of radiation if needed for adjuvant therapy. If the pelvic lymph node dissection demonstrates a positive node, the para-aortic and common iliac lymph nodes are usually sampled as well at the time of surgery because of the increased risk for positive para-aortic nodes when at least one pelvic node is positive.

For patients with stage Ib1 and IIa tumors that are less than 4 centimeters, a radical hysterectomy with pelvic lymphadenectomy can be performed. If there is at least one positive node, parametrial invasion, or positive margins, a patient usually will receive adjuvant pelvic radiation and concurrent chemotherapy, which will be discussed further in this chapter. Some gynecologic oncologists might recommend radiation therapy initially as primary therapy for those women with cervical tumors greater than 4 cm. For those patients whose tumors are greater than 4 centimeters, radiation can be given at a reduced dose for 4 to 6 weeks, followed by a hysterectomy and pelvic and para-aortic lymphadenectomy.

Stages IIb through stage IV are primarily treated with a combination of radiation and chemotherapy because surgery would not be curative due to the size of the tumor or the presence of metastatic disease.

Radiation Therapy

Radiation therapy has long been a standard of care for patients with a higher risk of recurrence following radical hysterectomy and pelvic lymphadenectomy. Patients with stage Ib disease who have extensive LVSI, at least one positive pelvic node, and high-risk histology and/or poorly differentiated tumors are usually candidates for adjuvant pelvic radiation therapy. These women will usually receive whole pelvis radiation therapy in a dose varying from 4000 to 5000 cGy over 4 to 6 weeks. In addition, a woman may be a candidate for vaginal brachytherapy in which a concentrated radiation dose is given by a high-dose-rate (HDR) machine to further decrease the chance of a tumor recurrence at the vaginal apex. These high-dose-rate implants have revolutionized the field of radiation oncology as the computerized dosimetry becomes more sophisticated to allow a more precise delineation of the radiation dose within the treatment field. Vaginal brachytherapy is now given on an outpatient basis via a high-dose-rate implant of iridium-192 over 10 to 20 minutes instead of the older cesium or radium implant, which was left inside the vagina for 36 to 48 hours. These HDR implants can be implemented using two to four applications, depending on the preference of the radiation and gynecologic oncologist. Usually the first brachytherapy is done after approximately 2000 cGy have been administered during the external beam therapy. This allows for any existing tumor to respond to therapy and allow for a lower tumor burden at the time of implant. Furthermore, the smaller the tumor burden, the more effective the radiation therapy will be. For some patients who have large, bulky or "barrel-shaped" tumors (stage Ib2, IIa, IIb) in which tumors are larger than 4 cm, external whole-pelvic radiation is given for 4 to 6 weeks, usually in conjunction with weekly chemotherapy, followed by hysterectomy to eliminate residual cancer.[52,53]

One of the most important standards recently developed in the field of gynecologic and radiation oncology is the concept of chemoradiation. Chemoradiation is the concomitant use of radiation therapy and chemotherapy as a radiation sensitizer to maximize radiation potential. Several studies have shown a statistically improved progression-free and disease-free survival for stage Ib and IIa patients undergoing radiation- and cisplatin-based therapy.[54,55] In addition, the locally advanced tumors of the cervix can benefit with increased response rates when both radiation and chemotherapy are given. Patients who have more locally advanced cancers in which there is significant bleeding or vaginal hemorrhaging can receive higher than normal daily doses of external beam radiation for 2 to 3 days to control bleeding.

For those patients who have pelvic, common iliac, or aortic node involvement, radiation can be given in an extended field as a "boost" to decrease the likelihood of recurrence with subsequent improved survival.[56] An additional alternative is to administer extended field radiation to patients who are at a high risk of having metastasis to the aortic nodes, such as existing positive pelvic nodes or a large tumor with LVSI.[57] Prior to extended field radiation, some gynecologic oncology centers would consider the resection of any large bulky nodes, particularly in the aortic region, before initiating therapy. Again, the smaller the tumor, the more effective the radiation therapy will be.

Although the survival rates for early stage cancers of the cervix are the same whether primary surgery or radiation therapy is used, most gynecologic oncologists prefer surgery rather than primary radiation therapy, particularly in young women who want to preserve ovarian function. However, there is an associated risk of vaginal stenosis and/or dyspareunia with radiation therapy, which is usually not a complication from a radical hysterectomy. Patients should understand the risks and benefits of any treatment to make an informed decision in their individual treatment plan. Radiation therapy also provides a treatment option for those patients who have comorbid diseases that preclude surgical intervention. For example, patients with severe cardiac or pulmonary disease may have less risk with outpatient radiation therapy than with general anesthesia.

Chemotherapy

Chemotherapy in cervical cancer has been widely studied over the last several decades with a multitude of different regimens that include combination with radiation therapy and multiple drug regimens. When chemoradiation began over the last decade, combinations of therapy including hydroxyurea, fluorouracil, and cisplatin were used to assess if adding a radiation sensitizer to potentiate the effectiveness of the radiation would actually improve survival. Several published studies indicated a statistically significant advantage in survival and disease-free interval for those patients receiving radiation and chemotherapy in comparison to women receiving radiation alone.[54,55,58] This prompted the National Cancer Institute (NCI) to announce an advisory to a change in standard of care to concurrent chemoradiation (concurrent radiation and chemotherapy) due to this statistically significant survival advantage. The drug of choice among most gynecologic oncologists has been cisplatin at a dose of 40 mg/m2 weekly while receiving whole-pelvic external beam therapy. Recent studies also show significant efficacy in the use of carboplatin concurrently with radiation.[59] Although fluorouracil (5-FU) in conjunction with radiation therapy also demonstrated increased survival, the standard is cisplatin at the dose of 40 mg/m2.

Primary chemotherapy has traditionally been used for advanced stage IV and recurrent cervical cancer with a variety of different agents. Cisplatin has been one of the most active agents showing response rates of at least 20% in first-line therapy. Recent studies have looked at cisplatin in combination with gemcitabine, paclitaxel, ifosfamide, vincristine, mitomycin C, and topotecan.[60–63] In 2006, the FDA approved the use of topotecan in combination with cisplatin in the treatment of stage IVb, recurrent, or persistent cervical cancer not amenable to curative treatment with surgery and/or radiation therapy. This was a result of the GOG 179 study, which for the first time showed significantly improved overall survival and progression-free survival in combination therapy when compared to cisplatin alone.[64] Further studies are addressing the combinations of different doublets with topotecan, such as paclitaxel/topotecan and bevacizumab/topotecan to see if there is a survival advantage in these high-risk patients.[65]

One of the treatment difficulties in recurrent or advanced cervical cancer is that patients who receive adjuvant radiation therapy and who recur within the radiation field do not usually benefit from the systemic chemotherapy because of the compromised blood supply. Consequently, this may inhibit effective and active distribution of most chemotherapy drugs within the irradiated field.

Neoadjuvant chemotherapy has also been studied to decrease the size of primary tumor prior to surgery or radiation therapy. Several chemotherapy agents have been utilized, including cisplatin, paclitaxel, and gemcitabine.[66] Choi et al. report response rates of 83% in mitomycin C, vincristine, and cisplatin (MVC) in patients with stages Ib2 and IIb cancers.[60] The role of neoadjuvant chemotherapy has not been clearly defined, and further studies are being evaluated to demonstrate not just efficacy but a distinct survival advantage if neoadjuvant chemotherapy is utilized. Betash et al. report no improvement in long-term overall survival of bulky early-stage cervical cancer when compared to primary radical surgery.[67]

Adjuvant chemotherapy following chemoradiation has also been recently studied to see if survival is improved by adding adjuvant chemotherapy with a variety of different agents including cisplatin, paclitaxel, carboplatin, and topotecan.

Recurrent Disease

Unfortunately, cervical cancer can recur or persist in spite of primary therapy irrespective of surgery, radiation, and chemotherapy. Recurrent cervical cancer will most likely occur within 2 years following the completion of primary therapy. If a woman is experiencing weight loss, pelvic, sacral or buttock pain, persistent cough, leg edema, vaginal bleeding, or sometimes even malaise, practitioners should attempt to discern whether there is a recurrence of cancer versus symptoms related to previous radiation, chemotherapy, or surgery. Generally, cervical cancer recurs in a local fashion, particularly at the vaginal apex or cuff. For those women who did not receive radiation therapy for their primary treatment, radiotherapy may be an effective and potentially curative option for disease occurring at the vaginal apex or cuff. Women can undergo vaginal brachytherapy with or without additional pelvic external beam therapy for palliation with a goal of prolonged remission but not cure. Local palliative radiation can also be given to the mediastinal area for a patient with increased dyspnea or coughing due to mediastinal node involvement or lung metastases.

When cervical cancer recurs, overall survival has been poor, with 1 year survival rates less than 20%. In addition to local recurrences, cervical cancer can recur in distant sites such as the lung, liver, or supraclavicular nodes. These patients must undergo systemic therapy to improve tumor response.

Combination chemotherapy with a platinum-based regimen is usually the choice in recurrent cervical cancer, particularly if the patient has received no prior chemotherapy or radiation therapy. Several studies have looked at different combinations with varying response rates, but the reality is that regardless of the combination utilized, overall survival has not been improved. Response rates for single and combination chemotherapy regimens have varied from 10% to 90% depending on the regimen, but the responses are short-lived with progression of disease usually occurring within 8 months.[68]

Total pelvic exenteration is a surgical option that is sometimes utilized with patients who have recurrent cervical cancer that occurs within the central pelvis without evidence of any distant disease. The central pelvis is usually defined as a recurrence within the cervix, vagina, bladder, rectum, or parametrium. A total pelvic exenteration involves a radical hysterectomy, pelvic lymphadenectomy or node dissection, and en bloc resection of the bladder and rectosigmoid colon. This procedure can vary with the degree of bladder and/or sigmoid surgery. An anterior pelvic exenteration involves the removal of the bladder and central pelvic tissues, but the rectosigmoid colon remains intact. A posterior pelvic exenteration involves the removal of a portion of the rectosigmoid colon and central pelvic tissues, but the bladder remains intact. Some patients can have an ileal conduit formed following the removal of the bladder, while some patients may be candidates for continent conduits such as the Kock or Indiana pouch. When patients undergo a rectosigmoid resection, it may be possible for the gynecologic oncologist to perform a low rectal reanastomosis to preserve rectal function without the need for an ostomy. In addition, some women can undergo vaginal reconstruction in which a neovagina is formed either from split thickness skin grafts from the buttock or leg. Sometimes colon or omentum can be utilized as well for the neovagina, but the neovagina can have more vaginal mucus from the colonic mucosa with this procedure.[69] It is imperative that candidates for these procedures be screened preoperatively to determine that there is no disease outside the central pelvic recurrence. Patients usually undergo a CT scan of chest, abdomen, and pelvis to assess lymph node status and distant organs such as the liver and chest.

At the time of laparotomy for the pelvic exenteration, a selective lymphadenectomy from the pelvis and para-aortic nodes, as well as random pelvic biopsies, are done to assure that there is no microscopic disease on frozen section before proceeding with any further surgery. If evidence of disease is found, the procedure is usually halted because the disease is no longer considered to be curable. It is noteworthy that the pelvic exenteration can cure up to 50% of patients.[69] However, patients should be counseled extensively prior to the pelvic exenteration due to the radical nature of the procedure. Many women will elect to have an exenterative procedure if it is their only chance for a cure. Because of the profound changes that can occur physically and psychologically, women may not fully realize the impact until postsurgery, even with the best of presurgical counseling. Complications such as fistulas, vaginal stenosis, fatigue, infections, and wound alterations are not uncommon and can strain even the best of coping mechanisms. Nurses and other members of the healthcare team must be diligent to address the physical, psychological, spiritual, and sociologic impact of this radical procedure with their patients.[70]

Symptom Management and Nursing Implications

Invasive cervical cancer and its treatment encompass a variety of nursing care issues unique to the gynecologic oncology patient. One area of nursing intervention relates to the bladder dysfunction that can be impacted by surgery and radiation. Following radical hysterectomy, nearly all women have some form of bladder dysfunction. This is attributed to the impact of surgery on the autonomic nerves serving the bladder sometimes due to the dissection of the bladder and/or ureters in removing the cervical cancer.[71] This dysfunction can vary in length of time and degree, but most patients require some form of bladder rest to prevent the bladder from becoming overdistended. A suprapubic catheter is sometimes placed at

the time of surgery, which provides drainage of the bladder postoperatively to prevent distention and then allows for women to undergo bladder training at a time deemed necessary by the gynecologic oncologist. The suprapubic catheter can be clamped for 3 to 4 hours to facilitate bladder function and allow for normal voiding. Women can usually void with some normalcy within a week or two following bladder training and/or bladder rest with a Foley catheter. Occasionally, bladder function does not return entirely prior to the initiation of adjuvant therapy, such as radiation therapy. In this population of women, patients can be taught self-catheterization techniques with catheters such as the pediatric Mentor catheter. This will allow a suprapubic catheter to be removed without impacting wound healing prior to the initiation of radiation therapy. In addition, sometimes ureteral stents are placed at the time of surgery to either identify the ureters at time of surgery or to prevent any potential ureteral obstruction. Most women will experience some hematuria following the stent procedure. The ureteral stents are removed usually 4 to 6 weeks postoperatively, depending on the discretion of the gynecologic oncologist. If a patient undergoes radiation therapy, sometimes the stents will be left in place until completion of radiation therapy. Nurses must educate patients regarding the potential for bladder dysfunction and its eventual return of function.

Bleeding is another expected side effect from treatment or at the presentation of cervical cancer. Following surgery, most women will have some vaginal bleeding or spotting for at least 2 to 4 weeks postoperatively. This usually requires a pad for comfort. If there is bright red bleeding or bleeding heavier than one pad an hour, patients must be instructed to call the gynecologic oncologist for follow-up. If a newly diagnosed cervical cancer also experiences extensive bleeding, it is not uncommon for the gynecologic oncologist to insert vaginal packing inside the vagina up against the cervix to stop bleeding. This is usually removed 12 to 24 hours later. Sometimes the bleeding can be severe enough to require blood transfusions, and nurses must be able to quantify and assess the amount of bleeding by pad counts and the monitoring of serial blood counts if necessary.

One of the most precarious issues following radical hysterectomy is the potential for deep vein thrombosis and/or pulmonary embolism. Gynecologic cancer patients are at risk for developing deep vein thrombosis.[72] Most gynecologic oncologists use either pneumatic calf compressors and/or low molecular weight heparin to help reduce this risk. If a postoperative radical hysterectomy patient has a sudden onset of chest pain, shortness of breath, or sudden decrease in oxygen saturation, the nurse should consider the possibility of a pulmonary embolism in this patient and get prompt medical attention.

Pain is an additional nursing issue when dealing particularly with advanced cervical cancer. If a cervical cancer grows posteriorly, the sacrum can become involved with tumor, and the sacral nerve plexus can be affected. Sciatic nerve pain related to tumor involvement can be very difficult to manage. It is not uncommon for these women to be on a patient-controlled analgesia system, as well as epidural pain medicine either through steroid blocks or via intrathecal pumps with continuous narcotic infusion. It is critical for nurses to assess the level of pain that each patient experiences and to understand that multiple modalities may be needed to improve quality of life and fear of pain, particularly in end of life care. Hospice is vital to the care of end-stage cervical cancer patients in providing the patient and family physical, emotional, and spiritual support.

The impact of surgery and radiation can induce acute and long-term effects, which are not always appreciated until after the treatment is completed. Women who are undergoing chemoradiation can present with urinary frequency and vaginal or rectal mucositis. Sometimes radiation and chemotherapy will be held for 1 to 3 days to help mitigate this irritation. Nursing remedies have included vaginal water-based lubrication to decrease burning upon urination or vaginal intercourse.

Diarrhea is also a known side effect with radiation as well as chemotherapy. Patients should be instructed on the use of a low residue diet and to avoid spicy foods and fruits (other than bananas and apples), which can increase the frequency of diarrhea. Patients should be encouraged to drink at least 1 liter of fluid daily while undergoing therapy. Sports drinks, such as Gatorade, can provide additional electrolytes for these patients and sometimes provide a pleasant taste instead of water.

Lymphedema can occur, particularly in patients who undergo radical hysterectomy, lymphadenectomy, and adjuvant radiation therapy. The lymphedema can occur in the leg or sometimes in the lower pelvis, such as the pubic area. Currently, there are lymphedema specialists, usually affiliated with freestanding cancer centers, that can assist the patient with manual stimulation of the collateral lymphatics in the affected area either through wrapping of the affected extremity or via pumps such as the Jobst stocking.

Bowel obstructions following surgery and radiation therapy are usually caused by the agglutination of the bowel via inflammation or intraperitoneal adhesions, particularly in patients who have had prior radiation therapy.[73] These obstructions will usually subside with bowel rest, such as with a nasogastric tube. Occasionally, surgery must be performed to relieve the obstruction, hopefully without the need of any ostomy.

Due to prior radiation and surgery, some women may develop fistulas between the bladder, rectum, and vagina. A vesicovaginal fistula will form either when a leak develops from the bladder through the top of the vagina, or when there has been a failed ureteral reimplantation. Sometimes these vesicovaginal fistulas will heal if a Foley catheter is inserted to divert the urine flow away from the fistula for a period of several weeks. In addition, percutaneous nephrostomy tubes can be inserted by interventional radiology to also provide rest for the fistula to heal. Some patients, however, will require surgical intervention for persistent fistulas, such as an ileal conduit or continent conduit such as an Indiana pouch. These surgeries usually cannot be reversed due to the compromised blood supply to the area from previous radiation. Nurses should be able to address the psychological issues that occur when fistulas develop. Enterstomal therapy nurses can be employed to help identify skin care products and odor control products for these patients who are awaiting a healing fistula. The true nursing challenge involves those patients with advanced disease who present with fistulas and may not be surgical candidates and must live with the management of multiple fistulas that may occur over time. For patients who develop rectovaginal fistulas in which stool can enter the vagina from the rectum located just underneath the vagina, maintaining hygiene can be a challenge.

Sometimes a rectovaginal fistula is present at the time of diagnosis of a bulky cervical cancer, and the gynecologic oncologist will perform a colostomy prior to the initiation of therapy. For patients with advanced disease, an ostomy may be indicated to improve quality of life, as most patients do not like the hygienic complications of discharge and odor that fistulas cause. It is vital that nurses caring for these patients with fistulas be able to provide care in a nurturing manner without facial grimacing because this sometimes conveys to the patient the known fact of the unpleasantness of the fistula.

Sexual sequelae can also result from surgery, radiation, and chemotherapy. Sometimes the vagina can be foreshortened after surgery if a portion of the vaginal apex is removed in the case of a bulky cancer infiltrating the vagina. Women will state that it is difficult to have vaginal intercourse following surgery and radiation due to changes in the elasticity of the vagina, diminished vaginal lubrication, or vaginal stenosis.[74,75,76] Women should be encouraged to utilize water-based lubricants to decrease friction during vaginal intercourse. Sometimes vaginal dilators are utilized to assist in decreasing the risk of vaginal stenosis.[77] It is also noteworthy that vaginal dilators have not yet been proven to decrease vaginal stenosis but are utilized with the intention of preventing vaginal agglutination over time. The Gynecologic Oncology Group is currently researching the use of vaginal dilators with its radiation protocols to address vaginal stenosis in these patients.

Psychologically, the impact of cancer can be devastating, particularly to young women undergoing surgery, radiation therapy, or chemotherapy. Issues such as medical disability, child care, loss of income, loss of health, and potentially the loss of fertility can be overwhelming for patients. Nurses must be able to address these issues with appropriate patient referrals to agencies to assist the patient, such as the American Cancer Society, which can provide transportation to and from radiation therapy appointments. Support groups for women undergoing cervical cancer treatment can sometimes be found at the local cancer center or community hospital. There are also support groups for children whose mothers have cancer. These groups facilitate the interaction with children and can open a dialogue between patients and their children to assist in coping with the disease of cervical cancer and its treatment.

Conclusion

Invasive cervical cancer can be highly curable when detected in early stages. With improved technology and proper screening, cervical cancer is detectable at early stages, sometimes even before invasion occurs. Treatment of invasive cervical cancer may depend on the size of the tumor, stage, grade, presence of lymphovascular invasion, node status, and other factors such as comorbid diseases. The treatment may include a combination of surgery, radiation, or chemotherapy, depending on each individual patient and the gynecologic oncologist's preference. It is important that further research is directed at the prevention of invasive cervical cancer by affecting disease progression in the preinvasive lesions of the cervix. The role of a prophylactic vaccine against high risk strains of human *Papillomaviruses*, such as HPV 16 and 18, has not been clearly defined, but the prophylactic vaccine will hopefully provide a step to decreasing the incidence, morbidity, and mortality associated with cervical cancer worldwide.

Suggested Readings

Burnett AF, Roman LD, O'Meara AT, Morrow CP. Radical vaginal trachelectomy and pelvic lymphadenectomy for preservation of fertility in early cervical carcinoma. Gynecol Oncol. 2003;88(3):419–423.

Fischer M. Gynecologic cancers. Cancer of the cervix. Semin Oncol Nurs. 2002;18(3):193–199.

Koutsky LA, Ault KA, Wheeler CM, et al. A controlled trial of a human papilloma virus type 16 vaccine. N Engl J Med. 2002:34(21):1645–1651.

Likes WM, Itano J. CJON writing mentorship program paper human papillomavirus and cervical cancer: not just a sexually transmitted disease. CJON. 2003;7(3):271–276.

Peters WA III, Liu PY, Barrett RJ II, et al. Concurrent chemotherapy and pelvic radiation therapy compared with pelvic radiation therapy alone as adjuvant therapy after radical surgery in high-risk early-stage cancer of the cervix. J Clin Oncol. 2000;18(8):1606–1613.

Shepherd JH, Mould T, Oram DH. Radical trachelectomy in early stage carcinoma of the cervix: outcome as judged by recurrence and fertility rates. BJOG. 2001;108(8): 882–885.

Spinelli A. Preinvasive disease of the cervix in HIV-infected women. J Gynecol Oncol Nurs. 1999;9(2):7–15.

Stier E. Cervical neoplasia and the HIV-infected patient. Hematol Oncol Clin North Am. 2003;17(3): 873–887.

Thomas GM. Concurrent chemotherapy and radiation for locally advanced cervical cancer: the new standard of care. Semin Radiat Oncol. 2000;10:44–50.

References

1. *ACS Cancer Facts &Figures—2008*. Atlanta, GA: American Cancer Society.

2. Monk BJ, Tewari KS, Koh WJ. Multimodality therapy for locally advanced cervical carcinoma: state of the art and future directions. *J Clin Oncol.* 2007;10;25(20):2952–2965.

3. Schiffman M, Castle PE, Jeronimo J, Rodriguez AC, Wacholder S. Human papillomavirus and cervical cancer. *Lancet.* 2007;370(9590):890–907.

4. Adewuyi SA, Shittu SO, Rafindadi AH. Sociodemographic and clinicopathologic characterization of cervical cancers in northern Nigeria. *Eur J Gynaecol Oncol.* 2008;29(1):61–64.

5. Deacon JM, Evans CD, Yule R, et al. Sexual behaviour and smoking as determinants of cervical HPV infection and of CIN3 among those infected: a case-control study nested within the Manchester cohort. *Br J Cancer.* 2000;83(11):1565–1572.

6. Peters RK, Thomas D, Hagan DC, et al. Risk factors for invasive cervical cancer among Latinas and non-Latinas in Los Angeles County. *J Ntl Cancer Inst.* 1986;77:1063.

7. Bornstein J, Rahat MA, Abramovici H. Etiology of cervical cancer: current concepts. *Obstet Gynecol Surv.* 1995;50:146.

8. McDougall JA, Madeleine NM, Daling JR, Li CI. Racial and ethnic disparities in cervical cancer incidence rates in the United States, 1992–2003. *Cancer Causes Control.* 2007;18(10):1175–1186.

9. Movva S, Noone AM, Banerjee M, et al. Racial differences in cervical cancer survival in the Detroit metropolitan area. *Cancer.* 2008;112(6):1264–1271.

10. Patel DA, Barnholtz-Sloan JS, Patel MK, Malone JM Jr, Chuba PJ, Schwartz K. A population-based study of racial and ethnic differences in survival among women with invasive cervical cancer: analysis of surveillance, epidemiology, and end results data. *Gynecol Oncol.* 2005;97(2):550–558.

11. Saraiya M, Ahmed F, Krishnan S, Richards TB, Unger ER, Lawson HW. Cervical cancer incidence in a prevaccine era in the United States, 1998–2002. *Obstet Gynecol.* 2007;109(2 Pt 1):360–370.

12. Kahn JA, Lan D, Kahn RS. Sociodemographic factors associated with high-risk human papillomavirus infection. *Obstet Gynecol.* 2007;110(1):87–95.

13. Apgar BS, Spitzer M, Brotozoman GL, Ignatavicius DD. *Colposcopy: Principles and Practice: An Integrated Textbook and Atlas.* Philadelphia, PA: Saunders; 2002.

14. Magnusson PK, Lichtenstein P, Gyllensten UB. Heritability of cervical tumors. *Int J Cancer.* 2000;88:698–701.

15. Alam S, Conway MJ, Chen HS, Meyers C. The cigarette smoke carcinogen benzo[a]pyrene enhances human papillomavirus synthesis. *J Virol.* 2008;82(2):1053–1058.

16. Trimble CL, Genkinger JM, Burke AE, et al. Active and passive cigarette smoking and the risk of cervical neoplasia. *Obstet Gynecol.* 2005;105(1):174–181.

17. Lacey JV, Frisch M, Brinton LA, et al. Associations between smoking and adenocarcinomas and squamous carcinomas of the uterine cervix (United States). *Cancer Causes Control.* 2001;12:153–161.

18. Tay SK, Tay KJ. Passive cigarette smoking is a risk factor in cervical neoplasia. *Gynecol Oncol.* 2004;93(1):116–120.

19. Waggoner SE, Darcy KM, Fuhrman B, et al. Gynecologic Oncology Group: association between cigarette smoking and prognosis in locally advanced cervical carcinoma treated with chemoradiation: a Gynecologic Oncology Group study. *Gynecol Oncol.* 2006;103(3):853–858.

20. McLachlin, CM. Human papillomavirus in cervical neoplasia. *Clin Laborat Med.* 2000;20:257–270.

21. Engels EA, Biggar RJ, Hall HI, et al. Cancer risk in people infected with human immunodeficiency virus in the United States. *Int J Cancer.* 2008;123(1):187–194.

22. Zunzunegui MW, King MC, Coria CF, Charlet J. Male influences on cervical cancer risk. *Am J Epidemiol.* 1986;123:302.

23. Spitzer M. Screening and management of women and girls with human papillomavirus infection. *Gynecol Oncol.* 2007;107(2 suppl 1):S14–S18.

24. Einstein MH, Goldberg GL. Human papillomavirus and cervical neoplasia. *Cancer Invest.* 2002;20:1080–1085.

25. Hakim AA, Lin PS, Wilczynski S, Nguyen K, Lynes B, Wakabayashi MT. Indications and efficacy of the human papillomavirus vaccine. *Curr Treat Options Oncol.* 2007;8(6):393–401.

26. Koutsky LA, Ault KA, Wheeler CM, et al. A controlled trial of a human papilloma virus type 16 vaccine. *N Engl J Med.* 2002;34(21):1645–1651.

27. Kaufmann AM, Nieland JD, Jochmus I, et al. Vaccination trial with HPV16 L1E7 chimeric virus-like particles in women suffering from high grade cervical intraepithelial neoplasia (CIN 2/3). *Int J Cancer.* 2007;121(12):2794–2800.

28. Paavonen J, Jenkins D, Bosch FX, et al. Efficacy of a prophylactic adjuvanted bivalent L1 virus-like particle vaccine against infection with human papillomavirus types 16 and 18 in young women: an interim analysis of a phase III double-blind, randomized controlled trial. *Lancet.* 2007;369(9580):2161–2170.

29. Joura EA, Leodolter S, Hernandez-Avila M, et al. Efficacy of a quadrivalent prophylactic human papillomavirus (types 6,11,16, and 18) L1 virus-like particle vaccine against high-grade vulvar and vaginal lesions: a combined analysis of three randomized clinical trials. *Lancet.* 2007;369(9574):1693–1702.

30. Villa LL, Costa RL, Petta CA, et al. High sustained efficacy of a prophylactic quadrivalent human papillomavirus types 6/11/16/18 L1 virus-like particle vaccine through 5 years of follow-up. *Br J Cancer*. 2006;95(11):1459–1466.

31. Merck & Co., Inc. Gardasil. http://www.gardasil.com. Accessed September 1, 2006.

32. Franco EL, Cuzick J, Hildesheim A, de Sanjose S. Issues in planning cervical cancer screening in the era of HPV vaccination. *Vaccine*. 2006;24(suppl 3): S171–S177.

33. Harper DM, Franco EL, Wheeler CM, et al. Sustained efficacy up to 4.5 years of a bivalent L1 virus-like particle vaccine against human papillomavirus types 16 and 18: follow-up from a randomized control trial. *Lancet*. 2006;367(9518):1247–1255.

34. GlaxoSmithKline plc. Cervarix http://www.gsk.com Accessed September 1, 2006.

35. Widdice LE, Kahn JA. Using the new HPV vaccines in clinical practice. *Cleve Clin J Med*. 2006;73(10):929–935.

36. Schiffman M, Castle PE. Human papillomavirus: epidemiology and public health. *Arch Pathol Lab Med*. 2003;127(8):930–934.

37. Morrow CP, Curtin JP. *Synopsis of Gynecologic Oncology*. 5th ed. New York, NY: Churchill Livingstone; 1998.

38. Kodama J, Seki N, Nakamura K, Hongo A, Hiramatsu Y. Prognostic factors in pathologic parametrium-positive patients with stage IB-IIB cervical cancer treated by radical surgery and adjuvant therapy. *Gynecol Oncol*. 2007;105(3):757–761.

39. Kamelle SA, Rutledge TL, Tillmanns TD, et al. Surgical-pathological predictors of disease-free survival and risk groupings for IB2 cervical cancer: do the traditional models still apply? *Gynecol Oncol*. 2004;94(2):249–255.

40. Ho CM, Chien TY, Huang SH, Wu CJ, Shih BY, Chang SC. Multivariate analysis of the prognostic factors and outcomes in early cervical cancer patients undergoing radical hysterectomy. *Gynecol Oncol*. 2004;93(2):458–464.

41. Sakuragi N. Up-to-date management of lymph node metastasis and the role of tailored lymphadenectomy in cervical cancer. *Int J Clin Oncol*. 2007;12(3):165–175.

42. Monk BJ, Tian C, Rose PG, Lanciano R. Which clinical/ pathologic factors matter in the era of chemoradiation as treatment for locally advanced cervical carcinoma? Analysis of two Gynecologic Oncology Group (GOG) trials. *Gynecol Oncol*. 2007;105(2):427–433.

43. Ayhan A, Al RA, Baykal C, Demirtas E, Ayhan A, Yuce K. Prognostic factors in FIGO stage IB cervical cancer without lymph node metastasis and the role of adjuvant radiotherapy after radical hysterectomy. *Int J Gynecol Cancer*. 2004;14(2):286–292.

44. Rob L, Strnad P, Robova H, et al. Study of lymphatic mapping and sentinel node identification in early stage cervical cancer. *Gynecol Oncol*. 2005;98(2):281–288.

45. Menell JH, Chi DS, Hann LE, Hricak H. The use of MRI in the diagnosis and management of a bulky cervical carcinoma. *Gynecol Oncol*. 2003;89(3):517–521.

46. Gold MA, Tian C, Whitney CW, Rose PG, Lanciano R. Surgical versus radiographic determination of paraaortic lymph node metastases before chemoradiation for locally advanced cervical carcinoma: a Gynecologic Oncology Group Study. *Cancer*. 2008;112(9): 1954–1963.

47. Landoni F, Parma G, Peiretti M, et al. Chemoconization in early cervical cancer. *Gynecol Oncol*. 2007;107(1 suppl 1):S125–S126.

48. Plante M, Roy M. Fertility-preserving options for cervical cancer. *Oncology*. 2006;20(5):479–488, 491–493.

49. Shepherd JH, Spencer C, Herod J, Ind TE. Radical vaginal trachelectomy as a fertility-sparing procedure in women with early stage cervical cancer-cumulative pregnancy rate in a series of 123 women. *BJOG*. 2006;113(6):719–724.

50. Shepherd JH, Mould T, Oram DH. Radical trachelectomy in early stage carcinoma of the cervix: outcome as judged by recurrence and fertility rates. *BJOG*. 2001;108(8):882–885.

51. Burnett AF, Roman LD, O'Meara AT, Morrow CP. Radical vaginal trachelectomy and pelvic lymphadenectomy for preservation of fertility in early cervical carcinoma. *Gynecol Oncol*. 2003;88(3):419–423.

52. Stehman FB, Ali S, Keys HM, et al. Radiation therapy with or without weekly cisplatin for bulky stage 1B cervical carcinoma: follow-up of a Gynecologic Oncology Group trial. *Am J Obstet Gynecol*. 2007;197(5):443–444.

53. Darus CJ, Callahan MB, Nguyen QN, et al. Chemoradiation with and without adjuvant extrafascial hysterectomy for 1B2 cervical carcinoma. *Int J Gynecol Cancer*. 2007; Oct 19.

54. Peters WA III, Liu Py, Barrett RJ II, et al. Concurrent chemotherapy and pelvic radiation therapy compared with pelvic radiation therapy alone as adjuvant therapy after radical surgery in high-risk early-stage cancer of the cervix. *J Clin Oncol*. 2000;18(8):1606–1613.

55. Keys HM, Bundy BN, Stehman FB, et al. Cisplatin, radiation, and adjuvant hysterectomy compared with radiation and adjuvant hysterectomy for bulky stage IB cervical carcinoma. *N Engl J Med.* 1999;340(15):1154–1161.

56. Denschlag D, Gabriel B, Mueller-Lantzsch C, et al. Evaluation of patients after extraperitoneal lymph node dissection for cervical cancer. *Gynecol Oncol.* 2005;96(3):658–664.

57. Rotman M, Choi K, Guse C, et al. Prophylactic irradiation of the para-aortic lymph node chain in stage IIB and bulky stage IB carcinoma of the cervix: initial treatment results of RTOG 7920. *Int J Radiat Oncol Biol Phys.* 1990;19:513.

58. Rose RG, Bundy BN, Watkins EB, et al. Concurrent cisplatin-based radiotherapy and chemotherapy for locally advanced cervical cancer. *N Engl J Med.* 1998;340:1144–1153.

59. Higgins RV, Nauman WR, Hall JB, Haake M. Concurrent carboplatin with pelvic radiation therapy in the primary treatment of cervix cancer. *Gynecol Oncol.* 2003;89(3):499–503.

60. Hirte HW, Strychowsky JE, Oliver T, Fung-Kee-Fung M, Elit L, Oza AM. Chemotherapy for recurrent, metastatic, or persistent cervical cancer: a systematic review. *Int J Gynecol Cancer.* 2007;17(6):1194–1204.

61. Moore KN, Herzog TJ, Lewin S, et al. A comparison of cisplatin/paclitaxel and carboplatin/paclitaxel in stage IVB, recurrent or persistent cervical cancer. *Gynecol Oncol.* 2007;105(2):299–303.

62. Choi CH, Kim TJ, Lee JW, Kim BG, Lee JH, Bae DS. Phase II study of neoadjuvant chemotherapy with mitomycin-c, vincristine, and cisplatin (MVC) in patients with stages IB2-IIB cervical carcinoma. *Gynecol Oncol.* 2007;104(1):64–69.

63. Park DC, Kim JH, Lew YO, Kim DH, Namkoong SE. Phase II trial of neoadjuvant paclitaxel and cisplatin in uterine cervical cancer. *Gynecol Oncol.* 2004;92(1):59–63.

64. Ackermann S, Beckmann MW, Thiel F, Bogenrieder T. Topotecan in cervical cancer. *Int J Gynecol Cancer.* 2007;17(6):1215–1223.

65. Tiersten AD, Selleck MJ, Hershman DL, et al. Phase II study of topotecan and paclitaxel for recurrent, persistent, or metastatic cervical carcinoma. *Gynecol Oncol.* 2004;92(2):635–638.

66. Duenas-Gonzalez A, Lopez-Graniel C, Gonzalez-Enciso A, et al. A phase II study of multimodality treatment for locally advanced cervical cancer: neoadjuvant carboplatin and paclitaxel followed by radical hysterectomy and adjuvant cisplatin chemoradiation. *Ann Oncol.* 2003;14(8):1278–1284.

67. Behtash N, Nazari A, Ayatollahi H, Modarres M, Ghaemmaghami F, Mousavi A. Neoadjuvant chemotherapy and radical surgery compared to radical surgery alone in bulky stage IB-IIA cervical cancer. *Eur J Surg Oncol.* 2006;32(10):1226–1230.

68. Kesic V. Management of cervical cancer. *Eur J Surg Oncol.* 2006;32(8):832–837.

69. Berek JS, Howe C, Lagasse LD, Hacker NF. Pelvic exenteration for recurrent gynecologic malignancy: survival and morbidity analysis of the 45-year experience at UCLA. *Gynecol Oncol.* 2005;99(1):153–159.

70. Lamb MA. Invasive cancer of the cervix. In: *Women and Cancer—A Gynecologic Oncology Nursing Perspective.* 2nd ed. Sudbury, MA: Jones & Bartlett; 2000.

71. Steed H, Rosen B, Murphy J, Laframboise S, De Petrillo D, Covens A. A comparison of laparascopic-assisted radical vaginal hysterectomy and radical abdominal hysterectomy in the treatment of cervical cancer. *Gynecol Oncol.* 2004;93(3):588–593.

72. Morgan MA, Iyengar TD, Napiorkowski BE, Rubin SC, Mikuta JJ. The clinical course of deep vein thrombosis in patients with gynecologic cancer. *Gynecol Oncol.* 2002;84(1):67–71.

73. Montz FJ, Holschnedier CH, Solh S, Schuricht LC, Monk BJ. Small-bowel obstruction following radical hysterectomy: risk factors, incidence, and operative findings. *Gynecol Oncol.* 1994;53(1):114–120.

74. Park SY, Bae DS, Nam JH, et al. Quality of life and sexual problems in disease-free survivors of cervical cancer compared with the general population. *Cancer.* 2007;110(12):2716–2725.

75. Burns M, Costello J, Ryan-Woolley B, Davidson S. Assessing the impact of late treatment effects in cervical cancer: an exploratory study of women's sexuality. *Eur J Cancer Care.* 2007:16(4):364–372.

76. Schover L, Fife M, Gershenson, D. Sexual dysfunction and treatment for early stage cervical cancer. *Cancer.* 1989;63(1):209–212.

77. Bruner DW, Iwamoto R. Altered sexuality. In: Groenwald S, Frogge M, Goodman M, Yarbro C, eds. *Cancer Symptom Management.* 2nd ed. Sudbury, MA: Jones and Bartlett; 1999.

Chapter 8

Vulvar and Vaginal Cancers

Amber Door, RN, BSN, OCN®

Cancers of the vulva and vagina make up approximately less than 5% of all new malignant gynecologic tumors,[1] with primary vaginal malignancies among the rarest of the malignant processes in the human body because the vaginal tissues are relatively immune to malignant change.[2] The American Cancer Society estimates that in 2008 there will be just under 3460 new cases of vulvar cancers and approximately 2210 new cases of vaginal/other female genital malignancies diagnosed in the United States.[1]

Management for these uncommon gynecologic cancers is multimodal, and when possible women should be cared for in tertiary care centers[3] or where there is access to gynecologic oncology, radiation oncology, and specialized care units. The primary treatment modalities used for vulvar and vaginal cancers are surgery and radiation therapy. In advanced disease, chemotherapy can be utilized in both the neoadjuvant and the palliative care role. When used to treat malignancies of the female genital tract, surgery and radiation therapy, with or without chemotherapy, have the potential to significantly impact quality of life secondary to the physical changes that occur. It is critical that women are educated regarding the disease, the expected and potential physical changes to their genital tract, and potential long-term sequelae of treatment.

Epidemiology/Risk Factors

Exact etiologies of vulvar and vaginal malignancies remain unknown but appear to be multifactorial. Both primary malignancies are most prevalent in women over the age of 60,[4-7] but they do occur in younger women. There continues to be debate over the role of bacterial and viral infectious processes, vulvar dystrophy, genetic cofactors, and chemical exposures in both malignant processes. The human *Papilloma* virus (HPV) is proving to have a role as a potential factor increasing the risk of vulvar and vaginal malignancies in younger women.

The development of vulvar cancer has been associated with risks factors[8-10] related to chronic medical illnesses, sexually transmitted disease/infections, chronic inflammatory diseases, and personal/lifestyle

Table 8-1 Possible risk factors for vulvar cancer.

Chronic medical illnesses
- Diabetes mellitus
- Hypertension
- Obesity
- Immunosuppression

Sexually transmitted disease/infections
- Granulomatous disease
- Syphilis
- Herpes simplex virus infection
- Human *Papillomavirus* infection

Chronic inflammatory diseases
- Lichen sclerosis
- Hypertrophic dystrophy

Personal/lifestyle factors
- Cigarette smoking
- Multiple sexual partners
- Prior genital tract neoplasia

Source: Burke T. Vulvar cancer. In: Barakat RR, Bevers MW, Gershenson DM, Hoskins WJ, eds. *Handbook of Gynecologic Oncology*. London: Martin Dunitz; 2000:208. Used with permission.

factors (see **Table 8-1**). The incidence of vulvar cancer appears to be rising secondary to the aging population[8] but at a much lower rate than preinvasive, or in situ disease.[4] Worldwide vulvar cancer is most often seen in the poor and elderly,[9] but reports over the last decade have shown an increase in invasive squamous cell carcinomas of the vulva in women younger than age 35 years.[11–14] This may be due in part to the fact that squamous cell carcinoma of the vulva, in particular, is a multifactorial disease with what appears to be two distinct pathways, one HPV dependent (predominantly HPV 16)[15] and one unrelated to HPV.[8,16,17] The subset associated with

HPV is most prevalent in the vulvar cancers diagnosed in younger women with a history of tobacco use.[8,11] These recent reports suggest that the presence of HPV-induced vulvar intraepithelial neoplasia (VIN) III may not only be a risk factor for vulvar carcinoma but may also be a positive prognostic factor,[18] although it is speculated that this difference could also be attributed to earlier diagnosis in a population more likely to do self-examination, seek care earlier, and have better follow up.[18] So, unlike the role of HPV as a precursor in the development of cervix cancer, its role in the development of vulvar cancer remains less clear,[8] but it is beginning to show a remarkable resemblance to cervical intraepithelial lesions.[16]

A primary carcinoma of the vagina is defined as a malignancy that arises in the epithelium of the vagina and does not involve the cervix or vulva.[5,19] The specific cause of this malignant change is still unknown. It is theorized that chronic irritation from substances "pooling" in the upper vagina, because this is the most common location for invasive vaginal malignancy,[20] may lead to malignant transformation. Other possible predisposing factors have been reported to include the use of vaginal pessaries, vaginal prolapse, syphilis, leukorrhea, and leukoplakia, but these factors have not been validated.[2] Vaginal intraepithelial neoplasia (VAIN) has been the subject of increasing attention as a precursor for vaginal cancer, although again, the true malignant potential of VAIN is not known because when diagnosed it is usually treated.[5] The treatment of VAIN 3 should potentially reduce the risk of developing an invasive carcinoma of the vagina, but this remains unproven as well due to the rare nature of the disease.[19] In addition, a great deal of attention has been focused on the development of clear cell adenocarcinomas of the vagina and cervix in women exposed to diethylstilbestrol (DES) in utero. DES and related drugs were used in the mid 1940s to 1950s to support high-risk pregnancies.[2] It has been suggested that DES exposure may be teratogenic with increased adenosis, a condition in which glandular epithelium is present in the vagina after development is complete and other uterine anomalies, but data do not substantiate that DES intrauterine exposure is a carcinogenic event.[2, 21] Primary adenocarcinomas are rare and occur most frequently in postmenopausal women, but in a series of 519 women with primary adenocarcinomas of the vagina exposed to DES in utero, 91% were diagnosed between the ages of 15 and 27 years.[21] In a retrospective review, DES-exposed daughters were 40 times more likely than women in the general population to develop clear cell adenocarcinoma of the vagina and cervix.[22] Because the use of DES was discontinued in 1971, the incidence of this has decreased markedly since 1975[2] and should continue to decrease as the cohort of women exposed to DES in utero continues to age.[2, 22]

Prevention and Detection

Because the etiology of both vulvar and vaginal malignancies are not known, there are no methods of prevention. Avoidance of potential risk factors may be beneficial but is not proven. Because of this, early detection is the key to less radical interventions and improved survival.

Vulvar cancer is a curable disease when diagnosed early. It is skin malignancy that is in an area that, in most cases, is easily evaluated. Long-term survival is dependent upon several prognostic factors, the most significant of which is the presence or absence of metastasis

to the lymph nodes at the time of diagnosis.[23] In 2007, the Surveillance, Epidemiology, and End Results Program (SEER) reported that in the United States between 1988–2001 there was a 14.6% difference in the 5-year survival between stage I (93.3%) and stage II (78.7%) vulvar cancers.[6] The survival differences between stages I–II and III–IV were 26% and 24%.[6] The presence of positive nodes and a primary lesion ≤ 2 cm decreased survival rates to 61%–62%.[6,24] Survival fell even further to 39.2%–43% if the lesion was > 2 cm with positive nodes.[6,24] Five-year survival in women with three or more unilateral or two or more bilateral nodes, regardless of the size of the primary tumor, fell to 29%.[24]

The most frequently noted symptom of vulvar carcinoma is pruritis. Other reported symptoms are burning, bleeding, pain, or an enlarging mass on the vulva. It is common for one or more of these symptoms to be present for 6–12 months prior to a pathologic diagnosis. Women often self-treat with over-the-counter medication or receive topical treatments from their medical professional based on reported symptoms without benefit of a vulvar examination or biopsy. Vulvar malignancies can present clinically as benign-appearing warty, condylomatous lesions, flat ulcerative lesions, or pigmented lesions. Malignant lesions are usually well demarcated in early stages and are most frequently unilateral. Assessment regarding vulvar symptoms should be part of a gynecologic nursing assessment, utilizing terminology that is understood by the patient. Visual examination, as well as colposcopic examination if possible, of the vulva with a biopsy of any visible lesion(s) at the onset of symptoms is critical to early detection and treatment. The lesion should be measured and its location to fixed structures, such as the urethra, clitoris, or anus should be clearly documented, particularly if the lesion is small.

Invasive cancers of the vagina, if detected and appropriately staged early, can be effectively treated with radical surgery, with or without radiation therapy.[20] As a rare malignancy, the published survival data for vaginal cancer in the last 20 years is based upon patient populations of 14–105 accrued from as early as the 1950s with mixed tumor histology. The overall survival for all stages ranged from 8%–56%.[2] Published data by Eddy, et al.[25] and Stock, et al.[26] showed survival for stage I of 67%–70%, stage II of 45%–53%, stage III of 0%–35%, and stage IV of 15%–28%, with an overall survival of 46%–50%. Most recently, the SEER survival monograph report on cancer of the vagina published 5-year survival data from 1988–2001 on 1041 women, showing survivals of 68.4% for stage I vaginal cancer, 54.3% for stage II, 35.5% for stage III, and 20.3% for stage IV.[7]

Vaginal malignancies often present with abnormal vaginal bleeding and/or watery or discolored vaginal discharge that is painless in early stage disease. Abnormal cytology on a Pap smear can detect early disease as well. Dyspareunia and changes in the bowel and bladder function, as well as pain, may be present in more advanced disease. Visual inspection of the entire vaginal canal is critical to detect abnormalities in the vagina. A thorough inspection requires that the vaginal speculum be rotated as it is withdrawn to allow for visualization of the anterior and posterior walls of the vagina, in addition to the lateral walls. Currently the ACS has no recommendations for vaginal cancer screening. Education is a key factor in early detection of vaginal cancer.[27]

Education of all female patients regarding the signs and symptoms of gynecologic abnormalities and encouragement to seek medical care early should be integrated into daily nursing practice. This is particularly important in women who have undergone hysterectomy for benign conditions and the elderly population who may be at increased risk for vaginal cancer but are no longer undergoing any form of gynecologic assessment or screening.

Histology/Pathology

Primary malignancies of the vulva and vagina are comprised of many different histologic types, each unique and requiring tailored treatment. The vulva and vagina are covered by squamous epithelium. In both sites, squamous cell carcinoma accounts for the overwhelming majority of malignant cases.[2,9,28,29]

Malignant melanomas of both the vulva and vagina are the second most common primary malignancies seen in both locations.[2,9,28,29]

Verrucous cell carcinomas, a distinct variant of squamous cell carcinoma, are large, locally invasive tumors that rarely metastasize. These are primarily seen on the vulva, but have been reported in the vagina.[2,28,29]

Basal cell carcinomas are found on the vulva and are treated with local excision because lymphatic spread is exceedingly rare.[9,28]

Adenocarcinoma can arise in both the vulva and the vagina. On the vulva, it can develop in the Bartholin gland, vulvar skin appendages, and anogenital glands. Primary adenocarcinomas and clear cell carcinomas of the vagina are rare and can arise in vaginal adenosis, and, as discussed previously, have been reported in women who were exposed to DES in utero.[2,9,21,29]

Extramammary Paget disease of the vulva, in rare cases, is an invasive disease. Paget disease of the vulva presents as an eczematoid, red, weeping area on the vulva. It is primarily seen in older Caucasian women. It is often misdiagnosed and treated as eczema or contact dermatitis for years without benefit of a biopsy. In approximately 15% of cases, it can be associated with an underlying adenocarcinoma. In addition to this, Paget disease can herald the development of an adenocarcinoma in another nonvulvar location, such as the breast, colon, rectum, and upper female genital tract.[9,28]

Sarcomas can be seen, although rarely, in both the vulva and vagina. In adults, they are predominantly leiomyosarcomas.[9,28] The botryoid variant of embryonal rhabdomyosarcoma is the most common malignant tumor of the vagina in infants and children, with 95% of cases being under the age of 5 years.[29]

Primary lymphomas can also be seen in the vagina and are most commonly of diffuse, large cell type. This tumor typically presents as a submucosal vaginal mass.[29]

Other rare tumors seen in the vulva are Merkel cell carcinomas, malignant schwannomas, carcinoma of the sweat glands, adenocystic carcinomas, adenosquamous carcinoma, and yolk sac tumors.[9,28]

Assessment

A complete assessment of the vulva and vagina should include both a visual inspection and a palpation of the tissue. All clinically evident lesions, even those that appear to be benign on the vulva, warrant a biopsy. This can be done using a local anesthetic and a punch biopsy instrument. In women with preinvasive changes on the vulva or dystrophies of the vulva, colposcopic examination of the vulva using a 3% acetic acid wash to the area may be helpful to the clinician in choosing a biopsy site. The biopsy should include, if possible, adjacent normal skin and the underlying dermis so that the pathologist can address depth of invasion. A punch biopsy of the lesion is preferred to excision of the lesion for establishing a diagnosis. This allows the gynecologic oncologist to tailor the surgical margins based on the size and location of the primary tumor.

The diagnosis of vaginal malignancies must include a thorough examination of the cervix (if present), vulva and vagina, visually as well as by palpation, with biopsies of any abnormal areas. This is to identify not only the primary site but the histology of the lesion as well. Pap smears may be helpful in the diagnosis of early vaginal cancer but will not detect a submucosal malignancy, as with adenocarcinomas or lymphoma. The use of colposcopy can also be helpful in identifying areas of abnormality of the vaginal mucosa.

Diagnosis/Staging

In 1988, FIGO (International Federation of Gynecology and Obstetrics) established a surgical staging system for carcinoma of the vulva. In 1994, this system was modified to subdivide stage I disease to A or B based on depth of invasion (see **Table 8-2**).[30] Prior to 1988, vulvar carcinoma was staged clinically based upon evaluation of the primary tumor, regional lymph nodes, and a limited search for distant metastasis. Microscopic lymph node metastasis is not clinically palpable, and inflammation may cause enlarged lymph nodes in the absence of metastatic disease. When compared

Table 8-2 FIGO STAGING FOR VULVAR CANCER *(2002).*

Stage 0	T_{is}	Carcinoma in situ, intraepithelial carcinoma
Stage I	$T_1N_0M_0$	Tumor $\leq$ 2 cm in greatest diameter, confined to the vulva or perineum; nodes are negative
IA	$T_{1a}N_0M_0$	As above with stromal invasion of $\leq$ 1.0 mm[a]
IB	$T_{1b}N_0M_0$	As above with stromal invasion of > 1.0 mm
Stage II	$T_2N_0M_0$	Tumor confined to the vulva/perineum, > 2 cm in greatest diameter; nodes are negative
Stage III	$T_1N_1M_0$ $T_2N_1M_0$ $T_3N_0M_0$ $T_3N_1M_0$	Tumor of any size with 1. Adjacent spread to the lower urethra and/or vagina and/or anus 2. Unilateral regional lymph node metastasis
Stage IVA	$T_1N_2M_0$ $T_2N_2M_0$ $T_3N_2M_0$ $T_4N_{any}M_0$	Tumor invades any of the following: Upper urethra, bladder mucosa, rectal mucosa, pelvic bone, or bilateral regional node metastasis
Stage IVB	$T_{any}N_{any}M_1$	Any distant metastasis, including pelvic lymph nodes

FIGO, International Federation of Gynecology and Obstetrics

[a] The depth of invasion is defined as the measurement of the tumor from the epithelial-stromal junction of the adjacent-most superficial dermal papilla to the deepest point of invasion.

Source: American Joint Commission on Cancer (AJCC). *AJCC Cancer Staging Manual.* 6th ed. Philadelphia, PA: Lippincott-Raven; 2002:247.

with surgical staging, the percentage of error in clinical staging increases from 18% for stage I disease to 44% in stage IV disease.[24] This change in staging has made it more difficult to compare outcomes in publications prior to 1988.

Although the histology of the malignant tumor impacts prognosis, the only risk factors, when considered together, that are associated with prognosis in vulvar cancer are the diameter of the primary lesion and the status of the lymph nodes at the time of diagnosis.[24] The age and the underlying medical condition of the patient have an impact on prognosis if they preclude the surgical resection of the primary lesion and lymph nodes.

Vulvar melanoma has been staged using a variety of systems. Clark's system for staging of cutaneous melanomas was developed in 1969.[31] It is based upon the depth of tumor invasion relative to the papillary dermis. Because the vulva and labia lack a well-defined papillary dermis, the use of Breslow's staging (see **Table 8-3**),[32] utilizing tumor

Table 8-3 CLARK, BRESLOW, AND CHUNG STAGING OF MELANOMA.

Level	Clark	Breslow	Chung
I	In situ: all tumor above the epidermal basement membrane	Tumor thickness < 0.76 mm	Same as Clark's
II	Tumor extends through the basement membrane into the papillary dermis	Tumor thickness 0.76–1.50 mm	Invasion ≤ 1 mm
III	Tumor fills papillary dermis and extends to the reticular dermis but does not invade into it	Tumor thickness 1.51–2.25 mm	Invasion 1–2 mm
IV	Tumor extends into the reticular dermis	Tumor thickness 2.26–3.0 mm	Invasion > 2 mm
V	Tumor extends into the subcutaneous fat	Tumor thickness > 3 mm	Same as Clark's

thickness—or Chung's staging, utilizing depth of invasion (see **Table 8-3**)[33]—may be a more accurate predictor of outcome.[34,35] In the only prospective study of vulvar melanoma patients conducted by the Gynecologic Oncology Group (GOG), it was concluded that the American Joint Committee on Cancer (AJCC) staging (see **Table 8-4**) should be used. In the absence of AJCC stage, Breslow's levels were the next most prognostic feature.[36,37]

Staging of vaginal cancer according to FIGO is done clinically, not surgically (see **Table 8-5**).[30] This is done utilizing physical examination, chest X-ray, intravenous pyelogram, cystoscopy, proctoscopy, and when indicated a barium enema and/or lymphangiogram. Further studies, such as CT scans or MRI may be utilized to individualize treatment but are not used for staging.

The primary prognostic indicator in vaginal cancer is the stage of disease at the time of diagnosis. Other factors that correlate with a poorer prognosis are: >60 years of age, any symptoms at diagnosis; a lesion in the middle or lower third of vagina; or a poorly differentiated tumor.[25,38] In addition, in squamous cell carcinoma, which initially spreads along the vaginal wall before invading the paravaginal tissue, the length of the vaginal wall involvement of the tumor has been found to correlate with survival and stage of disease.[39]

Primary Treatment

The primary treatment for invasive vulvar malignancies in operable patients has been a radical vulvectomy with groin dissection(s). This aggressive surgical approach has been associated with an operative mortality rate that approached 20% in early series.[40] In the last two decades, this has been reduced to 1%–2%.[6] The most frequently encountered complication

Table 8-4 AJCC PATHOLOGIC STAGING FOR SKIN MELANOMA (*2002*).

Staging	Groupings	Definitions
Stage 0	Tis N0 M0	Melanoma in situ
Stage IA	T1a N0 M0	Melanoma ≤ 1.0 mm thickness and Clark Level II or III, no ulceration
Stage IB	T1b N0 M0	Melanoma ≤ 1.0 mm thickness and Clark Level IV or V, with ulceration
	T2a N0 M0	Melanoma 1.01–2.0 mm in thickness, no ulceration
Stage IIA	T2b N0 M0	Melanoma 1.01–2.0 mm in thickness, with ulceration
	T3a N0 M0	Melanoma 2.01–4.0 mm in thickness, no ulceration
Stage IIB	T3b N0 M0	Melanoma 2.01–4.0 mm in thickness, with ulceration
	T4a N0 M0	Melanoma > 4.0 mm in thickness, no ulceration
Stage IIC	T4b N0 M0	Melanoma > 4.0 mm in thickness, with ulceration
Stage IIIA	T1-4a N1a M0	Melanoma any thickness, no ulceration, 1 Microscopic (+) node
	T1-4a N2a M0	Melanoma any thickness, no ulceration, 1 Macroscopic (+) node
Stage IIIB	T1-4b N1a-2a M0	Melanoma any thickness, with ulceration, 1–3 Microscopic (+) nodes
	T1-4a N1b-2b M0	Melanoma any thickness, no ulceration, 2–3 Microscopic/Macroscopic (+) nodes
	T1-4a-b N2c M0	Melanoma any thickness +/– ulceration, satellite or in-transit metastasis without nodal metastasis

(continues)

Table 8-4 AJCC PATHOLOGIC STAGING FOR SKIN MELANOMA (**2002**) *continued.*

Staging	Groupings	Definitions
Stage IIIC	T1-4b N1b-2b M0	Melanoma any thickness, with ulceration, 1–3 Macroscopic (+) nodes
	Any T N3 M0	Melanoma any thickness, +/− ulceration, 4+ regional (+) nodes, matted nodes or in-transit metastasis of satellite(s) with metastasis to regional nodes
Stage IV	Any T Any N M1	Melanoma any thickness, +/− ulceration, any nodes or in-transit metastasis, (+) distant metastasis
	M1a	Metastasis to skin, subcutaneous tissues, or distant lymph nodes
	M1b	Metastasis to lung
	M1c	Metastasis to all other visceral sites or any site associated with an elevated serum lactic dehydrogenase (LDH)

Source: American Joint Commission on Cancer (AJCC). *AJCC Cancer Staging Manual.* 6th ed. Philadelphia, PA: Lippincott-Raven; 2002:219–220.

of surgery remains wound breakdown and impaired wound healing, which in most series occurs in over 50% of patients.[9] Other potential postsurgical complications are lymphedema, formation of lymphocyst in the resected groin, and development of cellulitus. Because of the high-risk of wound-related complications, the trend in the last 2 decades is toward a more conservative surgical approach for early disease, with surgery tailored to cause less disfigurement of the genitals and fewer changes in sexual function and body image. The factors that have led to this change are concerns over postoperative morbidity and long hospitalizations that are associated with en bloc radical dissections (resection of the entire vulva, subcutaneous fat, contiguous skin, and regional inguinal/femoral lymph nodes); an increased number of younger women with smaller lesions; and an increased awareness of the psychosexual consequences of radical vulvectomy.[41] The use of radical or modified radical vulvectomy with separate groin incisions (triple incision approach) has been associated with decreased complications and similar survival and recurrence rates to en bloc approach.[42,43] In recent years, two further modifications to the surgical management of vulvar malignancies have been studied in an attempt to improve upon surgical complications that are most frequently associated with resection of groin lymph nodes. Those modifications are sentinel lymph node evaluation and mapping in an attempt to decrease the extent of the nodal dissection[44] and sparing of the saphenous vein during resection in an attempt to decrease the risk of long-term lymphedema

Table 8-5 FIGO STAGING FOR VAGINAL CANCER.

Stage 0	T_{is}	Carcinoma in situ, intraepithelial carcinoma
Stage I	T_1	Carcinoma is limited to the vaginal wall
Stage II	T_2	Carcinoma has involved the subvaginal tissue but has not extended onto the pelvic wall
Stage III	T_3	Carcinoma has extended onto the pelvic wall
Stage IV	T_4	Carcinoma has extended beyond the true pelvis or has involved the mucosa of the bladder or rectum; bullous edema or tumor bulge into the bladder or rectum is not acceptable evidence of invasion
IVA		Spread of the growth to adjacent organs and/or direct extension beyond the true pelvis
IVB		Any distant metastasis

FIGO, International Federation of Gynecology and Obstetrics
Source: American Joint Commission on Cancer (AJCC). *AJCC Cancer Staging Manual.* 6th ed. Philadelphia, PA: Lippincott-Raven; 2002:255.

and cellulitis.[45] The data appears promising in the reports done with small cohorts and selected practitioners.[44,46] Further investigation of these modifications and techniques are still needed. Studies are currently being conducted in an attempt to improve upon the short- and long-term complications of treatment.

Management of early stage disease should be individualized. The goal of treatment is for the most conservative surgical intervention that optimizes cure. The factors that need to be considered are size of the lesion, location on the vulva, depth of invasion, risk of groin node involvement, condition of the remaining vulva, and the patient's overall medical condition. The use of intraoperative lymphatic mapping and lymphoscintigraphy may assist the surgeon in tailoring treatment even further. Early results of lymphatic mapping for vulvar cancer has shown that it has the ability to detect sentinel lymph nodes in 86% of patients, and in no case was a nonsentinel lymph node found to be positive if the sentinel node was negative.[47] With careful patient selection and experience, sentinel node identification with blue dye alone has been permitted in more than 95% of patients with vulvar cancer.[47] Because of this, the use of sentinel node mapping is currently undergoing clinical investigation by the GOG.

Planning primary treatment for vaginal cancer is dependent on the stage at presentation, location of the lesion, and the presence or absence of the uterus. The maintenance of a functional vagina is an important factor to consider when planning treatment. Cases of squamous cell carcinoma of the vagina reported in the gynecologic literature have been treated primarily by radiotherapy,[2] largely due to the difficulty in attaining adequate surgical margins short of exenteration (resection of the vagina, bladder, and/or rectum). For stage I disease with lesions located on the upper vagina, radical surgical resection with pelvic lymph node dissection, and vaginal reconstruction if feasible, can be performed, followed by radiation therapy if resection margins are close or involved.[26,48] For early lesions in the lower third of the vagina, the inguinal lymph nodes must be included in the treatment field due to the lymphatic drainage. Radiation therapy is also used in place of radical surgery in early stage vaginal cancer.[2,26,49] In stage II vaginal cancer, combined external beam radiation therapy and brachytherapy is currently standard treatment.[2,49] The role of concomitant radiation therapy and chemotherapy is not clear but may play a role based on current data in squamous cell carcinoma of the cervix. Unfortunately, the rarity of vaginal carcinomas precludes it from being evaluated in any large phase III clinical trial.

Advanced or Recurrent Disease

As with early vulvar cancer, treatment in advanced and recurrent disease must be individualized. Treatment must be tailored, taking into account the overall medical condition of the patient, size and location of the tumor, as well as the treatment goal. In the case of recurrent disease, prior treatment must be taken into account as well. Treatment for stage III/IV disease is most often surgery combined with external beam radiation therapy.[50,51] Surgical resection with adequate margins may require fecal and/or urinary diversion in the form of an exenterative procedure if a radical resection is performed initially. Additionally, closure of large wounds may require reconstructive surgery utilizing cutaneous and myocutaneous flaps. In an attempt to decrease the morbidity and mortality of extensive surgical resections, the GOG evaluated patients with disease that would require this type of exenterative procedure. It was found that the use of preoperative chemoradiation, followed by a more conservative surgical resection in advanced vulvar malignancies, was feasible and reduced the need for more radical resections, to include pelvic exenteration. The chemotherapy agents used in the initial trial were cisplatin and 5-FU. The use of weekly cisplatin is currently under investigation to avoid the 4-day continuous infusion.[50,52–54] Unfortunately, there have been no adequate prospective studies comparing various therapies or combinations that are available for analysis.[9] Chemotherapy for distant recurrence/disease of the vulva has not been proven beneficial.[9,49,55] The goal of treatment should be focused on palliation of symptoms and local palliative measures.[50]

The treatment for advanced and recurrent vaginal carcinomas remains external radiation therapy and brachytherapy, both intracavitary and interstitial therapy with consideration for tailored surgery.[2,47] As with recurrent vulvar cancer, the primary treatment given must be taken into account when forming a plan for recurrent disease. Chemotherapy for advanced or recurrent disease does not have a significant role in disease management at this time,[3,47,51] and treatment should again be focused on local measures for palliation of symptoms.

Nursing Implications

Nursing care for women diagnosed with vulvar and vaginal carcinoma presents particular challenges. The first challenge is rarity of both vulvar and vaginal cancer. Women are frequently unaware that they can develop cancers of the vulva and vagina, which is often the reason that there is such a delay in diagnosis. Education regarding these malignancies is crucial to ensure early detection, thereby improving the chance of cure for women. Nurses must educate themselves regarding the diseases to educate the women they encounter about risk factors for both diseases. Women should be taught vulvar self-examination at an early age, just as self-examination of the breast is taught. Women should be encouraged to continue to have pelvic examinations even after hysterectomy and menopause. Most importantly, women should be encouraged and instructed to seek medical attention for a persistent sore, itch, rash, or change in the vulva or new vaginal discharge.

When the diagnosis of malignancy is made, nurses play a key role in the patient education and reinforcement regarding the disease, treatment options, and potential complications (see Table 8-6).[56] Information regarding postoperative care that is provided to the patient and caregivers preoperatively is an important tool for preparing the patient and others involved in her care and support. Written information is useful, but it must be easily understandable. Postoperatively, the primary concern is wound healing. Vulvectomy wounds are under tremendous stress due to multiple factors, primarily location. Both the groin and vulvar incisions are difficult to immobilize, placing an undue amount of tension on them. Additionally, the groin node dissection undermines the skin, leaving a pocket in which lymphatic fluid can collect, called a lymphocyst. A lymphocyst causes

a lack of tissue adherence to the underlying tissue, delaying wound healing and increasing risk of infection and wound breakdown. This complication is a frequent occurrence despite the use of drains postoperatively. It is hoped that in the future modifications to the standard surgical procedure will help further decrease the risk of development. As with other surgical procedures, postoperative infection is always a concern. The location of vulvar and groin incisions in proximity to the urethra and the rectum increases the risk of infection. Meticulous perineal care is required both pre- and postoperatively. This is often difficult and time consuming in the older population that is affected by vulvar cancer. Early assessment of the patient's home situation, as well as the functional and cognitive ability to care for perineal and groin wounds will facilitate early interventions to assist in wound healing. When a vulvar or groin wound is disrupted, the care becomes a challenge. Vulvar wounds by location do not allow for easy maintenance of a dressing. In the past, referral for whirlpool therapy to the vulva was often necessary for large wound breakdowns. Most recently, the use of a vacuum assisted closure dressing (VAC) on the vulva has been used to facilitate granulation and healing, but, as expected, maintaining vacuum suction on the perineum presents another set of challenges. Care of an open groin wound must be done with caution, particularly if debridement is necessary secondary to the underlying large vessels that are in the base of the wound. Lower extremities should be assessed for temperature changes and pulses on a regular basis to assure that there is adequate vascular flow.

Lymphedema of both the lower extremity and vulva is a potential long-term complication of surgical resection of inguinal lymph

Table 8-6 Nursing aspects of vulvar and vaginal cancers.

Consideration	Guideline/Teaching
Prevention and early detection	Identify at-risk patients: elderly, chronic medical illness, sexually transmitted disease history to include HPV, cervix cancer history, tobacco use, prior hysterectomy, prior radiation to genitals, DES exposure, chronic genital skin disorder history. Teach/instruct patient/primary caregiver in periodic examination of vulva and genitals. Encourage regular gynecologic examinations and Pap smears in all women. Prompt medical evaluation of persistent symptoms or new lesion of the genitals.
Preoperative	Ongoing pain assessment. Educate regarding disease, treatment, and plan of care. Education on appropriate skin care of lesion prior to surgery and skin care requirements postoperatively. Provide emotional support to patient and family. Nutritional assessment. Thrombolic prophylaxis.
Postoperative	Assess for pulmonary emboli and deep vein thrombosis. Ongoing pain assessments/pain management. Activity as ordered. Perineal care, sitz baths, and drying of perineum as ordered. Instruction of patient and caregiver with return demonstrations of perineal/incision care. Wound care of open wounds until healed by secondary intent. Nutritional assessment. Initiate early viewing of incision by patient and caregiver. Educate for signs and symptoms of infection. Education of drain management and drainage record if groin drains remain in place post-discharge. Facilitate appropriate referrals if needed after discharge.

(continues)

Table 8-6 Nursing aspects of vulvar and vaginal cancers *continued.*

Adjuvant treatment radiation/chemotherapy	Teach appropriate skin care of perineum—sitz bath, blow dryer. Potential need for urinary catheter care with radiation to perineum. Pain medication as necessary. Antiemetics as necessary with chemotherapy. Education regarding potential side effects of chemotherapy/radiation therapy. Education regarding management of vulvitis during radiation—iced Burrow solution, saline.
Long-term rehabilitation	Educate regarding potential lower extremity edema; support hose, leg elevation, activity, manual lymph drainage education referral when available; compression sleeves; potential need for long-term cellulitis prophylaxis. Sexual dysfunction—discuss alteration in sexual activity with patient and significant other – (correct) if patient desires, lubrication issues, vaginal dilation, positioning, change in genital appearance, referral for counseling if necessary. Urinary changes: change in urinary stream direction, conduit. Disfigurement: provide ongoing emotional support, referral for psychological counseling/assistance if necessary. Education for long-term follow up and signs and symptoms of recurrent disease.

nodes and/or radiation therapy to the pelvis and perineum for both vulvar and vaginal malignancies that occur in nearly 30% of patients in some studies.[57] Patients should be educated to the possibility of lymphedema preoperatively and be given instructions as to the management of lymphedema if it occurs. Prevention teaching should include wearing loose clothing with avoidance of tight garments around the groin, knee, or ankle; regular exercise to maintain muscle tone; the use of appropriately sized medical support stockings, particularly when standing for long periods is anticipated; and not sitting with knees crossed and hips bent for an extended time. It is important to reinforce this teaching with each contact because lymphedema is a long-term side effect and may not occur until months to years later. If lymphedema does occur, patients should be assessed for early referral to a manual lymph drainage specialist whenever possible.

Cellulitis is a potential problem for as many as 57% of patients undergoing lymph node dissection[57] occurring both as an early and a late complication. Patient education should include the signs and symptoms of cellulitis, which may include redness across the lower abdomen, groin, thigh, or vulva, or fever and pain. Prompt treatment with antibiotics is necessary and may require hospitalization because it can spread quickly. A long-term, low-dose, prophylactic antibiotic may be prescribed to decrease the chance of recurrence in the future. Education on avoiding infections in the lower extremities includes avoiding going barefoot; wearing shoes that fit properly; using an electric razor to shave legs; avoiding cuts and scrapes to legs, ankle, and feet; and avoiding cutting toenails too short.

Desquamation of the skin on the vulva and groin during radiation therapy[54] is a painful potential short-term complication of treatment. Although not life threatening or permanent, it is painful and distressing to the patient and often causes treatment delays. Reinforcing previous teaching regarding meticulous skin care is essential during radiation therapy. The area must be kept clean and dry, which is often difficult, utilizing vigilant pericare with mild soaps, warm water sitz baths, blow dryers, and if necessary, corticosteroid and antibiotic creams to decrease or prevent skin infections. If desquamation occurs, it may be necessary for patient comfort to place an indwelling catheter during vulvar radiation therapy, and the appropriate teaching for catheter management is needed.

For women who receive radiation therapy to the pelvis for vulvar or vaginal cancer, a major adverse effect is vaginal fibrosis from scarring secondary to the loss of blood supply and elasticity,[58] as well as narrowing of the vaginal introitus. This can cause significant sexual dysfunction. Currently, the general recommendation is for the use of a vaginal dilator or vaginal intercourse with the use of a water-soluble lubricant or estrogen cream, if necessary, two to three times per week for life. To date there have been no prospective randomized trials regarding the use of vaginal dilators to optimize vaginal length and caliber, although efforts are currently underway in the GOG to address this issue to optimize the care of women who are undergoing radiation therapy to the pelvis, vagina, and/or cervix. Surgical interventions can be performed, but the potential for poor wound healing and further complication of wound healing when operating on irradiated tissues make this less than appealing for most patients. Open discussion with both the patient and her significant other should occur. This should start at some level at the time of diagnosis and continue throughout the course of her treatment and in follow up, with early referral for counseling if necessary, can provide benefit for this long-term effects. (referring to long-term effect of vaginal fibrosis/narrowing of vaginal introitus, as stated in beginning of paragraph).

Patients should be encouraged to keep regular follow-up visits after treatment to ensure that in the event of recurrence, it will be detected early. The importance of this was documented in a large retrospective review that showed 65% of vulvar recurrences were found at the time of a routinely scheduled appointment, with only 50% of women reporting new symptoms.[59] Although self-report of changes is important, examination of the vulva and vagina is crucial for this population.

Conclusion

Vulvar and vaginal cancers are rare gynecologic malignancies that, if detected early, have the high possibility of cure. Treatments are often aggressive and radical to improve long-term survival. Access to multimodal treatment and specialists with expertise in all aspects of the care of these malignancies is critical. Radiation and surgery to the vulva and vagina can cause long-term physical changes in appearance; functional changes to the vulva, vagina, bladder, and bowel; lymphedema; and a change in sexual function. These physical changes, in addition to a malignant diagnosis, can lead to psychological and emotional changes as well. These issues must be addressed, and education of the patient and family should begin at the time of diagnosis. Communication across all disciplines of health care is necessary for the complete care that women with these uncommon malignancies require. A nurse educated in the treatment of these rare diseases and the management of the sequelae of treatment will aid the patient and her family in adapting to the changes that are likely to occur.

References

1. American Cancer Society. *Cancer Facts & Figures 2008*. Atlanta, GA: American Cancer Society; 2008:4.

2. Slomovitz BM, Coleman RL. Invasive cancer of the vagina and urethra. In: DiSaia DJ, Creasman WJ, eds. *Clinical Gynecologic Oncology*. 7th ed. St. Louis, MO: Mosby; 2007:265–281.

3. Beller U, Maisonneuve P, Benedict JL, et al. Carcinoma of the vulva. *J Epid Biostat*. 2001;6(1):153–174.

4. Judson PL, Habermann EB, Baxter NN, et al. Trends in the incidence of invasive and in situ vulvar carcinoma. *Obstet Gyn*. 2006;107(5):1018–1022.

5. Hacker NG. Vaginal cancer. In: Hacker NG, Berek JS, eds. *Practical Gynecologic Oncology*. 4th ed. Philadelphia, PA: Lippincott Williams & Wilkins; 2005:585–601.

6. Kosary CL. Cancer of the vulva. In: Ries LAG, Young GE, Eisner MP, et al, eds. *SEER Survival Monograph: Cancer Survival Among Adults: U.S. SEER Program, 1988–2001, Patient Tumor Characteristics*. National Cancer Institute, SEER Program, NIH Pub No. 07-6215. Bethesda, MD: National Cancer Institute; 2007:147–154.

7. Kosary CL. Cancer of the vagina. In: Ries LAG, Young GE, Eisner MP, et al, eds. *SEER Survival Monograph: Cancer Survival Among Adults: U.S. SEER Program, 1988–2001, Patient Tumor Characteristics*. National Cancer Institute, SEER Program, NIH Pub No. 07-6215. Bethesda, MD: National Cancer Institute; 2007:155–160.

8. Bloss JD, Liao SY, Wilczynski SP. Clinical and histologic features of vulvar carcinomas analyzed for human papillomavirus status: evidence that squamous cell carcinoma of the vulva has more than one etiology. *Human Pathol*. 1991;22(7):711–718.

9. Stehman FB. Invasive cancer of the vulva. In: DiSaia DJ, Creasman WJ, eds. *Clinical Gynecologic Oncology*. 7th ed. St. Louis, MO: Mosby; 2007:235–264.

10. Burke, T. Vulvar cancer. In: Barakat RR, Bevers MW, Gershenson DM, Hoskins WJ, eds. *Handbook of Gynecologic Oncology*. London: Martin Dunitz; 2000:208.

11. Al-Ghamdi A, Freedman D, Miller D, et al. Vulvar squamous cell carcinoma in young women: a clinicopathologic study of 21 cases. *Gynecol Oncol*. 2002;84(1):94–101.

12. Messing MJ, Gallup DG. Carcinoma of the vulva in young women. *Obstet Gynecol*. 1995;86(1):51–54.

13. Jones RW, Baranyai J, Sables S. Trends in squamous cell carcinoma of the vulva: the influence of vulvar intraepithelial neoplasia. *Obstet Gynecol*. 1997;90(3):448–452.

14. Losch A, Joura E. Vulvar neoplasia in young women (letter to editor). *Gynecol Oncol*. 1999;75:519.

15. Hillemanns P, Wang X. Integration of HPV-16 and HPV-18 DNA in vulvar intraepithelial neoplasia. *Gynecol Oncol*. 2006;100(2):276–282.

16. van de Avoort IA, Shirango H, Hoevenaars BM, et al. Vulvar squamous cell is a multifactorial disease following two separate and distinct pathways. *Int J Gynecol Pathol*. 2006;25(1):22–29.

17. Trimble CL, Hildesheim A, Brinton LA, et al. Heterogeneous etiology of squamous carcinoma of the vulva. *Obstet Gynecol*. 1996;87(1):59–64.

18. Rouzier R, Morice P, Haie-Meder C, et al. Prognostic significance of epithelial disorders adjacent to

invasive vulvar carcinoma. *Gynecol Oncol.* 2001;81(3): 414–419.

19. Helm CW, Chan KK. Vaginal cancer. In: Shingleton HM, Fowler WC, Jordan JA, Lawrence WD, eds. *Gynecologic Oncology Current Diagnosis and Treatment.* London; WB Saunders; 1996:109–116.

20. Creasman WT. Vaginal cancers. *Curr Opin Obst Gynecol.* 2005;17(1):71–76.

21. Melnick S, Cole P, Anderson D, et al. Rates and risks of diethylstilbesterol-related clear-cell adenocarcinomas of the vagina and cervix. An update. *N Engl J Med.* 1987;316(9):514–516.

22. Hatch EE, Palmer JR, Titus-Ernstoff L, et al. Cancer risk in women exposed to diethylstilbesterol in utero. *JAMA.* 1998;280(7):630–634.

23. Raspagliesi F, Hanozet F, Ditto A, et al. Clinical and prognostic factors in squamous cell carcinoma of the vulva. *Gynecol Oncol.* 2006;102(2): 333–337.

24. Holmsley HD, Bundy BN, Sedlis A, et al. Assessment of current International Federation of Gynecology and Obstetrics staging of vulvar carcinoma relative to prognostic factors for survival (A Gynecologic Oncology Group study). *Am J Obstet Gynecol.* 1991;164(4):997–1003.

25. Eddy GL, Marks RD Jr, Miller MC, et al. Primary invasive vaginal carcinoma. *Am J Obstet Gynecol.* 1991;165(2):292–298.

26. Stock RG, Chen AS, Seski J. A 30-year experience in the management of primary carcinoma of the vagina: analysis of prognostic factors and treatment modalities. *Gynecol Oncol.* 1995;56(1):45–52.

27. Smith RA, Cokkinides V, Eyre HJ. American Cancer Society guidelines for the early detection of cancer, 2003. *CA: Cancer J Clin.* 2003;53(1): 27–43.

28. Burke TW, Eifel PJ, McGuire WP, et al. Vulva. In: Hoskins WJ, Perez CA, Young RC, eds. *Principles and Practice of Gynecologic Oncology.* 3rd ed. Philadelphia, PA: Lippincott Williams & Wilkins; 2000: 775–810.

29. Perez CA, Gersell DJ, McGuire WP, et al. Vagina. In: Hoskins WJ, Perez CA, Young RC, eds. *Principles and Practice of Gynecologic Oncology.* 3rd ed. Philadelphia, PA: Lippincott Williams & Wilkins; 2000: 811–840.

30. American Joint Commission on Cancer (AJCC®). *AJCC Cancer Staging Manual.* 6th ed. Philadelphia, PA: Lippincott-Raven; 2002.

31. Clark WH, Frm L, Bernardina EA, et al. The histogenesis and biologic behavior of primary malignant melanomas of the skin. *Cancer Res.* 1969;29(3): 705–727.

32. Breslow A. Thickness, cross sectional areas, and depth of invasion in the prognosis of cutaneous melanoma. *Ann Surg.* 1970;172(5):902–908.

33. Chung AF, Woodruff JM, Lewis JL. Malignant melanoma of the vulva. *Obstet Gynecol.* 1975;45(6): 638–646.

34. Podratz KC, Gaffey TA, Symmonds RD, et al. Melanoma of the vulva: an update. *Gynecol Oncol.* 1983;16(2):153–168.

35. Trimble EL, Lewis JL, Williams LL, et al. Management of vulvar melanoma. *Gynecol Oncol.* 1992;45(3): 254–258.

36. Phillips GL, Bundy BN, Okagaki T, et al. Malignant melanoma of the vulva treated by radical hemivulvectomy: a prospective study of the Gynecologic Oncology Group. *Cancer.* 1994;73(10):2626–2632.

37. Irvin WP, Legallo RL, Stoler MH, et al. Vulvar melanoma: a retrospective analysis and literature review. *Gynecol Oncol.* 2001;83(3):457–465.

38. Kucera H, Vavra N. Radiation management of primary carcinoma of the vagina: clinical and histopathological variables associated with survival. *Gynecol Oncol.* 1991;40(1):12–16.

39. Dixit S, Singhal S, Baboo HA. Squamous cell carcinoma of the vagina: a review of 70 cases. *Gynecol Oncol.* 1993;48(1):80–87.

40. Way S. The surgery of vulvar carcinoma: an appraisal. *Clin Obstet Gynecol.* 1978;5(3):623–628.

41. Hacker NG. Vulvar cancer. In: Hacker NG, Berek JS, eds. *Practical Gynecologic Oncology.* 4th ed. Philadelphia, PA: Lippincott Williams & Wilkins; 2005:543–583.

42. Siller BS, Alvarez RD, Conner WD, et al. T2/3 vulva cancer: a case-control study of triple incision versus en bloc radical vulvectomy and inguinal lymphadenopathy. *Gynecol Oncol.* 1995;57(3): 335–339.

43. Magrina JF, Gonzalez-Bosquet J, Weaver AL, et al. Primary squamous cell cancer of the vulva: radical versus modified radical vulvar surgery. *Gynecol Oncol.* 1998;71(1):116–121.

44. Moore RG, Robinson K, Brown AK, et al. Isolated sentinel lymph node dissection with conservative management in patients with squamous cell

carcinonoma of the vulva: a prospective trial. *Gynecol Oncol.* 2008;109(1):65–70.

45. Frumovit M, Levenback CF. Lymphatic mapping and sentinel node biopsy in vulvar, vaginal, and cervical cancers. *Oncology.* 2008;22(5):529–536.

46. Dardarian TS, Gray HJ, Morgan MA, et al. Saphenous vein sparing during inguinal lymphadenectomy to reduce morbidity in patients with vulvar carcinoma. *Gynecol Oncol.* 2006;101(1):140–142.

47. Levenback C, Coleman RL, Burke TW, et al. Intraoperative lymphatic mapping and sentinel node identification with blue dye in patients with vulvar cancer. *Gynecol Oncol.* 2001;83(2):276–281.

48. Rubin SC, Young J, Mikuta JJ. Squamous carcinoma of the vagina: treatment, complications, and long-term follow-up. *Gynecol Oncol.* 1985;20(3): 346–353.

49. Kirkbride P, Fyles A, Rawlings GA, et al. Carcinoma of the vagina: experience at the Princess Margaret Hospital (1974–1989). *Gynecol Oncol.* 1995;56(3):435–443.

50. Stehman FB, Look KY. Carcinoma of the vulva. *Obstet Gynecol.* 2006;107(3):719–733.

51. Thomas GM, Dembo AJ, Bryson SC, et al. Changing concepts in the management of vulvar cancer. *Gynecol Oncol.* 1991;42(1):9–21.

52. Moore DH, Thomas GM, Montana GS, et al. Preoperative chemoradiation for advanced vulvar cancer: a phase II study of the Gynecologic Oncology Group. *Int J Radiat Oncol Biol Phys.* 1998;42(1): 79–85.

53. Montana GS, Thomas GM, Moore DH, et al. Preoperative chemo-radiation for carcinoma of the vulva with N2/N3 nodes: a gynecologic oncology group study. *Int J Radiat Oncol Biol Phy.* 2000;48(4):1007–1013.

54. Downs LS, Ghosh K, Dusenbery KE, et al. Stage IV carcinoma of the bartholin gland managed with primary chemoradiation. *Gynecol Oncol.* 2002;87(2): 210–212.

55. Roberts WS, Hoffman MS, Kavanagh JJ, et al. Further experience with radiation therapy and concomitant intravenous chemotherapy in advanced carcinoma of the lower female genital tract. *Gynecol Oncol.* 1991;43(3):233–236.

56. Door A. Less common gynecologic malignancies. *Semin Oncol Nurs.* 2002;18(3):207–222.

57. Gould N, Kamelle S, Tillmanns T, et al. Predictors of complications after inguinal lymphadenectomy. *Gynecol Oncol.* 2001;82(2):329–332.

58. Guarnier C, Klemm PR. Vulvar and vaginal cancer. In: Yarbro CH, Frogge MH, Goodman M, Groenwald S, eds. *Cancer Nursing Principles and Practice.* 5th ed. Sudbury, MA: Jones and Bartlett; 2000:1511–1525.

59. Oonk MH, de Hullu JA, Hollema H, et al. The value of routine follow-up in patients treated for carcinoma of the vulva. *Cancer.* 2003;98(12):2624–2629.

Chapter 9

Gynecologic Sarcomas

Amber Door, RN, BSN, OCN®

Sarcomas are rare malignant tumors that can occur in all sites of the female genital tract but are most common in the uterus. Until recently, it was thought that uterine sarcomas represented approximately 2%–4% of all uterine malignancies.[1] The most recent Surveillance, Epidemiology, and End Results Program (SEER) analysis showed that from 1989–1999, approximately 8% of uterine malignancies were diagnosed as sarcomas.[2,3] A sarcoma is a malignant tumor arising from connective or stromal tissue. Sarcomas can be either pure, consisting of only malignant stoma (i.e., leiomyosarcoma [LMS], endometrial stromal sarcoma; see **Table 9-1**), or mixed, consisting of both malignant stromal and malignant epithelial tissue (i.e., carcinosarcoma, also known as malignant mixed mesodermal tumor or mixed müllerian tumor; see **Table 9-2**).

Because of the low incidence of these tumors, it has proven difficult even for large cooperative clinic trial groups to perform prospective studies to determine effective treatments for each tumor type. This also makes it difficult to interpret data regarding therapy and outcomes for individual histologic subtypes and disease sites. Surgery is used as the primary treatment modality for these rare tumors. Surgery can vary from a local excision, as in the case of some low-grade adenosarcomas, or it may require total abdominal hysterectomy, bilateral salpingoophorectomy, and extended staging. Current knowledge regarding adjuvant therapy is based on relatively small samples of patients or retrospective studies and in some cases includes mixed histology. This is problematic because the need for and type of further therapy is dependent upon the type of sarcoma encountered. Chemotherapy, radiation therapy, and hormonal therapy are all used in the treatment of sarcomas, but the true benefit of currently available treatments is still less than entirely clear in all uterine sarcomas.

Epidemiology/Risk Factors

The exact cause of gynecologic sarcomas is unknown. The triad of factors commonly associated with endometrial cancer, marked obesity, exogenous estrogen use, and nulliparity, have also been described as risk factors for uterine sarcoma, particularly

---

Table 9-1 Pure nonepithelial tumor classifications.

Endometrial stromal tumors
- Stromal nodule
- Low-grade stromal sarcoma
- High-grade stromal sarcoma

Smooth-muscle tumors
- Leiomyoma
- Cellular
- Epithelioid
- Bizarre (symplastic, pleomorphic)
- Lipoleiomyoma

Smooth-muscle tumor of uncertain malignant potential
- Leiomyosarcoma
- Epithelioid
- Myxoid

Other smooth-muscle tumors
- Metastasizing leiomyoma
- Intravenous leiomyomatosis
- Diffuse leiomyomatosis

Mixed endometrial stromal and smooth-muscle tumors
- Adenomatoid tumor

Other soft-tissue tumors (benign and malignant)
- Homologous
- Heterologous

Source: Reprinted with permission from Hoskins WJ, Perez CA, Young RC, eds. *Principles and Practice of Gynecologic Oncology.* 3rd ed. Philadelphia, PA: Lippincott Williams & Wilkins; 2000:962.

carcinosarcomas.[1,3,4] The use of tamoxifen has also been reported as a factor that increases the risk of developing a uterine sarcoma.[5] Race also is a risk factor for tumor development. SEER registries and other large retrospective reviews have consistently shown that the rate of both carcinosarcomas and leiomyosarcomas in black women are twice that of white women and more than twice that of women of other races.[2,6] The reason for this is not currently known.

The risk of developing a sarcoma varies by histology, with age being a factor. Carcinosarcomas are more prevalent in women over the age of 40 years and have the highest incidence in black women between the ages of 65 and 74 years. Uterine leiomyosarcomas occur at an earlier age than carcinosarcomas and have the highest incidence in women in their mid 50s.[1–3] Endometrial stromal sarcomas occur greater than 50% of the time in premenopausal women, with the median age range at diagnosis of 42–53 years.[7,8]

Table 9-2 MIXED EPITHELIAL-NONEPITHELIAL TUMOR CLASSIFICATION.

Benign
- Adenofibroma
- Adenomyoma
- Atypical polypoid adenomyoma

Malignant
- Adenosarcoma
- Homologous
- Heterologous

Carcinosarcoma (malignant mixed mesodermal tumor; malignant mixed müllerian tumor)
- Homologous
- Heterologous
- Carcinofibroma

Soure: Reprinted with permission from Hoskins WJ, Perez CA, Young RC, eds. *Principles and Practice of Gynecologic Oncology*. 3rd ed. Philadelphia, PA: Lippincott Williams & Wilkins; 2000:962.

The risk factor for the development of primary, mixed sarcomas (carcinosarcomas and adenosarcomas) that currently has the strongest evidence in the literature is a history of prior irradiation. Women who have a history of pelvic radiation, regardless of the reason for the treatment, have a higher incidence of uterine sarcoma. Sarcomas have been documented to develop in this patient population from 2–21 years posttreatment with incidences ranging from 0%–29%.[1,9,10]

Prevention/Detection

Because the specific etiology of gynecologic sarcoma development is not known, with the possible exception of prior radiation, there are no screening recommendations. Early detection, as with other malignancies, may be the key to improved survival.

Histology

The term "sarcoma" covers a wide variety of histologically unique tumors. In order of decreasing frequency, malignant uterine sarcomas are: carcinosarcomas (malignant mixed mesodermal tumor/malignant müllerian tumors/MMMT), leiomyosarcomas (LMS), endometrial stromal sarcomas, and müllerian adenosarcoma. Sarcomas are classified as either pure tumors or mixed tumors. A pure sarcoma is made up of only malignant mesenchymal tissue, such as leiomyosarcomas and endometrial stromal sarcomas. Mixed sarcomas have both malignant mesenchymal element and epithelial element, with the epithelial element being either benign or malignant. If the epithelial element of the tumor is malignant, the tumor is classified as a carcinosarcoma. If the epithelial element is benign, the tumor is classified as an adenosarcoma. Sarcomas are further classified as either homologous or heterologous. A homologous tumor is one that is comprised of tumor cells that would normally be found in the site of origin. A homologous sarcoma of the uterus would be a leiomyosarcoma, endometrial stromal sarcoma, adenosarcoma, or angiosarcoma.

A heterologous tumor would have features of tissue that are considered to be foreign to the site of origin. Thus, a chondrosarcoma (bone), rhabdomyosarcoma (muscle), or liposarcoma (fat) would be a heterologous sarcoma in the uterus. These heterologous tumors are rarely seen in the uterus in their pure form and are most frequently seen in mixed carcinosarcomas.[1,3,8]

Assessment

The majority of women, 77%–95% with uterine sarcomas, present with abnormal or postmenopausal bleeding.[1,3,8] Other potential presenting symptoms are pelvic/abdominal discomfort or pain associated with either a rapidly enlarging (doubling in 3–6 months or less) uterine mass, foul vaginal discharge, urinary and bowel changes, bone pain associated with bone metastasis, shortness of breath, or cough secondary to pleural effusions or lung metastasis.[1,11]

All women with abnormal uterine bleeding or postmenopausal bleeding should undergo evaluation for possible malignant etiology. When a malignant diagnosis is established, a two-view chest X-ray should be obtained to evaluate for lung lesions. Ultrasonography is widely used in the community setting to evaluate abnormal uterine bleeding. Although this may be helpful in detecting a uterine mass or fibroid, ultrasound cannot provide a pathologic diagnosis and should not take the place of or delay a pelvic examination and uterine sampling. Additionally, the use of magnetic resonance imaging (MRI), computed tomography (CT) scan, and nuclear medicine bone scans can be helpful, when the diagnosis is made, to evaluate for the presence of metastatic disease and assist in treatment planning both pre- and postoperatively.[12]

Diagnosis/Staging

The diagnosis of a gynecologic sarcoma, regardless of the primary site, is made following histologic evaluation of the tumor. In the case of uterine tumors that reside within the uterine cavity (endometrium), this would require, at minimum, an endometrial sampling or dilatation and curettage. In some cases, a patient will present after passing necrotic tissue or a viable tumor vaginally. For tumors that reside within the uterine wall (myometrium), obtaining tissue is more problematic. This is evidenced by the fact that a leiomyosarcoma is often found incidentally at the time of hysterectomy for what was thought to be symptomatic (pain, bleeding, or enlarging uterus) fibroids.[13] In young women, the tumor may be found at the time of a myomectomy, done for a presumed enlarging fibroid. In these cases, further surgery is warranted because the risk of residual tumor is high,[14] particularly if the resection was performed laparoscopically and/or the tumor was morcelated prior to removal.

Gynecologic sarcomas are surgically staged using the FIGO (International Federation of Gynecology and Obstetrics) staging for the site of origin (see specific disease site chapters for staging).

Primary Treatment

The standard treatment for uterine sarcomas involves surgical resection of the tumor. The extent of the surgery is dictated by the histology of the sarcoma. For some tumors, such as adenosarcomas, surgical resection may be the only treatment that is recommended. But, for the majority of sarcomas, surgical resections consist of total abdominal hysterectomy, bilateral salpingoophorectomy, lymph node dissection/sampling (per uterine staging), pelvic and upper abdominal washing, careful inspections of all peritoneal surfaces, and possible extended staging. Aggressive surgical debulking is not likely to influence disease outcome, yet it may provide palliation of pain and potential bowel obstruction.[1,3,15] Additionally, consideration should be given to having the tumor evaluated for estrogen and progesterone receptors[1] because this may provide the option of an adjuvant treatment with minimal side effects.

There are currently no guidelines or standards regarding the use of radiation therapy following the surgical resection and staging for uterine sarcomas. The use of pelvic radiation therapy to date has not been shown to improve overall survival, but it does seem to have an impact on local pelvic control and recurrence patterns.[16] Despite this lack of data, adjuvant pelvic radiation therapy is still recommended by clinicians based upon the information about patterns of relapse. Because of the propensity for intra-abdominal spread of disease, the role of whole abdominal radiation therapy in the adjuvant setting has been looked at for sarcomas.[17,18] The Gynecologic Oncology Group study comparing whole pelvic radiation therapy versus combination chemotherapy (ifosfamide and cisplatin), found that although there was no significant advantage in recurrence or survival when whole abdominal radiation therapy was compared to chemotherapy in women with stage I–IV uterine carcinosarcomas, the observed differences favor the use of combination chemotherapy in future trials.[18]

The use of systemic chemotherapy for sarcomas is appealing because of the high risk of recurrence (as high as 50% even in stage I disease),[19] in addition to the tendency for early distant metastases to the upper abdomen, liver, bone, and lungs. Yet again, because these tumors are often heterogeneous in nature and histologically unique, each should be looked at separately for response. Because of these factors and overall poor prognosis, a myriad of chemotherapeutic agents have undergone investigation in both carcinosarcomas and leiomyosarcomas because these are the most common gynecologic sarcomas that are encountered.

The active agents for carcinosarcomas include doxorubicin, ifosfamide, and cisplatin[20,21] with the highest response rate with single agent ifosfamide demonstrating a 35% response in the untreated patient.[21] Other agents, such as etoposide, aminothiadiazole, paclitaxel, and trimetrexate, have demonstrated minimal activity,[22–26] again as single agent treatment. Because of this, women should be encouraged to participate in ongoing clinical trials when they are eligible.

In the treatment of leiomyosarcomas, the active agents have been doxorubicin[27,28] and, to a lesser extent, ifosfamide[29] or a combination of the two drugs.[30] Gemcitabine has also demonstrated activity.[31] Most recently, data from the Gynecologic Oncology Group reports that the use of combination docetaxel and gemcitabine achieves a high response rate in front line therapy for metastatic disease.[32] The use of multiagent combinations in gynecologic sarcomas, using three to five drug regimens, have offered added toxicity and cost with minimal to no significant improvement in response or survival.[33–36] Further investigation is definitely needed, and issues, such as FDA-approved drug status for the disease being treated, impact how the aging population is to be treated in the future. Again, as in the case of carcinosarcomas, women with leiomyosarcomas should be encouraged to participate in clinical trials when they are eligible.

The use of a multimodal adjuvant therapy approach may provide benefit for some patients with advance uterine sarcoma. Utilizing both chemotherapy and whole pelvic radiation in a sequential manner has, in at least one retrospective review, shown to provide the highest median 5-year survival rate when compared with single modality adjuvant therapy.[37] Although it is suggested that further exploration of this combination treatment be undertaken, the rarity of the disease makes this a difficult endeavor.

Hormonal therapy has not been evaluated extensively in the treatment of mesenchymal tumors of the uterus, but estrogen receptors and progesterone receptors have been found to be present in a mixed group of uterine sarcomas that have been tested.[38,39] The knowledge regarding the presence or absence of hormone receptors in an individual tumor may provide the clinician and patient the option of a relatively nontoxic treatment option in a group of malignancies where a true standard of adjuvant care does not yet exist. The sarcoma that may be impacted most significantly by hormonal therapy is low-grade endometrial stromal sarcoma (LGESS). LGESS has been shown to have high levels of both estrogen and progesterone receptors leading to the recommendation of ovarian resection in this population.[1] It has also been suggested that progestin therapy be routinely considered as adjuvant therapy because of the high risk of recurrence in women who are given estrogen replacement following surgical resection.[40]

Recurrent Disease

There is currently no standard treatment for recurrent uterine sarcomas. In some cases of low-grade tumors, further surgical excision may extend survival but does not offer a cure. When eligible, patients should be encouraged to participate in ongoing clinical trials to further define the role of emerging therapies and new chemotherapeutic agents.

Symptom Management/ Nursing Implications

Gynecologic sarcomas can be highly aggressive tumors and carry poor prognosis even in early stages. Because there is currently no standard adjuvant therapy, particularly in the face of advanced or recurrent sarcomas, the primary nursing goal should be quality of life. Since the individual defines quality of life, it is critical that each patient's definition be assessed. This will assist in caring for the patient and her support system throughout the course of her disease.

To determine how the disease and subsequent treatments will impact the quality of life for the patient, education regarding the nature of the disease along with the current knowledge regarding adjuvant treatment, in addition to the expected response, is necessary for the patient and her support system to make an informed decision. The information that is provided may be overwhelming and will require reinforcement with further review at subsequent visits as the patient and her support persons process the information and formulate questions. Because gynecologic sarcomas are rare tumors, patients should be offered treatment on clinical trial if they meet entry criteria. Because the majority of clinical trials for gynecologic sarcomas are Phase II studies that look at agents that have not yet been proven to be beneficial for their disease, the decision to enter a treatment regimen out of her and her physician's control can be fraught with uncertainty for a patient who is facing a new or recurrent cancer diagnosis. Nurses have a key role in assuring that the information provided is understandable and that the desires of the patient are understood and respected by all the members of the healthcare team, as well as the members of her support system.

Because of the propensity of gynecologic sarcoma to metastasize, the signs and symptoms of metastasis to the distant sites, such as the lung, peritoneal cavity, vagina, liver, skin, bone, subcutaneous tissue, and brain should be reviewed (see **Table 9-3**). An assessment of all potential sites of metastasis should be made at each encounter. Further education regarding management of symptoms as they present will be required. This may require potential referrals for palliative treatments of bone metastasis, chemotherapy, pain management, and hospice care.

Table 9-3 SIGNS AND SYMPTOMS OF RECURRENT SARCOMA.

	Signs and Symptoms of Disease Recurrence/Metastasis
Lung	Shortness of breath Cough Hemoptysis Chest discomfort/pain
Peritoneal cavity	Increased abdominal girth Early satiety Abdominal pain/discomfort Change in bowel function Nausea/vomiting Bowel obstruction
Vagina	Vaginal bleeding Vaginal pain/discomfort Dyspareunia
Liver	Upper abdominal pain Early satiety Upper abdominal mass Nausea/vomiting Abnormal liver functions Jaundice
Bone	Pain Bone fracture
Skin/subcutaneous tissue	New palpable mass Pain
Brain	Neurologic change Headache

Conclusion

Although the women who are diagnosed with gynecologic sarcomas present many challenges to the healthcare team, nurses have the ability to educate and promote quality of life for patients throughout the course of their disease. Because these tumors are infrequent and can occur in all areas of the female genital tract, although they most commonly occur in the uterus, nurses require knowledge regarding the specific malignant process that is diagnosed. This is essential to effectively provide the intensive education, as well as timely and offensive symptom management, that is likely to be required for the patient, support system, and other healthcare professionals who are involved in the care of the individual patient.

References

1. Sutton G, Kavanagh JJ, Wolfson A, et al. Corpus: mesenchymal tumors. In: Hoskins WJ, Perez CA, Young RC, et al, eds. *Principles and Practice of Gynecologic Oncology*. 4th ed. Philadelphia, PA: Lippincott Williams & Wilkins; 2005:873–894.

2. Brooks SE, Zhan M, Cote T, et al. Surveillance, epidemiology, and end results analysis of 2677 cases of uterine sarcoma 1989–1999. *Gynecol Oncol*. 2004;93(1):204–208.

3. DiSaia DJ, Creasman WJ. Sarcoma of the uterus. In: *Clinical Gynecologic Oncology*. 7th ed. St. Louis, MO: Mosby; 2007:185–199.

4. Zelmanowicz A, Hildesheim A, Sherman ME, et al. Evidence for a common etiology for endometrial carcinomas and malignant mixed müllerian tumors. *Gynecol Oncol*. 1998;69(3):253–257.

5. Lavie O, Barnett-Griness SA, Narod SA, Rennert G. The risk of developing uterine sarcoma after tamoxifen use. *Int J Gynecol Cancer*. 2008;18(2):352–356.

6. Harlow BL, Weiss NS, Lofton S. The epidemiology of sarcomas of the uterus. *J Natl Cancer Inst*. 1986;76(3):399–402.

7. Chang LK, Crabtree GS, Lim-Tan SK, et al. Primary uterine endometrial stromal neoplasms. A clinicopathologic study of 117 cases. *Am J Surg Path*. 1990;15(5):415–438.

8. Anciaux D, Lawrence WD. Malignant uterine tumors. In: Shingleton HM, Fowler WC, Jordan JA, Lawrence WD, eds. *Gynecologic Oncology Current Diagnosis and Treatment*. London: WB Saunders; 1996:130–145.

9. Norris HJ, Taylor HB. Post irradiation sarcomas of the uterus. *Obstet Gynecol*. 1965;26(5):689–694.

10. Meredith RF, Eiser DR, Kaka Z, et al. An excess of uterine sarcomas after pelvic irradiation. *Cancer*. 1986;58(9):2003–2007.

11. Salazar OM, Bonfiglio TA, Patten SF, et al. Uterine sarcomas: natural history, treatment and prognosis. *Cancer*. 1978;42(3):1152–1160.

12. Page JE, Constant O, Parsons C. The role of abdominal computed tomography in the assessment of patients with malignant tumours of the cervix and body of the uterus. *Clin Radiol*. 1988;39(3):273–277.

13. Leibsohn S, d'Ablaing G, Mishell DR Jr, et al. Leiomyosarcoma in a series of hysterectomies performed for presumed uterine leiomyomas. *Am J Obstet Gynecol*. 1990;162(4):968–974.

14. Berchuck A, Rubin SC, Hoskins WJ, et al. Treatment on endometrial stromal tumors. *Gynecol Oncol*. 1990;36(1):60–65.

15. Peters WA 3rd, Kumar NB, Fleming WP, et al. Prognostic features of sarcomas and mixed tumors of the endometrium. *Obstet Gynecol*. 1984;63(4):550–556.

16. Omura GA, Blessing JA, Major FJ, et al. A randomized clinical trial of adjuvant adriamycin in uterine sarcomas: a Gynecologic Oncology Group study. *J Clin Oncol*. 1985;3(9):1240–1254.

17. Loeffler JS, Rosen EM, Niloff JM, et al. Whole abdominal irradiation for tumors of the uterine corpus. *Cancer*. 1988;61(7):1332–1335.

18. Wolfson AH, Brady MF, Rocereto TF, et al. A Gynecologic Oncology Group randomized trial of whole abdominal irradiation (WAI) vs cisplatin—ifosfamide+mesna (CIM) as post-surgical therapy in Stage I-IV carcinosarcoma (CS) of the uterus [abstract]. *Gynecol Oncol*. 2007;107(2):177–185.

19. Major FJ, Blessing JA, Silverberg SG, et al. Prognostic factors in early-stage uterine sarcoma: a Gynecologic Oncology Group study. *Cancer*. 1993;71(suppl 4):1702–1709.

20. Omura GA, Major FJ, Blessing JA, et al. A randomized clinical trial of adriamycin with and

without dimethyl triazenoimidazole carboxamide in advanced uterine sarcomas. *Cancer*. 1983;52(4): 626–632.

21. Sutton GP, Blessing JA, Homesley HD, et al. A phase II trial of ifosfamide and mesna in patients with advanced or recurrent mixed mesodermal tumors of the ovary previously treated with platinum-based chemotherapy: a Gynecologic Oncology Group study. *Gynecol Oncol*. 1994;53(1):24–26.

22. Slayton RE, Blessing JA, Angel C, et al. Phase II trial of etoposide in the management of advanced and recurrent leiomyosarcomas of the uterus: a Gynecologic Oncology Group study. *Cancer Treat Rep*. 1987;71(12):1303–1304.

23. Currie JL, Blessing JA, McGehee R, et al. Phase II trial of hydroxyurea, dacarbazine (DTIC), and etoposide (VP-16) in mixed mesodermal tumors of the uterus: a Gynecologic Oncology Group study. *Gynecol Oncol*. 1996;61(1):94–96.

24. Fowler JM, Blessing JA, Burger RA, et al. Phase II evaluation of oral trimetrexate in mixed mesodermal tumors of the uterus: a Gynecologic Oncology Group study. *Gynecol Oncol*. 2002;85(2):311–314.

25. Smith HO, Blessing JA, Vaccarello L. Trimetrexate in the treatment of recurrent or advanced leiomyosarcomas of the uterus: a phase II study of the Gynecologic Oncology Group. *Gynecol Oncol*. 2003;84(1): 140–144.

26. Curtain JP, Blessing JA, Soper JT, et al. Paclitaxel in the treatment of carcinosarcomas of the uterus: a Gynecologic Oncology Group study. *Gynecol Oncol*. 2001;83(2):268–270.

27. Rose PG, Boutselis JG, Sachs L. Adjuvant therapy for stage I uterine sarcoma. *Am J Obstet Gynecol*. 1987;156(3):660–662.

28. Hannigan EV, Freedman RS, Elder KW, et al. Treatment of advanced uterine sarcoma with adriamycin. *Gynecol Oncol*. 1983;16(1):101–104.

29. Sutton GP, Blessing JA, Barrett RJ, et al. Phase II trial of ifosfamide and mesna in leiomyosarcoma of the uterus: a Gynecologic Oncology Group study. *Am J Obstet Gynecol*. 1992;166(2):556–559.

30. Sutton G, Blessing JA, Malfetano JH. Ifosfamide and doxorubicin in the treatment of advanced leiomyosarcomas of the uterus: a Gynecologic Oncology Group study. *Gyn Onc*. 1996;62(2): 226–229.

31. Look KY, Sandler A, Blessing JA, et al. Phase II trial of gemcitabine as second-line chemotherapy of uterine leiomyosarcoma: a Gynecologic Oncology Group study. *Gynecol Oncol*. 2004;92(2):644–647.

32. Hensley ML, Blessing JA, Mannel R, Rose PG. Fixed-dose gemcitabine plus docetaxel as first line therapy for metastatic uterine leiomyosarcoma: a Gynecologic Oncology Group study. *Gynecol Oncol*. 2008;109(3):329–334.

33. Pearl ML, Inagami M, McCauley DL, et al. Mesna, doxorubicin, ifosfamide, and dacarbazine (MAID) chemotherapy for gynecologic sarcomas. *Int J Gynecol Cancer*. 2002;12(6):745–748.

34. Pautier P, Genestie C, Fizazi K, et al. Cisplatin based chemotherapy regimen (DECAV) for uterine sarcomas. *Int J Gynecol Cancer*. 2002;12(6):749–754.

35. Edmonson JH, Blessing JA, Cosin JA, et al. Phase II study of mitomycin, doxorubicin, and cisplatin in the treatment of advanced uterine leiomyosarcomas: a Gynecologic Oncology Group study. *Gynecol Oncol*. 2002;85(3):507–510.

36. Sutton GP, Brunetto VL, Kilgore L, et al. Phase III trial of ifosfamide with or without cisplatin in carcinosarcoma of the uterus: a Gynecologic Oncology Group study. *Gynecol Oncol*. 2000;79(2):147–153.

37. Menczner J, Levy T, Piura B, et al. A comparison between different postoperative treatment modalities of uterine sarcoma. *Gynecol Oncol*. 2005;97(1): 166–170.

38. Sutton GP, Stehman F, Michael H, et al. Estrogen and progesterone receptors in uterine sarcomas. *Obstet Gynecol*. 1986;68(5):709–714.

39. Ansink AC, Cross PA, Scorer P, et al. The hormone receptor status of uterine carcinosarcomas (mixed müllerian tumours): an immunohistochemical study. *J Clin Pathol*. 1997;50(4):328–331.

40. Chu MC, Mor G, Lim C, et al. Low-grade endometrial stromal sarcoma: hormonal aspects. *Gynecol Oncol*. 2003;90(1):170–176.

Chapter 10

Cancer Genetics

Sheri Babb, MS, CGC

Judith A. Parham, RN, MSN

Introduction

Advances in molecular biology and genomics are greatly impacting the practice of medicine. As a result of the Human Genome Project, we are now able to map human genetic makeup. This information, along with improved computer technology, has allowed us to explore the genetic makeup of cancer.[1,2]

Cancer, uncontrolled cell growth, can be attributed to a breakdown in the genetic material of our body. Genetic changes may be inherited or acquired. Either way, cancer is the result of a failure of DNA to replicate reliably, resulting in a malfunction of our genetic checks and balances, that leads to cell mutation and unregulated cell reproduction.

Approximately 10% of all cancers are believed to be due to inherited cancer predisposition genes.[3] Inherited conditions are due to genetic alterations passed on to offspring from one or both parents.[4] These genetic alterations can cause a precancerous condition, cancer, or a susceptibility to environmental agents that can result in a cancer.[3] BRCA1 and BRCA2 are examples of genes associated with hereditary cancer predisposition. Mutations in these genes

are estimated to increase a woman's lifetime risk of developing ovarian cancer to between 15%–40%.[5]

Acquired genetic alterations account for the majority of cancers. Alterations can be acquired as a result of an environmental exposure. This could be from exposure to radiation, certain viruses, or chemicals resulting in DNA damage.[6]

In this chapter we will review normal cell biology, the biology of cancer, hereditary gynecologic cancer syndromes, genetic risk assessment, genetic counseling, and the nurse's role in cancer genetics.

Normal Cell Biology—Basic Cell Components

The human cell is made up of three core components: cell membrane, cytoplasm, and nucleus. The cell membrane is the outer boundary of a cell, providing support and regulation for the transport of substances in and out of the cell. Cytoplasm is the liquid substance inside the cell membrane. The nucleus is inside the cytoplasm and contains deoxyribonucleic acid (DNA). DNA guides protein synthesis within the cell and contains the body's genetic material.[3,7]

Figure 10-1 A DNA molecule.

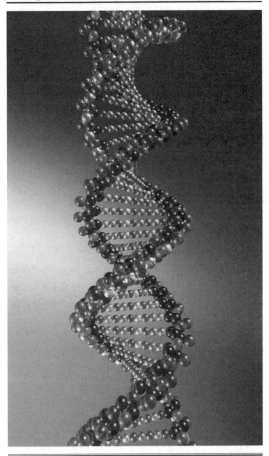

Figure 10-2 Chromosome 17.

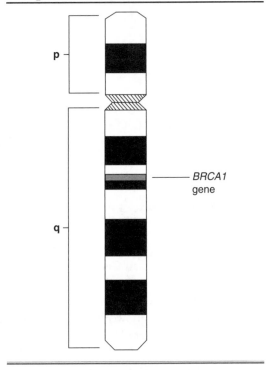

Source: From Loescher, #7.

DNA is a large, complex, double-helix molecule consisting of antiparallel strands of nucleotides (see Figure 10-1). Nucleotides are made of a phosphoric acid, a sugar (deoxyribose), and a nitrogenous base. The backbone of DNA is made of a sugar and phosphoric acid. Nitrogenous bases compose the stranding, or steps, between the backbones. Bases consist of cytosine and thymine (pyrimidine bases) and guanine and adenine (purine bases). These bases, abbreviated as C, T, G, and A, form the genetic alphabet. Adenine on one side of the double helix links to thymine on the parallel side. Guanine and cytosine link to each other. This is known as base pairing. The order in which the bases are arranged along one side of the helix backbone is called DNA sequence. Two sides of the DNA are held together by weak hydrogen bonds. The weak bonding enables the DNA to be easily separated into single strands for the process of replication.[3,7,8]

Chromosomes are composed of a large DNA molecule and other proteins. There are 23 pairs of chromosomes in the human species. One chromosome of each pair is inherited from the mother, the other from the father. Each chromosome has an individual appearance, by means of size, staining qualities, or morphologic characteristics. They have a short (p) and a long (q) segment divided by a constricted area (centromere). Each chromosome has a specific banding pattern (see Figure 10-2). The ends of the chromosomes are referred to as telomeres. Telomeres are felt to have a role in cell aging.[3] Chromosomes are found in the nucleus of the cell. The human genome, the genetic blueprint of a human, is contained in these 23 pairs of chromosomes.[7]

Genes are small molecules within the DNA that consist of sequences of nucleotides that code for specific proteins. Genes are the core units of inherited information. Each gene may contain as many as 1000 pairs for nucleotides and have a specific location on a specific chromosome. Because one chromosome of each paired chromosome is acquired from each parent, there may be an alternate form of genes (alleles) in the pair. If both paired chromosomes have the same alleles, the person is homozygous for that trait. If the paired chromosomes have different alleles, the person is considered to be heterozygous for that trait.

Gene Expression

Gene expression is the process of protein synthesis, which is comprised of two steps: transcription and translation. DNA stores the genetic code for proteins. Codons consist of triplets of bases that specify sequencing of amino acids for certain proteins. There are 64 possible codons, of which 61 are codons for amino acids and three are stop codons.[9]

In the translation process, the DNA double strand loosens and unwinds. The codon for the protein being synthesized is attached to ribonucleic acid (RNA) and replicated, creating messenger RNA (mRNA). This occurs in the nucleus of the cell. The mRNA, which contains a copy of the instructions to create the protein, then moves out into the cytoplasm to signal the next step in protein synthesis: translocation. In the cytoplasm, the mRNA attaches to ribosomes. Transfer RNA, ribosomal RNA, and enzymes then work to produce sequenced chains of amino acids to form proteins[6,7] (see Figure 10-3).

Figure 10-3 Gene expression in the human cell.

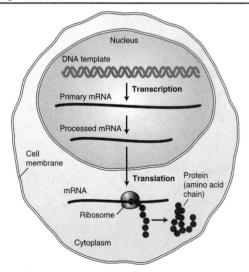

Source: From Loescher, #17.

When errors occur in this process, the result can be genetic mutations. These mutations can lead to alterations in growth, reproduction, and cell death.

Cell Life Cycle

Normal cell reproduction is an orderly process of steps with numerous checks and balances to ensure accuracy of replication. G0 is the inactive stage or resting stage. In the synthesis (S) phase, the DNA is replicated and the chromosomes are duplicated. During gap2 (G2), the cell prepares for mitosis (M). In the M phase, the chromosomes and other cell components segregate to create two daughter cells, each with a full complement of chromosomes. This process is called cytokinesis. The cells then proceed to the gap1 (G1) phase, when the cell prepares to divide again or leave the cycle to differentiate. Throughout this process cell growth is occurring, usually in response to growth signals. Checkpoints are in place during this process to identify replication errors and to give proliferative and antiproliferative signals.[4,7] Pauses may occur in the G1 or G2 phases to allow repair enzymes to correct genetic information, thereby preventing genetically damaged cells from proceeding to duplication.[7]

Cancer Biology—Carcinogenesis Stages

The mechanism by which a normal cell develops into a malignant cell can simply be described as "cell replication gone awry."[10] It is the result of two or more events or exposures that led to cancer development.[2,6,7,11] This process can be described as "stages of carcinogenesis."

1. *Initiation*: Initiation is the genetic mutation within a single cell. This may be an inherited mutation or a somatic (acquired) mutation. Most are somatic. Not all initiated cells will develop into an active cancer. The body's normal checks and balances will destroy some mutated cells, while others will remain in a nonneoplastic state. The time frame for an initiated cell to develop into a detectable tumor is highly variable.

2. *Promotion*: The initiated cells gain a selective growth advantage. This happens as a result of a random error during cell division or as the result of exposures to a carcinogen. If this error goes uncorrected, cells will continue to mutate and multiply in the carcinogenic pathway.

3. *Progression*: The carcinogenic characteristics of the cells become irreversible. Rapid, continuous cell division occurs, and genetic mutations continue to occur.

4. *Metastasis*: Cancerous cells separate from the primary tumor and attach to new tissue sites. Not all metastatic cells successfully attach in a new location. Those that successfully attach in a new location will multiply and create new tumors at that site.

Checkpoint Alterations

The cellular signal transduction pathway is the method by which cells are given signals to replicate. There are many steps in this pathway, involving numerous genes and leaving room for error to occur. As mentioned earlier, there are several checkpoints in cell replication where mutations can be identified and corrected or disposed of. A variety of genes are involved in this regulatory system: proto-oncogenes, tumor suppressor genes, DNA-repair genes, and apoptosis genes. An alteration in the performance of these genes can have major effects on the function and integrity of the cell.[2,6,7,11]

Proto-oncogenes act as regulated cell growth promoters. Oncogenes are mutations of proto-oncogenes caused by changes in gene structure or changes in gene expression regulation.[6] Oncogenes typically occur at the somatic level. A single mutation in a proto-oncogene, resulting in an oncogene, can cause unregulated cell growth, causing overproduction. Proto-oncogenes are located at various points in the signaling pathway and perform specific functions at each location. Major classifications of proto-oncogenes are as follows:

1. *Growth factors*: Most growth factors are extracellular. They have an important role in the mediation of cell proliferation, differentiation, and survival.[9] They send a signal across the cell membrane, initiating the signal transduction pathway. Mutations of these proto-oncogens cause constant stimulation of adjacent cells to multiply.

2. *Growth factor receptors*: Many growth factor receptors are tyrosine kinases located in the cell membrane. They bind to growth factors to initiate the transduction pathway. Mutations in growth factor receptors result in overproduction of receptors. Cellular response is to continually divide until no available receptors are present. Examples include HER2 and EGFR. Overexpression of HER2 is found in 25% to 30% of breast cancers.[7] It has also been found to be overexpressed in some ovarian cancer tumors.[8] EGFR has been found to be overexpressed in breast and ovarian cancers and in some squamous cancers of the cervix.[7,11]

3. *Cytoplasmic tyrosine kinases*: Cytoplasmic tyrosine kinases are intracellular messengers of growth signals that do not require a receptor. They are located in the cytoplasm or nucleus. Examples are the SRC and ABL genes. SRC activity is increased in breast adenocarcinoma. Mutated messenger genes can give misinformation to the nucleus, resulting in enhanced growth and proliferation.[7,11]

4. *Signal transducers*: Signal transducers are found on the inner membrane of the cell and act as messengers for the cell-surface growth-factor receptors. RAS is the most common signal transducer. Mutations of RAS result in cell proliferation, even when not initiated by a growth factor receptor.

5. *Nuclear transcription factors*: Nuclear transcription factors are proteins at the end of the signaling pathway that bind to DNA. Mutations in transcription factors can drive the malignant process by perpetuating cell growth independent of extracellular factors.[7,11]

Tumor Suppressor Genes

Tumor suppressor genes act as negative regulatory controllers of cell division by encoding proteins that inhibit the action of growth-promoting proteins. It is when this negative regulatory mechanism is impaired that a malignant process is allowed to proceed.[10] Suppressor genes are frequently mutated or missing in cancer patients.[1] Both tumor suppressor alleles must be inactivated to result in deregulated cell growth. The initial inactivation of a tumor suppressor allele can happen at the germline or somatic level. The second allele inactivation occurs at the somatic level.[11]

The tumor suppressor gene TP53 is one of the most studied suppressor genes. Mutations or deletions of TP53 are found in a variety of cancers, including breast and ovarian cancer.[2] Functions include control of the cell cycle, initiation of apoptosis (cell death), and maintenance of the genome integrity. If DNA damage is identified, cell cycle arrest will be initiated to allow for DNA repair. If DNA repair is not possible, apoptosis is induced by TP53.[11]

Other tumor suppressor genes associated with increased risk for breast and ovarian cancer are BRCA1 and BRCA2. BRCA1 and BRCA2 also seem to have a role in DNA repair. The scientific community continues to define the role of hereditary cancer predisposition genes that could be used to develop new prevention and treatment options for hereditary cancer.[12]

DNA-Repair Genes

DNA-repair genes are not part of cell–regulatory pathways; rather they prevent genetic instability.[2] Their major function is identification and repair of DNA nucleotide errors. Inactivation of these genes will lead to a less effective repair system, resulting in an accumulation of DNA errors. If these errors occur in proto-oncogenes or tumor suppressor genes, cancer can develop. The DNA-repair genes, therefore, have an indirect role in tumorgenesis.[11]

Mismatch repair genes have the function of correcting DNA errors occurring during replication. At numerous places in the genome, there are sequences of DNA nucleotide repeats called microsatellite DNA. Such sequences appear to be susceptible to errors during DNA replication. Defective mismatch repair genes can result in "stutters" of the microsatellite DNA, leading to altered lengths of repeated DNA sequences or microsatellite instability.[11]

MLH1, MSH2, MSH6, and PMS2 are examples of DNA mismatch repair genes. Mutations of these genes are associated with Lynch syndrome, also known as hereditary nonpolyposis colorectal cancer (HNPCC). Individuals with Lynch syndrome are at greater risk for developing colorectal and endometrial cancer, as well as a variety of other cancers. MSH6 mutation has been shown to be associated with 1.6% of endometrial cancers.[13]

Hereditary Cancer

Approximately 10% of all cancers are due to hereditary factors. Conversely, this means that 90% of all cancers occur sporadically or by chance. Oncology health professionals can take the lead in identifying individuals and families at increased risk for hereditary cancer. The goal is to begin thinking of the *possibility* of hereditary cancer risk when an individual presents with gynecologic cancer and a personal or family history of benign or malignant tumors associated with particular hereditary syndromes.

The purpose of this section is to: (1) review the indications of hereditary cancer and five hereditary syndromes that include gynecologic cancer, (2) discuss the importance of obtaining an accurate cancer family history for risk assessment and medical management, and (3) discuss general strategies for genetic counseling and genetic testing in hereditary cancer families.

Indications of hereditary cancer when reviewing cancer family history include:[14]

1. Early age of onset of cancer as compared to the general population
2. Multiple primary cancer diagnoses in one individual

3. Bilateral cancers
4. Presence of rare tumor
5. Multiple generations affected
6. Physical features suggestive of particular hereditary cancer syndrome

Hereditary Cancer Predisposition Syndromes Associated with Gynecologic Cancers

Gynecologic cancer is present in a multitude of hereditary cancer syndromes. Our understanding of the specific types of tumors associated with different hereditary cancer syndromes is evolving. **Table 10-1** provides a summary of the cancers associated with the hereditary cancer syndromes presented in this chapter. The two most common hereditary cancer syndromes that predispose to gynecologic malignancies are hereditary breast and ovarian cancer (HBOC) and Lynch syndrome. Other rare syndromes that include gynecologic cancer as part of the tumor spectrum are introduced in this chapter but are not covered in detail.

Lynch Syndrome

Lynch syndrome accounts for approximately 2% all colorectal cancers.[15,16] Colon and uterine cancer (endometrial) are the most common types of cancer in families with Lynch syndrome.[17] The term "nonpolyposis" is used to describe the fact that individuals with Lynch syndrome typically have few colon polyps as compared to individuals with the familial adenomatous polyposis (FAP) syndrome, who have multiple polyps throughout the colon.[18] Other cancers associated with Lynch syndrome include ovarian, stomach, urinary tract, small bowel, hepatobiliary, and brain.[19–21]

Table 10-1 HEREDITARY CANCER SYNDROMES THAT INCLUDE GYNECOLOGIC CANCER.

Hereditary Syndrome	Most Common Associated Cancers
Hereditary nonpolyposis colon cancer	Primarily colorectal and endometrial cancer. Also ovarian, urinary tract, stomach, small bowel, hepatobiliary tract, and brain cancer.
Hereditary breast/ovarian cancer	Primarily breast and ovarian cancer. Possible associations with small increased risk for other cancers.
Li-Fraumeni syndrome	Primarily osteosarcoma; soft tissue sarcomas; breast, brain, and adrenocortical carcinoma; and acute leukemia. Later reports suggest association with other cancer sites, including ovary and gonadal germ cell tumors.
Peutz-Jeghers	Cancer associations include: gastrointestinal, pancreas, breast, ovarian, uterine, cervix, testicular, and gallbladder cancer. Benign ovarian sex cord tumor is also seen.
Cowden syndrome	Primarily breast, thyroid, and endometrial cancer.

Table 10-2 LIFETIME CANCER RISKS IN HNPCC.

Type of cancer	Persons with HNPCC (%)	General Population (%)
Colorectal	80%–82%	5%–6%
Endometrial (women)	50%–60%	2%–3%
Gastric	13%	1%
Ovarian (women)	12%	1%–2%
Small bowel	1%–4%	0.01%
Bladder	4%	1%–3%
Brain	4%	0.6%
Kidney, renal, pelvis	3%	1%
Biliary tract	2%	0.6%

Source: From {Chung, 2003 #28} with permission.

Lifetime risks for cancer in individuals with Lynch syndrome as compared to the general population are shown in **Table 10-2**.

The mean age of onset of colorectal cancer in Lynch syndrome families is 45 years of age, with approximately two-thirds occurring in the ascending colon or right side of the colon.[22]

Prior to the availability of clinical genetic testing, diagnosis of Lynch syndrome was based upon family history assessment only. Specific diagnostic criteria were published in 1991 and are referred to as the Amsterdam Criteria.[23] Revised Amsterdam Criteria (Amsterdam II) were published in 1999 to include the extra-colonic cancers associated with HNPCC.[21] The Amsterdam I and Amsterdam II criteria are shown in **Table 10-3**.

Cancer surveillance guidelines have been published for individuals with Lynch syndrome.[24–27] People with Lynch syndrome tend to develop cancers earlier than the general population, and cancer screening is recommended at younger ages than for individuals at average risk. It is recommended that full colonoscopy begin at age 20 to 25 years (or 10 years younger than the youngest diagnosis in the family) and be repeated every 1 to 2 years. Additional screening that is recommended for individuals from Lynch syndrome families includes annual trans-vaginal ultrasound of the uterus and ovaries, and endometrial sampling starting at age 30 to 35 years (or 5–10 years younger than the earliest age of diagnosis of these cancers in the family) and annual CA 125 along with transvaginal ultrasound to screen for ovarian cancer; consideration of annual urinalysis and blood tests for liver function to screen for urinary tract and hepatobiliary cancers; and upper endoscopy to screen for gastric cancer. Continued research, ongoing clinical trials, and long-term follow-up of hereditary cancer families are needed to gain knowledge regarding the efficacy of cancer surveillance and prevention options for the other cancers associated with Lynch syndrome.[26] Prophylactic hysterectomy and bilateral salpingo-oophorectomy is a

---

Table 10-3 AMSTERDAM I AND AMSTERDAM II CRITERIA.

Amsterdam I Criteria

Three or more relatives with histologically verified colorectal cancer:
    One must be a first-degree relative to the other two
    Two or more generations affected with colorectal cancer
    One or more diagnosed with colorectal cancer at less than 50 years old
    Familial adenomatous polyposis must have been excluded

Amsterdam II Criteria

Three or more relatives with colorectal or HNPCC-associated cancer (endometrial, ovarian, stomach, hepatobiliary, small bowel, brain, and transitional cell carcinoma of the renal pelvis or ureter):
    One must be a first-degree relative to the other two
    Two or more generations affected with an HNPCC-associated cancer
    One or more HNPCC-associated cancer diagnosed at less than 50 years old
    Familial adenomatous polyposis must have been excluded

Source: From {Vasen, 1991 #23;Vasen, 1999, #21}.

risk-reducing option for women who have completed childbearing.[24–27]

Lynch syndrome is inherited as an autosomal dominant condition with incomplete penetrance. This means an individual with a germline mutation has a 50% chance of passing that mutation on to each child, but not all individuals who inherit a mutation for Lynch syndrome will develop cancer. Lynch syndrome is caused by inherited mutations in DNA mismatch repair genes, most commonly MSH2, MLH1, or MSH6.[22,28,29] These genes are involved in correcting errors of DNA replication. MLH1 and MSH2 account for approximately 90% of all mutations identified in families with HNPCC.[18] Families with MSH6 mutation often present with a different clinical picture than MLH1 or MSH2 families, with a greater association with endometrial cancer.[30,31]

Clinically, there are several strategies to help establish a diagnosis of Lynch syndrome. One approach is to obtain a blood sample from an individual suspected to have Lynch syndrome and perform gene sequence studies of MSH2, MLH1, and MSH6. However, a mutation cannot be identified in some families even when they meet Amsterdam Criteria. Therefore, absence of a known mutation does not necessarily rule out hereditary cancer.

A second approach used for clinical genetic testing for someone suspected of having Lynch syndrome is to "screen" the colon or endometrial tumor for microsatellite instability (MSI) and the presence of the proteins made by the genes with a test called immunohistochemistry (IHC).[15,32,33] Tumors can be tested for the expression of a mutation in mismatch repair genes by looking at small repetitive genetic sequences throughout the DNA called microsatellites that are prone to errors during DNA replication. In Lynch syndrome, the MSI occurs because the inherited defective gene is not working and cannot fix an error during DNA replication, resulting in an accumulation of areas of genetic instability called microsatellite instability (MSI).[34] Colon tumors in families with Lynch syndrome express MSI approximately 90% of the time, while sporadic colon tumors express MSI approximately 10%–15% of the time.[34,35] In sporadic endometrial tumors, high MSI occurs approximately 20% of the time, mostly because a mismatched repair gene (MLH1) is chemically silenced or methylated.[36] Research is ongoing to assess the relationship between MSI in extracolonic tumors in HNPCC and underlying germline defects in mismatch repair genes.

IHC looks for the presence of the proteins made by MSH2, MLH1, MSH6, and PMS2. The absence of a particular protein suggests there is a mutation within that specific gene, thus guiding the decision for gene sequencing of that particular gene only. A tumor that shows high MSI due to methylation of the MLH1 protein will have absent MLH1 with the IHC testing, but this is not associated with hereditary disease because the methylation shuts down the protein production. Both MSI and IHC are available for clinical studies through several commercial and academic laboratories. Research and discussion in the literature continue to determine the best strategy to identify patients at risk for Lynch syndrome and to define the optimal cancer surveillance and prevention options.[15,26,32,33]

Hereditary Breast and Ovarian Cancer Syndrome

Hereditary breast and ovarian cancer syndrome (HBOC) primarily predisposes an individual to breast and ovarian cancer. The majority of families with hereditary breast and/or ovarian cancer are believed to have mutations in either Breast Cancer Gene 1 (BRCA1) or Breast Cancer Gene 2 (BRCA2).[37]

The lifetime risk of breast cancer in a woman with a BRCA1 or BRCA2 mutation ranges from 45% to 87%, and the lifetime risk of ovarian cancer in a woman with a BRCA1 or BRCA2 mutation ranges from 16% to 60%, depending upon the population studied.[24,37–40] For women who have already had breast cancer, the lifetime chance of developing a second breast cancer is significantly increased. Cancer risks and subsequent medical management primarily focus on cancer of the breast and ovary for BRCA mutation carriers. Research continues to define the spectrum of tumors and lifetime risks associated with BRCA mutations. Data has shown increased risk for male breast cancer, prostate cancer, melanoma, and pancreatic cancer, with possible small increased risks for other cancers.[39,40]

A critical review published in 2004 provides criteria based upon family history to identify individuals and families that would benefit from cancer risk assessment services.[41] The 2008 NCCN Practice Guidelines present diagnostic criteria for HBOC. Published diagnostic criteria rely on either a known mutation in the family or a significant personal and family history of breast and ovarian cancer. In general, the criteria to warrant referral for cancer risk assessment include a member of a family with a known BRCA mutation; personal history of breast cancer or ovarian cancer and Ashkenazi Jewish ancestry; personal history of breast or ovarian cancer with close male blood relative with breast cancer; personal history of early onset breast cancer and/or ovarian cancer; personal history of breast or ovarian cancer and two or more relatives on the same side of the family with breast or ovarian cancer; three or more relatives on the same side of the family with breast and/or ovarian cancer; and two or more cases of ovarian cancer in first- or second-degree relatives on the same side of the family.

Medical management for BRCA mutation carriers includes recommendations for surveillance and prevention of breast and ovarian cancer.[38,42] **Table 10-4** outlines these recommendations. Research continues to evaluate the efficacy of screening and prevention methods for individuals known to have a BRCA mutation.

Prophylactic oophorectomy (also called risk-reducing salpingo-oophorectomy or RRSO) is recommended for women when childbearing is complete to reduce the risk for ovarian cancer and breast cancer.[8,38,42] Reports of foci of malignant tumors discovered at the time of prophylactic oophorectomy have led to the recommendation that the fallopian tubes and ovaries should be submitted entirely to pathology and be evaluated in serial sections by a pathologist with expertise in gynecologic cancer.[42–45]

Table 10-4 BREAST AND OVARIAN CANCER SURVEILLANCE OPTIONS FOR WOMEN WITH BRCA1 OR BRCA2 MUTATIONS.

Intervention	Provisional Recommendation
Breast Cancer (surveillance)	
• Breast self-examination	• Education regarding monthly self-examination starting at age 18 years
• Clinical breast examination	• Semiannually beginning at age 25 years
• Mammography and breast MRI screening	• Annually beginning at age 25–35 years; alternating MRI and mammography every 6 months
Breast cancer (prevention)	
• Bilateral prophylactic mastectomy	• Discussion of prophylactic mastectomy on case-by-case basis
• Consideration of chemoprevention options	
• Bilateral prophylactic oophorectomy	
Ovarian cancer (surveillance)	
• Transvaginal ultrasound with color Doppler and CA 125 level	• Semiannually, beginning at age 25–35 years
Ovarian cancer (prevention)	
• Bilateral prophylactic oophorectomy	• Between 35 and 40 years or upon completion of childbearing
• Consideration of chemoprevention options	

Source: Burke W, Daly M, Garber J, et al. (1997). Recommendations for follow-up care of individuals with an inherited predisposition to cancer. Ii. BRCA1 and BRCA2. Cancer genetics studies consortium [see comments]. *JAMA*. 1997;277(12):997–1003. Domchek SM, Weber BL. Clinical management of BRCA1 and BRCA2 mutation carriers. *Oncogene*. 2006;25(43):5825–5831. NCCN. Clinical practice guidelines in oncology—v.1.2008: genetic/familial high-risk assessment: breast and ovarian. Clinical practice guidelines in oncology v.1.2008. http://www.nccn.org. Published 2008.

HBOC follows a pattern of dominant inheritance with reduced penetrance. BRCA mutations can be inherited from either the mother or the father.

Clinical genetic testing is available for BRCA1 and BRCA2, and genetic testing is typically ordered for both genes simultaneously when there is suspicion for hereditary breast and ovarian cancer. It is estimated that approximately 2% of individuals of Ashkenazi Jewish ancestry have a mutation in BRCA1 or BRCA2.[46] There are three common mutations (two mutations in BRCA1 and one mutation in BRCA2) that are responsible for the majority of hereditary breast and ovarian cancer in individuals of Ashkenazi Jewish ancestry.[46–49] These mutations have also been observed in non-Jewish breast and ovarian cancer families, but less commonly. It is possible to request testing only for the three common Ashkenazi Jewish mutations in BRCA1 and BRCA2, and proceed with additional BRCA1 and BRCA2 screening if the results of the first tests were negative.

Li-Fraumeni Syndrome

Li-Fraumeni syndrome is a rare cancer predisposition syndrome caused by mutations in the p53 gene. P53, also called TP53, is a tumor suppressor gene inherited in an autosomal dominant fashion. The original Li-Fraumeni tumor spectrum included osteosarcomas, soft-tissue sarcomas, premenopausal onset breast cancer, brain tumors, adrenal cortical tumors, and acute leukemia.[50,51] Other tumor sites associated with germ-line p53 mutations include: lymphoma, melanoma, stomach, colorectal, pancreas, lung, ovary, endometrial, thyroid, and gonadal germ cell tumors.[52,53]

The lifetime risk of cancer in individuals with a p53 mutation is up to 90% by age 70 years.[54,55] According to Nichols et al.,[52] nearly one-third of cancers are diagnosed prior to the age of 20 years and another one-third are diagnosed in the third and fourth decades of life.

The classic diagnostic criteria for Li-Fraumeni syndrome were defined in 1969.[51] These were modified in 1994 and called Li-Fraumeni-like syndrome.[53] **Table 10-5** outlines these diagnostic criteria.

Table 10-5 LI-FRAUMENI AND LI-FRAUMENI-LIKE DIAGNOSTIC CRITERIA.

Li-Fraumeni Diagnostic Criteria (1969)

- Individuals with a sarcoma less than age 45 years AND

- One first-degree relative diagnosed with cancer less than age 45 years AND

- A first-degree or second-degree relative diagnosed with either sarcoma at any age or other cancer under the age of 45 years

Li-Fraumeni-like Diagnostic Criteria (1994)

- Individuals with any childhood cancer, sarcoma, brain tumor, or adrenocortical tumor less than age 45 years AND

- One first-degree relative diagnosed with a typical cancer associated with Li-Fraumeni syndrome (sarcoma, breast, brain, adrenal cortical tumor, or leukemia) at any age AND

- A first-degree or second-degree relative diagnosed with any cancer less than age 60 years

Source: {Li, 1969 #51; Birch, 1994 #53}.

Medical management of at-risk individuals should be carried out by medical professionals familiar with Li-Fraumeni syndrome and current screening and prevention recommendations for this rare syndrome.

Clinical molecular genetic testing for germline p53 mutations is available.

Peutz-Jeghers syndrome (PJS) is characterized by multiple hamartomatous polyps in the small intestine, stomach, and large bowel.[56–58] Characteristic melanin spots of the lips, buccal mucosa, eyes, nostrils, perianal area, and hands and feet usually develop during the first decade of life.[56,57] Individuals with Peutz-Jeghers also are predisposed to benign ovarian sex chord tumors with annular tubules and an increased risk for cancer, including gastrointestinal, pancreas, breast, ovarian, uterine, cervix, testicular, and gallbladder.[56,57,59,60]

Reports of cancer risks in individuals with Peutz-Jeghers syndrome range from 22%–93%.[58,61–64]

Giardiello et al.[60] proposed a definition of PJS to include: histopathologic confirmation of hamartomatous gastrointestinal polyps and two of the following three features: (1) small-bowel polyposis, (2) family history of PJS, and (3) pigmented macules of the buccal mucosa, lips, fingers, and toes. Tomlinson and Houlston[56] suggest that a diagnosis can be made if an individual fulfills one of the following criteria: (1) two or more PJS polyps in the gastrointestinal tract, or (2) one PJS polyp in the gastrointestinal tract, together with either classical PJS pigmentation or a family history of PJS.

Medical management of at-risk individuals should be carried out by medical professionals familiar with PJS and current screening and prevention recommendations for this rare syndrome. PJS is associated with mutations in the STK11 gene.[64] Clinical genetic testing is available.

Cowden Syndrome is characterized by multiple hamartomas of the skin, intestine, breast, and thyroid, and an increased risk for cancer of the thyroid and breast.[59,66,67] Criteria published by the International Cowden Consortium outline Pathognomonic Criteria, Major Criteria and Minor Criteria.[67,68] The most common skin manifestation is a benign tumor of the hair shaft called a trichilemmoma.[59] A diagnosis of Cowden syndrome is made when an individual presents with a combination of physical manifestations that fit this criteria. Endometrial cancer, breast cancer, and thyroid cancer (non-medullar), as well as macrocephay (>95th centile) and Lhermitte-Dublos disease, are included in the major diagnostic criteria for Cowden syndrome. Minor manifestations of Cowden syndrome include thyroid lesions, mental retardation, GI hamartoma, lipomas, fibromas, GU tumors or malformation, and fibrocystic breast disease. Renal cell carcinoma and melanoma have also been suggested to be possibly associated with Cowden syndrome.[68] Women with Cowden syndrome have a 30–50% risk for developing breast cancer and a 5–10% risk for endometrial cancer; men and women with Cowden syndrome have an approximate 10% risk for developing epithelial thyroid cancer.[59,68]

Surveillance recommendations for individuals with Cowden syndrome primarily focus on screening options for breast cancer, thyroid cancer, and endometrial cancer.[24,68,59]

Cowden syndrome is inherited as an autosomal dominant condition with high penetrance. Cowden syndrome is one of a group of PTEN hamartoma syndromes associated with mutations the PTEN gene.[59,66,67] Clinical genetic testing is available for PTEN.

The Cancer Family History

The increase in genetic information and the impact of the Human Genome Project is changing the practice of medicine. This explosion of genetic information has already made a significant impact in the detection, prevention, and treatment of cancer. Oncology health professionals are at the forefront of identification of those families at increased risk for hereditary or familial cancer. The cancer family history is the fundamental tool for identifying individuals at risk. The collection and interpretation of family history information has been identified as a core skill necessary for healthcare providers.[70–73]

The importance of gathering one's medical family history was brought to national attention in 2005 when the US Surgeon General, in cooperation with other agencies within the US Department of Health and Human Services (HHS), launched a national public health campaign, called the US Surgeon General's Family History Initiative, to encourage all American families to learn more about their family health history.[74] The National Society of Genetic Counselors (www.nsgc.org) provides an online family history tool to assist in gathering medical family history and a searchable database of genetic counselors providing cancer genetic counseling services.

Documentation of the medical history for first- and second-degree relatives allows for a quick glance at the cancer family history to determine the necessity of expanding portions of the family history and/or referral to an appropriate cancer genetic professional. Personal interviews are time-consuming and costly in terms of staff time. Paper interviews (questionnaires) may not provide sufficient intake information to appraise the family history to determine the appropriate-

ness of further evaluation. There is no good data to define the most appropriate questions for an optimum *screening* family history. Research continues to determine the most efficient method of obtaining a screening family history at initial intake.[75–77]

Schneider[78] recommends 10 general strategies and provides examples of questions to ask to elicit a thorough cancer family history (see **Table 10-6**).

Drawing the cancer family history in a pedigree format allows for visualization of the pattern of cancer development within the family for clues to hereditary cancer. Prior to 1995, there were no standard pedigree symbols, and the usage of pedigree symbols was inconsistent among genetic professionals and publications in medical journals, genetics journals, and medical genetic textbooks.[79] A proposed standard for pedigree symbols was published in 1995[80] and is the accepted standard among genetics professionals.[81,82]

Figure 10-4 illustrates a five-generation mock pedigree with relationships to the proband noted. The proband is the individual through whom the family history is obtained and is indicated by an arrow. It is standard practice to draw the male partner on the left and the female partner on the right. Siblings are typically presented from left to right in descending birth order (oldest to youngest). First-degree relatives (parents, full siblings and children) share one-half of their DNA. Second-degree relatives (grandparents, aunts/uncles, nieces/nephews, and half-siblings) share one-fourth of their DNA. Third-degree relatives (i.e., first cousins, great-aunts, great-uncles, great-grandparents) share one-eighth of their DNA. Therefore, if an individual has a known mutation in a cancer predisposition gene, all first-degree relatives

Table 10-6 SAMPLE FAMILY HISTORY QUESTIONS TO ASK.

- What type of cancer was diagnosed?
- Do you know the exact diagnosis?
- Where was your relative diagnosed and/or treated?
- Did the relative develop any other types of cancer?
- Do you know whether the second cancer spread from the original tumor?
- How old was your relative at diagnosis?
- What year was the cancer diagnosed?
- Is your relative still living? If yes, how old is your relative now? If no, what year and at what age did your relative die?
- What was your relative's occupation?
- Did your relative smoke cigarettes?
- Was your relative exposed to any other harmful agents that might have caused cancer?

Source: {Schneider, 2002 #82} [printed with permission].

have a 50% chance of having the same mutation, second-degree relatives have a 25% chance, and third-degree relatives have a 12.5% chance of having the same mutation.

Obtaining a detailed family history and verification of the cancer diagnoses are essential for appropriate risk assessment and medical management based upon the cancer family history. Inaccurate reporting can lead to a misclassification of the cancer family history. Multiple studies have documented the inaccuracy of a verbal cancer family history, both in the clinical and the research settings.[83–88] The closer the biological relationship to the proband, the more accurate the reported cancer site and age of diagnosis within 5 years. Metastatic sites are often reported as the primary tumor site. Individual cancer sites of the female pelvic organs are notoriously reported incorrectly.

It is important to verify the age and histology of the cancer diagnoses in the family history by review of medical records. A signed medical record release is required to obtain confirmatory records. The pathology report is the optimum source for verification of both the age of diagnosis and histology. The operative report and discharge summary may provide additional details about the personal medical history and family history. A death certificate is not the optimum source for confirmation of a cancer diagnosis. The cancer diagnosis may not be listed on the death certificate if the cause of death was unrelated to the cancer, or the cancer diagnosis documented on the death certificate may be the metastatic site, not the primary tumor.[87,89]

Genetic Counseling and Genetic Testing

Genetic counseling is the process of helping people understand and adapt to the medical, psychological, and familial implications of

Figure 10-4

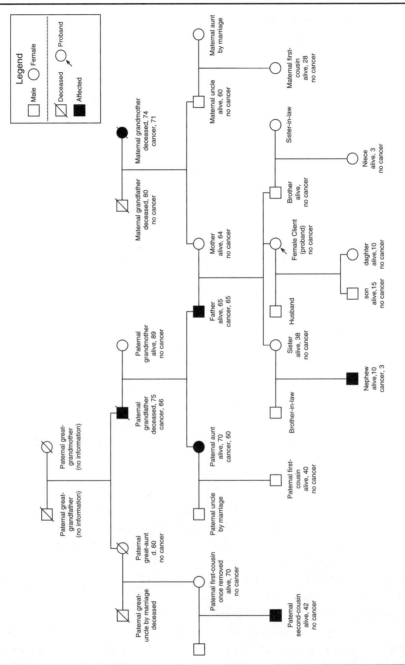

Source: Adapted with permission from Schneider, 2002, #82.

genetic contributions to disease. This process integrates the following: interpretation of family and medical histories to assess the chance of disease occurrence or recurrence; education about inheritance, testing, management, prevention, resources, and research; and counseling to promote informed choices and adaptation to the risk or condition.[90]

The American Society of Clinical Oncologists (ASCO) recommends that genetic counseling and testing be offered when: (1) the individual has a personal or family history suggestive of a genetic cancer susceptibility condition, (2) the genetic test can be adequately interpreted, and (3) the test results will aid in the diagnosis or influence the medical or surgical management of the patient or family members at hereditary risk of cancer.[91]

ASCO also outlines the basic elements of informed consent for cancer susceptibility testing.[91] This includes: (1) information on the specific test being performed, (2) implications of both positive and negative results, (3) possibility that the test will not be informative, (4) options for risk estimation without genetic testing, (5) risk of passing a mutation to children, (6) technical accuracy of the test, (7) fees involved in testing and counseling, (8) psychological implications of test results (benefits and risks), (9) risks of insurance or employer discrimination, (10) confidentiality issues, (11) options and limitations of medical surveillance and strategies for prevention following testing, and (12) importance of sharing genetic test results with at-risk relatives so that they may benefit from this information.

Cancer genetic counseling is often provided in high-risk multidisciplinary clinics. A detailed discussion of the practice of cancer genetic counseling is beyond the scope of this chapter and is a field of medical specialty in itself. The National Society of Genetic Counselors (www.nsgc.org) provides a searchable database of genetic counselors who provide cancer genetic counseling services. There are numerous reference books and journal articles for health professionals seeking information regarding the provision of cancer genetic services[82,92,93] covering a wide range of topics relating to hereditary cancer, such as the cancer family history; genetic counseling and risk assessment; the medical, psychosocial, and ethical ramifications of identifying at-risk individuals through cancer risk assessment with or without genetic testing; and surveillance and prevention options.

Greco[72] discusses the impact of genetic information on the various roles of different levels of oncology nursing practice: the general oncology nurse, the advanced practice oncology nurse, and the advanced practice oncology nurse with a subspecialty in genetics. There will be an increasingly important role in case finding, risk assessment, education, counseling, psychosocial support, health advocacy, and coordination of services and referral for cancer risk management.[72,73]

Conclusion

Cancer genetics is a rapidly evolving field and will continue to change the practice of medicine and have an impact on the field of oncology nursing. New cancer treatments will be evolving to target cellular genetics. Oncology nurses need to understand the basis of these treatments and provide patient education to those receiving genetic therapy. MacDonald[73] states that oncology nurses have many opportunities to promote health by educating others about cancer prevention, early detection, and risk avoidance behaviors. Oncology nurses can make a significant impact by incorporating cancer genetic information in their health education and through identification and referral of high-risk families.

References

1. Loud J, et al. Applications of advances in molecular biology and genomics to clinical cancer care. *Cancer Nursing*. 2002;25(2):110–122.

2. Jenkins J, Masny A. Why should oncology nurses be interested in genetics. In: Tranin AS, Masny A, Jenkins J, eds. *Genetics in Oncology Practice: Cancer Risk Assessment*. Pittsburgh, PA: Oncology Nursing Society; 2003:1–8.

3. Lashley FRC. Cancer. In: *Clinical Genetics in Nursing*. New York: Springer Publishing Company; 1998: 425–448.

4. Peters J, et al. Cancer genetics fundamentals. *Cancer Nursing*. 2001;24(6):446–461.

5. Wooster R, Weber BL. Breast and ovarian cancer. *N Engl J Med*. 2003;348(23):2339–2347.

6. Volker DL. Normal cell biology and the biology of cancer. In: Rieger PT, ed. *Biotherapy: A Comprehensive Overview*. Sudbury, MA: Jones and Bartlett Publishers; 2001:65–84.

7. Loescher LJ, Whitesell L. The biology of cancer. In: Tranin AS, Masny A, Jenkins J, eds. *Genetics in Oncology Practice: Cancer Risk Assessment*. Pittsburgh, PA: Oncology Nursing Society; 2003:23–56.

8. Wooster R, Weber BL. Breast and ovarian cancer. *N Engl J Med*. 2003;348:2339–2347.

9. Spencer-Cisek PA. The role of growth factors in malignancy: a focus on the epidermal growth factor receptor. *Seminars in Oncology Nursing*. 2002;18 (2, suppl 2):13–19.

10. Offit K. Cancer as a genetic disorder. In: *Clinical Cancer Genetics: Risk Counseling and Management*. New York: Wiley-Liss; 1998:39–65.

11. Schneider K. Cancer biology. In: *Counseling About Cancer: Strategies for Genetic Counseling*. New York: Wiley-Liss; 2002:51–71.

12. Gudmundsdottir K, Ashworth A. The roles of BRCA1 and BRCA2 and associated proteins in the maintenance of genomic stability. *Oncogene*. 2006;25(43):5864–5874.

13. Goodfellow PJ, et al. Prevalence of defective DNA mismatch repair and MSH6 mutation in an unselected series of endometrial cancers. *PNAS*. 2003;100(10):5908–5913.

14. Bale A, Li F. Principles of cancer management: cancer genetics. In: Devita VT, Hellman S, Rosenberg S, eds. *Cancer: Principles and Practice of Oncology*. Philadelphia, PA: Lippincott-Raven; 1997:285–293.

15. Hampel H, et al. Screening for the Lynch syndrome (hereditary nonpolyposis colorectal cancer). *N Engl J Med*. 2005;352(18):1851–1860.

16. Lawes DA, SenGupta SB, Boulos PB. Pathogenesis and clinical management of hereditary nonpolyposis colorectal cancer (review). *British Journal of Surgery*. 2002;89(11):1357–1369.

17. Aarnio M, et al. Cancer risk in mutation carriers of DNA-mismatch-repair genes. Int J Cancer, 81(2) 214–218.

18. Lynch HT, de la Chapelle A. Hereditary colorectal cancer. *N Engl J Med*. 2003;348(10):919–932.

19. Aarnio M, et al. Cancer risk in mutation carriers of DNA-mismatch-repair genes. *Int J Cancer*. 1999;81(2):214–218.

20. Aarnio M, et al. Life-time risk of different cancers in hereditary non-polyposis colorectal cancer (HNPCC) syndrome. *Int J Cancer*. 1995;64(6):430–433.

21. Vasen HF, et al. New clinical criteria for hereditary nonpolyposis colorectal cancer (HNPCC, Lynch syndrome) proposed by the International Collaborative Group on HNPCC. *Gastroenterology*. 1999;116(6):1453–1456.

22. Lynch HT, de la Chapelle A. Hereditary colorectal cancer (comment). *N Engl J Med*. 2003;348(10): 919–932.

23. Vasen HF, et al. The International Collaborative Group on Hereditary Non-Polyposis Colorectal Cancer (ICG-HNPCC). *Dis Colon Rectum*. 1991;34(5): 424–425.

24. NCCN. Clinical practice guidelines in oncology, v. 1. 2008: Genetic/familial high-risk assessment: breast and ovarian. http://www.nccn.org. Accessed June 1, 2008.

25. Burke W, et al. Recommendations for follow-up care of individuals with an inherited predisposition to cancer. II. BRCA1 and BRCA2. Cancer Genetics Studies Consortium. *JAMA*. 1997;277(12):997–1003.

26. Lindor NM, et al. Recommendations for the care of individuals with an inherited predisposition to Lynch syndrome: a systematic review. *JAMA*. 2006;296(12):1507–1517.

27. NCCN. Clinical practice guidelines in oncology, v. 1. 2008: Colorectal screening. http://www.nccn.org. Accessed April 23, 2008.

28. Chung DC, Rustgi AK. The hereditary non-polyposis cancer syndrome: genetics and clinical implications. *Annals of Internal Medicine.* 2003;138(7):560–570.

29. Mitchell RJ, et al. Mismatch repair genes hMLH1 and HMSH2 and colorectal cancer: a HuGE review. *American Journal of Epidemiology.* 2002;156(10): 885–902.

30. Goodfellow PJ, et al. Prevalence of defective DNA mismatch repair and MSH6 mutation in an unselected series of endometrial cancers. *Proc Natl Acad Sci USA.* 2003;100(10):5908–5913.

31. Peltomaki P. Role of DNA mismatch repair defects in the pathogenesis of human cancer. *J Clin Oncol.* 2003;21(6):1174–1179.

32. Baudhuin LM, et al. Use of microsatellite instability and immunohistochemistry testing for the identification of individuals at risk for Lynch syndrome. *Fam Cancer.* 2005;4(3):255–265.

33. Hampel H, et al. Screening for Lynch syndrome (hereditary nonpolyposis colorectal cancer) among endometrial cancer patients. *Cancer Res.* 2006;66(15):7810–7817.

34. Boland CR, et al. A National Cancer Institute Workshop on Microsatellite Instability for cancer detection and familial predisposition: development of international criteria for the determination of microsatellite instability in colorectal cancer. *Cancer Res.* 1998;58(22):5248–5257.

35. Wheeler JM, Bodmer WF, Mortensen NJ. DNA mismatch repair genes and colorectal cancer. *Gut.* 2000;47(1):148–153.

36. Simpkins SB, et al. MLH1 promoter methylation and gene silencing is the primary cause of microsatellite instability in sporadic endometrial cancers. *Hum Mol Genet.* 1999;8(4):661–666.

37. Ford D, et al. Genetic heterogeneity and penetrance analysis of the BRCA1 and BRCA2 genes in breast cancer families: the Breast Cancer Linkage Consortium. *Am J Hum Genet.* 1998;62(3):676–689.

38. NCCN. Clinical practice guidelines in oncology, v. 1 2008: Genetic/familial high-risk assessment: breast and ovarian. http://www.nccn.org. accessed April 23, 2008.

39. Thompson D, Easton DF. Cancer incidence in BRCA1 mutation carriers. *J Natl Cancer Inst.* 2002;94(18):1358–1365.

40. BCLC. Cancer risks in BRCA2 mutation carriers: the Breast Cancer Linkage Consortium. *J Natl Cancer Inst.* 1999;91(15):1310–1316.

41. Hampel H, et al. Referral for cancer genetics consultation: a review and compilation of risk assessment criteria. *J Med Genet.* 2004;41(2):81–91.

42. Domchek SM, Weber BL. Clinical management of BRCA1 and BRCA2 mutation carriers. *Oncogene.* 2006;25(43):5825–5831.

43. Leeper K, et al. Pathologic findings in prophylactic oophorectomy specimens in high-risk women. *Gynecol Oncol.* 2002;87(1):52–56.

44. Lu KH, et al. Occult ovarian tumors in women with BRCA1 or BRCA2 mutations undergoing prophylactic oophorectomy. *J Clin Oncol.* 2000;18(14):2728–2732.

45. Paley PJ, et al. Occult cancer of the fallopian tube in BRCA-1 germline mutation carriers at prophylactic oophorectomy: a case for recommending hysterectomy at surgical prophylaxis. *Gynecol Oncol.* 2001;80(2):176–180.

46. Tonin P, et al. Frequency of recurrent BRCA1 and BRCA2 mutations in Ashkenazi Jewish breast cancer families. *Nat Med.* 1996;2(11):1179–1183.

47. Struewing JP, et al. The risk of cancer associated with specific mutations of BRCA1 and BRCA2 among Ashkenazi Jews. *N Engl J Med.* 1997;336(20): 1401–1408.

48. Abeliovich D, et al. The founder mutations 185delAG and 5382insC in BRCA1 and 6174delT in BRCA2 appear in 60% of ovarian cancer and 30% of early onset breast cancer patients among Ashkenazi women. *Am J Hum Genet.* 1997;60(3):505–514.

49. Moslehi R, et al. BRCA1 and BRCA2 mutation analysis of 208 Ashkenazi Jewish women with ovarian cancer. *Am J Hum Genet.* 2000;66(4):1259–1272.

50. Li FP, et al. A cancer family syndrome in twenty-four kindreds. *Cancer Res.* 1988;48(18):5358–5362.

51. Li FP, Fraumeni Jr. JF. Soft-tissue sarcomas, breast cancer, and other neoplasms: a familial syndrome? *Ann Intern Med.* 1969; 71(4):747–752.

52. Nichols KE, et al. Germ-line p53 mutations predispose to a wide spectrum of early-onset cancers. *Cancer Epidemiol Biomarkers Prev.* 2001;10(2):83–87.

53. Birch JM, et al. Prevalence and diversity of constitutional mutations in the p53 gene among 21 Li-Fraumeni families. *Cancer Res.* 1994;54(5):1298–1304.

54. Schneider K, Li F. GeneReviews: Li-Fraumeni syndrome. http://www.genetests.org. Accessed April 23, 2008.

55. Schneider K, Li F. GeneReviews: Li-Fraumeni syndrome. http://www.genetests.org. Accessed September 5, 2006.

56. Tomlinson IP, Houlston RS. Peutz-Jeghers syndrome (review). *Journal of Medical Genetics.* 1997;34(12):1007–1011.

57. Lindor N, Greene M. The concise handbook of family cancer syndromes. *Journal of the National Cancer Institute.* 1998;90(14):1039–1071.

58. Giardiello FM, Trimbath JD. Peutz-Jeghers syndrome and management recommendations. *Clin Gastroenterol Hepatol.* 2006;4(4):408–415.

59. Wirtzfeld DA, Petrelli NJ, Rodriguez-Bigas MA. Hamartomatous polyposis syndromes: molecular genetics, neoplastic risk, and surveillance recommendations (review). *Annals of Surgical Oncology.* 2001;8(4):319–327.

60. Giardiello FM, et al. Increased risk of cancer in the Peutz-Jeghers syndrome. *N Engl J Med.* 1987;316(24):1511–1514.

61. Boardman LA, et al. Increased risk for cancer in patients with the Peutz-Jeghers syndrome. *Ann Intern Med.* 1998;128(11):896–899.

62. Giardiello FM, et al. Very high risk of cancer in familial Peutz-Jeghers syndrome. *Gastroenterology.* 2000;119(6):1447–1453.

63. Spigelman AD, Murday V, Phillips RK. Cancer and the Peutz-Jeghers syndrome. *Gut.* 1989;30(11):1588–1590.

64. Vasen HF. Clinical diagnosis and management of hereditary colorectal cancer syndromes (review). *Journal of Clinical Oncology.* 2000;18(21, suppl):81S–92S.

65. Nelen MR, et al. Localization of the gene for Cowden disease to chromosome 10q22–23. *Nat Genet.* 1996;13(1):114–116.

66. Zbuk K, Stein J and Eng C. PTEN GeneReviews: PTEN hamartoma tumor syndrome (PHTS). http://www.genetests.org. Accessed on April 23, 2008.

67. Pilarski R, Eng C. Will the real Cowden syndrome please stand up (again)? Expanding mutational and clinical spectra of the PTEN hamartoma tumour syndrome. *J Med Genet.* 2004;41(5):323–326.

68. Eng C. Will the real Cowden syndrome please stand up: revised diagnostic criteria. *J Med Genet.* 2000;37(11):828–830.

69. Eng C. Cowden syndrome. *Journal of Genetic Counseling.* 1997;6(2):181–192.

70. NCHPEG, N.C.f.H.P.E.i.G. Core competencies in genetics essential for all healthcare professionals. *Genetics in Medicine.* 2001;3(2):155–159.

71. Lea D, et al. *Genetics and Cancer Care: A Guide for Oncology Nurses.* Pittsburgh, PA: Oncology Nursing Society; 2002.

72. Greco K. Cancer genetic nursing: impact of the double helix. *Oncology Nursing Forum.* 2000;27 (9, suppl):29–36.

73. MacDonald D. The oncology nurse's role in cancer risk assessment and counseling. *Seminars in Oncology Nursing.* 1997;13(2):123–128.

74. HHS, U.S.D. *U.S. Surgeon General's Family History Initiative;* 2007 http://www.hhs.gov/familyhistory Accessed April 23, 2008.

75. Gilpin CA, Carson N, Hunter AG. A preliminary validation of a family history assessment form to select women at risk for breast or ovarian cancer for referral to a genetics center. *Clin Genet.* 2000;58(4):299–308.

76. Leggatt V, Mackay J, Yates JR. Evaluation of questionnaire on cancer family history in identifying patients at increased genetic risk in general practice. *BMJ.* 1999;319(7212):757–758.

77. Theis B, et al. Accuracy of family cancer history in breast cancer patients. *Eur J Cancer Prev.* 1994;3(4):321–327.

78. Steinhaus KA, et al. Inconsistencies in pedigree symbols in human genetics publications: a need for standardization. *American Journal of Medical Genetics.* 1995;56(3):291–295.

79. Bennett RL, et al. Recommendations for standardized human pedigree nomenclature: Pedigree Standardization Task Force of the National Society of Genetic Counselors (comment). *American Journal of Human Genetics.* 1995;56(3):745–752.

80. NSGC, N.S.o.G.C. Position statements: standard pedigree symbol position statement. http://www.nsgc.org/about/position.asp. Accessed April 23, 2008.

81. Gould R. *Cancer and Genetics: Answering Your Patient's Questions.* Huntington, NY: PRR, Inc. and the American Cancer Society; 1997.

82. Schneider K. *Counseling About Cancer: Strategies for Genetic Counselors.* New York: Wiley-Liss; 2002.

83. Aitken J, et al. How accurate is self-reported family history of colon cancer? *American Journal of Epidemiology.* 1995;141(9):863–871.

84. Bondy ML, et al. Accuracy of family history of cancer obtained through interviews with relatives of patients with childhood sarcoma. *Journal of Clinical Epidemiology.* 1994;47(1):89–96.

85. Husson G, Herrinton LJ. How accurately does the medical record capture maternal history of

cancer? *Cancer Epidemiology, Biomarkers & Prevention.* 2000;9(7):765–768.

86. Ivanovich J, et al. Evaluation of the family history collection process and the accuracy of cancer reporting among a series of women with endometrial cancer. *Clinical Cancer Research.* 2002;8:1849–1856.

87. Ziogas A, Anton-Culver H. Validation of family history data in cancer family registries. *Am J Prev Med.* 2003;24(2):190–198.

88. Love RR, Evans AM, Josten DM. The accuracy of patient reports of a family history of cancer. *J Chronic Dis.* 1985;38(4):289–293.

89. Novakovic B, Goldstein A, Tucker M. Validation of family history of cancer in deceased family members. *Journal of the National Cancer Institute.* 1996;88(20):1492–1493.

90. Resta R, et al. A new definition of genetic counseling: National Society of Genetic Counselors' Task Force report. *J Genet Couns.* 2006;15(2):77–83.

91. ASCO, A.A.o.C.O. American Society of Clinical Oncology policy statement update: genetic testing for cancer susceptibility. *Journal of Clinical Oncology.* 2003;21(12).

92. Colditz GA, Stein CJ. *Handbook of Cancer Risk Assessment and Prevention.* Sudbury, MA: Jones and Bartlett Publishers; 2004.

93. Offit K. *Clinical Cancer Genetics.* New York: Wiley-Liss; 1998.

Chapter 11

Sexuality Issues

Evelyn H. Larrison, RN, BSN

Introduction

The foundation of Maslow's hierarchy includes physiological needs of survival and stimulation. Sex and sexuality are essential and basic components of all our human needs. Every gynecologic cancer impacts sex and sexuality in some way and yet is often overlooked and under-treated by healthcare professionals who work with these women and their partners. Continued education and encouragement of our peers to be proactive in meeting the sexuality needs of our patients is important.

Scope of the Problem

Sexuality reflects an individual's personality and lifestyle. It is more than just the ability to have sex. It is a complex system, incorporating biological, psychological, interpersonal, and behavioral elements. There is a wide range of normal sexual functioning. For cancer patients, the ability to feel "sexy" verifies that they are returning to some degree of prediagnosis normalcy. Sexuality is a quality of life issue that is often overlooked[1] or underestimated. Estimates of sexual dysfunction after a diagnosis of cancer can range from 31%–88%.[2] Ongoing research suggests that sexual dysfunction is a long-term process that lasts years after diagnosis and treatment.[3] Degree of sexual dysfunction is related to the site of the cancer and subsequent treatments.[4,5] Self-esteem and body image, which are integral to sexuality, are areas that are impacted by a diagnosis and treatment for cancer.

Definition of Sexuality

Sexuality can have many meanings to patients and healthcare providers. The World Health Organization[5] defined it as "the integration of the somatic, emotional, intellectual, and social aspects of communication and love." In 2002 the definition was refined to include sex, gender identities and roles, sexual orientation, eroticism, pleasure, intimacy, and reproduction. Most healthcare providers, patients, and their partners define sexuality as the ability to want, have, and enjoy sexual expressions.

Review of Literature

Shell[6] reviewed published articles, books, and practice standards from 1980–2000 for evidence-based practice on sexual dysfunction in adults with cancer. She concluded that although there was an abundance of literature related to interventions for sexual dysfunction, few were from randomized controlled clinical trials. Davis[7] noted that while female sexuality has historically received little scientific study, there appears to be an increased interest in the field. In 1990[8] it was estimated that 76% of women experience some type of sexual dysfunction. The absence of empirical data, combined with varying definitions of sexual dysfunction, prevents a clear understanding of the prevalence of women's sexual problems. However, based on research on male erectile dysfunction, physicians are beginning to understand female sexual problems.[9] Interventional studies are emerging in professional literature. Lay publications abound with articles on how to improve one's sex life. An extensive Internet search of articles related to sexuality and cancer revealed that much in the way of the current literature is missing, however. Many of the articles and books were written in the 1990s, and those articles tend to be repetitive. The articles written since 2000 do not offer much new information. There continues to be a lack of research published on cancer and sexuality, especially for women. It is encouraging to note that there are clinical investigations that are incorporating a sexuality component.

Clinical Nursing Implication

Many nurses feel uncomfortable about providing sexual advice, despite the trusting relationships they often develop with their patients.[10] Assessment models can guide nurses in obtaining a sexual history that can be useful. The most common models used are Kaplan's, Triphasic, PLISSIT, and ALARM.[11] A newer model, BETTER, is similar to the PLISSIT model. While the PLISSIT model provides a framework for initiating sexuality discussions, the BETTER model focus is on guiding assessment of sexuality.[12] The May 2007 newsletter of the Houston ONS chapter[13] lists 10 tips for improving sexuality assessment. The topics listed are:

1. Expand your concept of sexuality.
2. Do not make patients ask.
3. Ask yourself "why" when feeling discomfort.
4. Get to know your personal worldview.
5. Eliminate "form-dependent" practice.
6. Use practice standards to guide sexuality assessment.
7. Form nurse–patient relationships by addressing sexuality.
8. Avoid any assumptions that sexuality is a low-priority concern.
9. Meet professional responsibility for sexuality education.
10. If nurses do not ask, they must tell.[14]

The expansion of each topic is an excellent guide for developing sexual assessment tools. Nurses need to understand how surgery and treatment affects sexual functioning, be nonjudgmental and accepting of lifestyle choices, and recognize when referral to mental health services for a serious sexual problem is needed.[14] One way to become comfortable discussing sexuality with patients and their partners is to start with a less threatening topic. Start by saying "many women who have undergone surgery/chemotherapy/radiation therapy report that they notice vaginal changes and painful intercourse. Have you experienced any of these changes?" This opens a dialogue that can be comfortable for both the patient and the nurse.

Causes of Sexual Dysfunction

Both physical and psychological factors cause changes in sexuality. Functional damage secondary to treatments, fatigue, and pain are physical factors. Add the direct physiological effects of treatment, and it is of little wonder that sexual dysfunction develops. Compounding the problems are the psychological effects, such as fallacies about the origin of cancer, the guilt associated with these beliefs, depression, and body image changes.

Surgery

Any surgery for gynecologic cancers involves the sexual organs of a woman. While each surgical procedure has specific results, they all affect sexuality in some way.

HYSTERECTOMY

The scar from a total abdominal hysterectomy with bilateral salpingo-oophorectomy (TAH/ BSO) may be sensitive and painful to pressure during face-to-face sexual positioning. The removal of the major estrogen-producing organs can cause the vagina to become dry and friable and may make intercourse painful. Some women find that a hysterectomy affects their self-image.

RADICAL HYSTERECTOMY

A radical hysterectomy removes the upper one-third of the vagina, which may make intercourse uncomfortable after surgery. This discomfort abates with time. The horizontal Pfannenstiel incision is less apt to cause discomfort during intercourse.[13] Decreased lubrication and genital swelling during sexual activity have been reported following treatment for cervical cancer.[15] Jensen et al. compared women who had undergone a radical hysterectomy with a control group and reported severe orgasmic problems and uncomfortable intercourse during the 6-month postoperative period. While the discomfort decreased over time, the women still reported decreased sexual desire and lubrication difficulties up to 2 years after the surgery.[14] A later report showed an increase in fatigue, anxiety, and depression up to 5 years after the end of treatment.[16]

Uterine Cancer

Historical studies have reported that women experienced dyspareunia or loss of orgasmic capacity following a radical hysterectomy.[15] In a subsequent study by Jensen et al.[14] comparing women who had undergone a radical hysterectomy with a control group found severe orgasmic problems and uncomfortable intercourse during the 6-month postoperative period. While the discomfort decreased over time, the women still reported decreased sexual desire and lubrication difficulties up to 2 years after the surgery. The development of safer and less invasive surgical procedures, such as laparoscopically assisted vaginal hysterectomy (LAVH) is both cost effective and offers less patient morbidity. Laparoscopic hysterectomies have been used in the treatment of early stage cervical and endometrial cancers. Studies suggest this surgical approach offers correct staging without compromising overall patient survival.[16–19]

Vulvectomy

One of the most sexually significant gynecologic oncology surgeries is a vulvectomy, performed for vulvar cancer. A total radical vulvectomy removes the clitoris, labia, and distal one-third of the vagina with exploration of the groin lymph nodes. The construction of a neovagina for these patients provides a means for intercourse, but the neovagina has little sensation, no natural lubricant, and atrophy is common. The incidence of wound breakdown is as high as 50%, resulting in lengthened recovery and more scarring. Sexually, the patient may experience dyspareunia due to the lack of lubrication and elasticity. Clitoral orgasm is no longer possible, and subsequent lower extremity edema and decreased range of motion makes intercourse uncomfortable. Changes in body image can also be significant.[20] Older women and larger excision areas have been correlated with poorer sexual function and quality of life. Because this study only included 43 women, a larger study is needed to understand the impact of vulvar cancer on sexuality.[21]

Total Pelvic Exenteration

A total pelvic exenteration removes the uterus, ovaries, and vagina (with reconstruction) and includes a radical cystectomy and rectosigmoid resection resulting in a colostomy and urostomy. Pelvic adhesions or scarring may contribute to dyspareunia. Each of these procedures has sexual side effects. Dyspareunia is also caused by the same factors that exist in a vulvectomy and hysterectomy. The sexual side effects of ostomies are associated with body image changes and the opportunity to visualize body waste during the sexual act. With the advent of shorter hospitalizations and less support staff, such as enterostomal therapists, the responsibility for ostomy education may fall to the bedside nurse. There are local and national support groups, such as United Ostomy Associations of America, Inc., that provide support and information.

Treatments

It is not only the surgical sexual side effects our patients must deal with. All of the adjuvant treatments also carry the potential for adverse sexual side effects.

Chemotherapy

Many chemotherapy agents have sexual side effects. Alkylating agents (doxorubicin) may cause amenorrhea and ovarian and erectile dysfunction.[10] Antiestrogen agents may cause decreased libido, decreased orgasmic response, and vaginal changes. Side effects of biological response modifiers, such as fatigue, mucositis, and flulike symptoms, can cause sexual disinterest and libido changes. In general, the side effects associated with chemotherapy, such as nausea, vomiting, diarrhea, constipation, and altered taste and smell, and the physical changes, such as alopecia and edemas, may leave women feeling asexual. Hormone replacement that would alleviate some of these side effects may not be indicated due to the relationship between some cancers and estrogen.

Radiation Therapy

Radiation to the pelvis can cause cessation of ovulation. The ovarian failure results in decreased vaginal lubrication and thinning and atrophy of the vaginal lining. These changes can make sexual intercourse uncomfortable. In a Denmark study of 118 women undergoing radiotherapy for cervical cancer, persistent sexual dysfunction was reported up to 2 years after treatment.[14] Patients who are disease free after radiation therapy continue to have a high risk of experiencing persistent sexual and vaginal problems.[22]

Medications

Several medications used for symptom management can impact sexuality. Antiemetics, sedatives, and tranquilizers can cause sedation, decreased libido, and decreased orgasm intensity. Antihistamines can dry up vaginal mucosa, decreasing elasticity. Sexual dysfunction is a common side effect of antidepressant therapy. Rates of sexual dysfunction observed may be higher than those reported in product information. Published studies suggest that as high as 60% of SSRI-treated patients may experience some form of sexual dysfunction.[23] Commonly used drugs like cimetidine, metronidazole, and spironolactone may cause decreased libido.[24]

Fatigue

The fatigue that cancer patients experience is frequently life consuming. The cause of cancer-related fatigue is multifactorial. Anemia is only one. Fatigue in the cancer patient may be caused by the tumor itself, rather than the therapy. Medications, such as opioids, dehydration, and inadequate nutrition can cause fatigue as well as abnormalities in blood work (low sodium, high calcium). Cancer patients may not sleep well because of pain, depression, anxiety, or excessive resting during the day.[25] The hallmark of cancer-related fatigue is that it is not relieved by rest. Patients do not have the stamina and energy to perform sexually and have diminished interest in sexual activity.

Psychological Effects

Self image is an integral part of our psyche and sexuality. How we see ourselves affects how we act and feel. If we feel "ugly," it is difficult to respond to overtures of affection. This feeling may also lead to self doubt.

Self-Image Changes

Diagnosis and treatment of gynecologic cancer can impact a woman's self-image on many levels. The scars and physical changes of surgery and treatment are visible reminders of what cancer has done to their lives. Women often feel unattractive and less self-confident.[26] Inability to work, continue with normal household routines, or maintain a social schedule affects the self and sexual self-esteem. Patients have reported feelings of social isolation.

Fear and Anxiety

Fear and anxiety are common reactions to a diagnosis of cancer. There is fear of the disease itself, fear of recurrence, and fear of death. Partners may fear catching cancer and distance themselves from contact. Prior diagnosis sexual functioning may influence postdiagnosis morbidity and coping strategies.

Interventions for Sexual Dysfunction

Interventions for sexual problems can be psychological, medical, and physical. Some patients may require more than one intervention. While nurses should assess each patient for sexual dysfunction, their comfort and skill in dealing with the subject is variable. Healthcare personnel who are uncomfortable with or inexperienced in sexual counseling can refer patients to healthcare practitioners who focus on sexuality.[27] You can find a registered sexual therapist by contacting the American Association of Sexuality Educators, Counselors and Therapists (AASECT).

Psychological Interventions

Psychological aspects of sexual dysfunction are the more difficult aspects to treat. Sexual desire begins in the mind. By finding ways to relax, a woman may feel more receptive to sexual activity. Suggest changing the scene, arranging for time alone with her partner, relaxation, or changing the time of day to when she feels her best. Planning ahead impacts the spontaneity of the occasion, but some trade-offs can be made. Scars, ostomies, edemas, and other physical changes may impact how a woman feels about herself and impair her sexual functioning. She may feel more attractive by wearing certain types of clothing, such as teddies or short gowns. Wigs and scarves can be secured with wig tape. Sexual positions that remove scars and ostomies from direct visual contact (side lying or from behind) may make her more comfortable. A supportive mate will help relieve these concerns. Many patients find comfort and help in peer support groups. Nurses often act as facilitators of these groups and should introduce the subject of sexuality. The Mautner Project offers support services for lesbian patients and their partners (see Suggested Patient Resources at the end of this chapter).

Medication Interventions

It may be possible to change medication schedules to decrease their effects. Keep in mind that some medications need to be tapered off, and patients should be counseled as such. Clinical trials of Viagra for female sexual problems have been inconclusive. Viagra did appear to increase blood flow to the clitoris, but did not significantly improve overall sexual satisfaction.[25] Other pharmacotherapy agents currently under investigation are L-arginine, prostaglandin E_1, phentolamine, and apomorphine.[11] Lay literature and television now carry ads for products such as Avlimil and ProSensual. The majority of these products have not been proven in randomized clinical trials. Other products undergoing investigation are apomorphine HCL, ESTRATEST Tablets, LibiGel, and Vasofem.[28] Intrinsa is a transdermal testosterone patch under clinical development for increasing sexual desire and satisfaction in women. Data from these studies found a significant increase in both of these elements.[28] However, in a 2007 study the increased testosterone level related to the patch did not translate into improved libido, which might have been related to the depleted estrogen levels in the women who were studied (150 female cancer survivors) Follow-up studies of the transdermal testosterone patch FDA advisory committee hearing on Intrinsa declined approval of the transdermal patch because of problems with the clinical trials.

Physical Interventions

Patients can be encouraged to experiment with vibrators as part of foreplay or to achieve orgasm. Dyspareunia (painful intercourse) often results from the loss of estrogen due to aging, surgery, or treatment. Patients should be instructed to use a water-soluble lubricant with good staying power. Lubricant can be applied to her partner as part of foreplay and to her vaginal opening. They may need to reapply lubricant during intercourse. Instead of applying more lubricant, a few drops of tepid water will reactivate it.

Lubricants are available in vaginal applicators (Replens), tubes, and applicator bottles (K-Y). A face-to-face position, where a woman places her thighs together after her partner achieves penetration, will offer more control of depth of penetration. Other sexual positions that reduce depth of penetration are side lying and with the woman in the dominant position. If she is experiencing discomfort with abdominal pressure, these positions will reduce the pressure on the abdomen. Rear entry allows for the greatest depth of penetration, which may cause a greater degree of discomfort. Patients should be advised to use this position slowly at first. Sexual positions are only limited by a woman's ability to bend and move. Patients should experiment to find a sexual position that works for them. Vaginal estrogens are also used to relieve vaginal changes. Vagifem is a preloaded applicator containing one tablet of 25 mcg estradiol. The same type of vaginal estrogen is available in a ring (ESTRING).[30] The ring is inserted in the same manner as a diaphragm and may be removed during intercourse if her partner finds it uncomfortable. These estrogens are localized to the vaginal area and have not been shown to increase systemic estrogen levels.[31] Vaginal estrogen creams are also used to decrease atrophic vaginits.[32] Vaginal dilators are used to maintain vaginal patency, both for sexual activity and for future pelvic exams. Patients are instructed to apply a water-soluble lubricant to the dilator and insert it in the vagina for a specified period of time, usually 10 minutes. Dilators come in all shapes and sizes. Candles and calf nipples (available at farm supply stores) are economical options to the medical models.[13] A small handheld vacuum, Eros Therapy, has undergone clinical trials in the treatment of radiation-induced sexual dysfunction.[33,34] The device, manufactured by UroMetrics, showed improved lubrication, orgasm, and sexual satisfaction compared to normal subjects. A matter-of-fact approach to these subjects will help ease the discomfort for the healthcare team and patients. (See Suggested Patient Resources at the end of this chapter for further information.)

Special Considerations

Sexual activity for the woman with an ostomy has special challenges. Patients should work with an enterostomal therapist to alleviate these concerns. Some of the things that can be discussed are pouch management, odor control, and sexual positions that prevent direct pressure on the ostomy site. A folded towel placed above the ostomy will act as a bridge to prevent direct contact on the ostomy itself.

Alternative Sexual Practices

Healthcare professionals are often reluctant to discuss alternate sexual practices. Women who have had major vulvar or vaginal surgery may be unable to participate in penetration sexual activity. Masturbation may be included in foreplay or the sexual act itself. Intact clitoral function is necessary to achieve a clitoral orgasm during masturbation. Vibrators can be used as part of the masturbation activity. Friction on the penis from a woman's closed thighs may be sufficient to produce an orgasm in the male. Anal sex is becoming more prevalent in American society. Anal sex is a high-risk activity, and patients should be instructed to use lots of water soluble lubrication, and a condom is suggested. It may be desirable to use a Fleet Enema prior to anal sex.[35] Oral sex is a common sexual practice. However, women may have reservations about the taste of semen. It can be suggested that they use a flavored condom with a good-tasting lubricant. The use of a dental dam will also impede the exchange of bodily fluids. Assessment of an individual's needs and abilities should be considered before introducing the subject of alternate sexual practices.

Internet Concerns

The Internet has become a major source of information for healthcare providers, patients, and their families. Using the Internet to find sexual information carries the risk of receiving unwanted and pornographic material. For that reason, it should be used with caution. It is possible to use protection programs to avoid this unwanted content. Use computer functions to remove "cookies" and temporary files, and to establish parental controls.

Conclusion

Sexuality does not disappear with a diagnosis of cancer. Today's society is more sexually open, but sexuality continues to be a "silent subject" in the treatment of cancer. Shell concludes that we need reliable and valid interventions to promote sexual function and practice guidelines based on research.[6] Patients wait for healthcare providers to introduce the subject, and they in turn wait for the patient to make the initial inquiry.[1] Nursing education on issues of sexuality will remove barriers and improve communication about sexual issues. It is our responsibility to start the discussion and recognize when to refer a patient for advanced counseling. Above all, we have to work as a team with patients and their partners.

Suggested Professional Resources

American Association of Sexuality Educators, Counselors and Therapists
P. O. Box 1960
Ashland, VA 23005–1960
www.aasect.org

Burke CC. *Psychosocial Dimension of Oncology Nursing Care.* Oncology Nursing Society; 1998. 1-866-257-4ONS.

Katz A. The sounds of silence: sexuality information for cancer patients. *J Clin Oncol.* 2005;23(1):238–241. http://jco.ascopubs.org/cgi/content/full/23/1/238.

Moore-Higgs G, ed. *Women and Cancer: A Gynecologic Oncology Nursing Perspective.* 2nd Ed. Sudbury, MA: Jones and Bartlett; 2000.

Suggested Patient Resources

American Cancer Society. Sexuality and cancer: for the woman who has cancer and her partner. 1-800-ACS-2345.

Conner K, Langford L. *Ovarian Cancer: Your Guide to Taking Control.* Sebastopol, CA: O'Reilly & Associates.

Gynecologic Cancer Foundation. Renewing intimacy and sexuality after gynecologic cancer. http://www.thegcf.org/pubs/gyne_sexuality.pdf. 1-312-644-6610.

Mautner Project: www.mautnerproject.org; 1-866-628-8637.

OncoLink. Abramson Cancer Center of the University of Pennsylvania. Coping with Cancer: Sexuality & Fertility. http://oncolink.com/coping/coping.cfm?c=4.

United Ostomy Associations of America, Inc.: www.uoaa.org

References

1. Mestel R. Cancer disability changes sex life. *The Capitol Times,* August 3; 2000.
2. Basen-Engquist K. Dialog: sexuality after gynecologic cancer. *OncoloLog.* 2004;49(10).

3. University of Chicago Medical Center. Sexual problems of long-term cancer survivors merit more attention. *ScienceDaily.* 2007 July 30.

4. Susman E. Recognizing female sexual dysfunction as a complication of chemotherapy. *Oncology Times.* 2001;XXIII:46.

5. World Heath Organization. Gender and reproductive rights glossary. WHO Draft Working Definition. 2002 October.

6. Shell A. Evidence-based practice for symptom management in adults with cancer: sexual dysfunction. *ONF.* 2002;(29)1:53–65.

7. Davis AR. Recent advances in female sexual dysfunction. *Curr Psychiatry Rep.* 2000;2(3):211–214.

8. Spector I, Carey M. Incidence and prevalence of the sexual dysfunctions: a critical review of the empirical literature. *Arch Sex Behav.* 1990;19:389–408.

9. Berman J, Berman L, Goldstein I. Female sexual dysfunction: past, present and future. *Med Aspects Hum Sex.* 1998;1(5):15–20.

10. Gossfeld L, Cullen M. Sexuality and fertility issues. In: Moore-Higgs G, ed. *Women and Cancer: A Gynecologic Oncology Nursing Perspective.* 2nd ed. Sudbury, MA: Jones & Bartlett; 2000:470–473.

11. Larrison E. Causes and treatment of sexual dysfunction in the gynecologic oncology patient. *Women's Oncol.* 2002;Rev 2:135–142.

12. Hughes MJ, Cohen M. Sexuality and cancer: how oncology nurses can address it better. *Oncol Nurs Form.* 2003;30:153.

13. Mick J. Ten tips to improve sexuality assessment. http://houston.vc.ons.org/. Published 2007.

14. Jensen P, Groenvold M, Klee M, Thranow I, Peterson M, Machin D. Longitudinal study of sexual function and vaginal changes after radiotherapy for cervical cancer. *Int J Radiat Oncol Bio Phys* 2003;56(4):937–949.

15. Lindau ST, Gavrilova N, Anderson D. Sexual morbidity in very long term survivors of vaginal and cervical cancer: a comparison to national norms. *Gynecol Oncol.* 2007;106(2):413–418.

16. Pomel C, Atallah D, et al. Laparoscopic radical hysterectomy for invasive cervical cancer: 8-year experience of a pilot study. *Gynecol Oncol.* 2003;91(3):534–539.

17. Steed H, Rosen B, Murphy J, et al. A comparison of laparscopic-assisted radical vaginal hysterectomy and radical abdominal hysterectomy in the treatment of cervical cancer. *Gynecol Oncol.* 2004;93(3):588–589.

18. Obermair A, Manolitsas, TP, et al. Total laparoscopic hysterectomy for endometrial cancer: patterns of recurrence and survival. *Gynecol Oncol.* 2004;92(3):789–793.

19. Frigerio L, Gallo A, Ghezzi F, et al. Laparoscopic-assisted vaginal hysterectomy versus abdominal hysterectomy in endometrial cancer. *Int J Gynaecol Obstet.* 2006;93(3):209–213.

20. Green M, Eilo M, Nauman R. The impact of vulvar surgery on sexual function. *Med Aspects Hum Sex.* 1998;1:7–12.

21. Likes WM, Stegbauer, C, et al. Correlates of sexual function following vulvar excision. *Gynecol Oncol.* 2007;105(3):600–603.

22. Jensen P, Groenvold M, Klee M, et al. Early-stage cervical carcinoma, radical hysterectomy, and sexual function: a longitudinal study. *Cancer.* 2004;100(1):97–106.

23. Gregorian RS, Golden KA, et al. Antidepressant-induced sexual dysfunction. *Ann Pharmacother.* 2002;36(10):1577–1589.

24. Crenshaw T, Goldberg J. *Sexual Pharmacology.* New York, NY: W.W. Norton & Co.; 1996: 355–366.

25. Cavalcanti AL, Bagnoli VR, et al. Effect of slidenafil on clitoral blood flow and sexual response in postmenopausal women with orgasmic dysfunction. *Int J Gynaecol Obstet.* In press.

26. Alison A, Michale K. Sexual function in gynecologic cancer survivors. *Obstet Gynecol.* 2008;3(3):331–337.

27. Gallo-Silver L. The sexual rehabilitation of persons with cancer. *Cancer Pract.* 2000;8(1):10–15.

28. Buster JE, Kingsberg SA, et al. Testosterone patch for low sexual desire in surgically menopausal women: a randomized trial. *Obstet Gynecol.* 2005;105:944–952.

29. Barton D, Wender J, et al. Randomized controlled trial to evaluate transermal testosterone in female cancer survivors with decreased libido: North Central Cancer Treatment Group Protocol NO2C3. *J Nat Cancer Inst.* 2007;99:672–679.

30. ESTRING Pharmacia & Upjohn Product Monologue. www.pharmacia.com. Published May 7, 2002.

31. Aynton RA, Darling GM, et al. A comparative study of safety and efficacy of continuous low dose oestradiol released from a vaginal ring compared with conjugated equine oestrogen vaginal cream in the

treatment of postmenopausal urogenital atrophy. *Br J Obstet Gynaecol*. 1996;103(4):351–358.

32. Rikous J, Devlin M, Gelfand M, et al. 17 estradiol vaginal tablet versus conjugated equine estrogen vaginal cream to relieve menopausal atrophic vaginitis. *Menopause*. 2000;7(3):7156–7161.

33. Goodman A. In small study, hand-held device offers hope for alleviating radiation-induced sexual dysfunction in women. *Onc Times*. 2002;24(12):44–45.

34. Shroder M, Mell LK, et al. Clitoral therapy device for treatment of sexual dysfunction in irradiated cervical cancer patients. *Int J Radiat Oncol Bio Phys*. 2005;61(4):1078–1086.

35. George S, Caine K, eds. *A Lifetime of Sex: The Ultimate Manual on Sex, Women and Relationships for Every Stage of a Man's Life*. Emmatus, PA: Rodale Press; 1998:168–180.

Chapter 12

Infertility Issues

Mary Lou Cullen,
RNP, MS

Nurses who care for cancer patients have a responsibility to provide holistic care to enhance the quality of life of their patient population. Frequently, because of high emotional stress and the rush to provide cancer treatment, issues such as infertility are overlooked. Fertility problems are often linked to a substantial amount of stress, a range of impairments to marital functioning, reduced quality of life, societal repercussions, and issues with spirituality.[1] Loss of fertility, in addition to the diagnosis of cancer, is monumental for most women, often placing a major burden on one's emotional well-being. Studies have shown that providing pretreatment psychological counseling increases reports of personal well-being and interpersonal functioning.[2] Advances in cancer therapy have resulted in an increased number of long-term cancer survivors, and these survivors want to have a family. The desire to reproduce children is a basic human instinct.[3]

The nurse, working with a woman who has potential for or actual fertility problems, has the potential to make an impact not only on the quality of her life but also the evolution of her family. Inherent in this opportunity is a responsibility to ensure that such influence is, ideally, helpful but at least not harmful.[4] Thus, the nurse must be well informed and realistic regarding options available to the woman. Local and state regulations may have an impact on the options that are available in the community or state. Consideration must also be given to patient and family desires, expectations, and goals.

Overview of Assisted Reproductive Technologies

A number of assisted reproductive technologies (ART) are available. With basic knowledge and referral information about these, the oncology nurse is prepared to suggest realistic alternatives to the woman with fertility problems. Furthermore, referral to an infertility practice for further information and potential treatment can be timelier. The ability of the cancer patient to seek information *prior* to any cancer treatment cannot be stressed enough; this will allow the patient to have adequate information to make an informed decision regarding what options may be available to her. **Table 12-1** provides an outline of fertility options available for women with different gynecologic cancers.

Table 12-1 Potential fertility options for women with gynecologic cancers.

Site	Stage/Histopathology	Fertility Options
Ovary	Stage Ia	Only one ovary removed, theoretically normal
	Favorable histological type	If one ovary is functioning but tube is not, IVF
	Borderline or well-differentiated epithelial ovarian cancer	If both ovaries removed and uterus remains, IVF with donor oocytes
	Young woman of low parity	
	Cancer encapsulated and unruptured	
	No surface excrescences or adhesions	
	No invasion of capsule or mesovarium	
	Negative peritoneal washings	
	Negative staging operation: omental biopsy, peritoneal biopsy, pelvic and periaortic node sampling, biopsy of opposite ovary	
	Reliable follow-up	
	Germ cell tumors (require chemotherapy)	
Cervix	Stage Ia1, Ia2, Ib1 s/p cone biopsy (less than 3 mm invasion with no lymphovascular space involvement)	Desires children: cone biopsy with close follow-up versus radical vag. trachelectomy versus simple hysterectomy
	Stage Ib, IIa, s/p radical hysterectomy with pelvic lymph node dissection (ovaries remain) versus radiation therapy	IVF with gestational carrier possible for ovary transposition (if radiation therapy indicated)
	Stage Ib, III, and IV Radiation and/or chemotherapy	Frozen embryo (IVF) (prior to treatment), implantation in gestational carrier Cryopreservation of ovarian tissue and oocytes
Gestational trophoblastic disease	Chemotherapy Hysterectomy	Normal IVF with gestational carrier

In-Vitro Fertilization

The concept of in-vitro fertilization (IVF) dates back to animal research in 1935, but it was not until 1978 that Edwards and Steptoe reported the first live birth of a human baby, Louise Brown, conceived by IVF in England. The Jones Institute in Norfolk, Virginia, reported the first live IVF birth in the United States in 1981. In 2006 alone, according to the most recent United States data available, approximately 50,000 babies were born as a result of IVF.[5] It has been estimated that over 3 million IVF babies have been born since 1978.

Initially, IVF was designed to provide a reproductive mechanism for women who had no fallopian tube function.[6] Due to increased knowledge and success, the process is now treating other forms of infertility. Some examples include: endometriosis, unexplained infertility, male infertility, immunological factors, cervical factors, and cancer-related infertility. IVF and related technologies allow access to the microenvironment of the human oocyte, the subtleties of gamete interaction, and the intricacies of syngamy and early embryonic development.[7]

The procedure of IVF is relatively simple and commonly done in an outpatient setting with mild sedation and minimal risk to the woman (**Figure 12-1**). After stimulation with ovulation-inducing medications, the woman's oocytes are collected from her ovaries through transvaginal ultrasound-directed aspiration and fertilized in the laboratory with her partner or donor's sperm. Following early development, the embryo(s) are placed into the uterus via the cervix. This procedure, called *embryo transfer* (ET), is performed using a fine catheter attached to a sterile syringe containing the embryo(s) and culture media. If

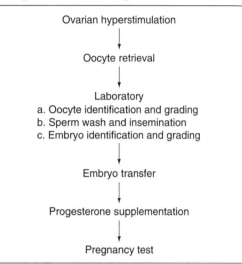

Figure 12-1 The procedure of IVF.

Ovarian hyperstimulation

↓

Oocyte retrieval

↓

Laboratory
a. Oocyte identification and grading
b. Sperm wash and insemination
c. Embryo identification and grading

↓

Embryo transfer

↓

Progesterone supplementation

↓

Pregnancy test

pregnancy ensues, the embryo(s) continues to develop naturally in the mother's uterus. The 2005 clinical pregnancy statistics reported by the American Society for Reproductive Medicine (ASRM) for IVF are approximately 30%, with a take-home baby rate of 25%.[5]

Gamete Intrafallopian Transfer

Gamete intrafallopian transfer (GIFT) is a technique that was developed in 1984 by Dr. Ricardo Asch. In this procedure, after ovarian stimulation, oocytes are aspirated from the woman's ovaries via laparoscopy. The oocytes are then loaded into a transfer catheter with sperm that have gone through a wash process and are immediately transferred into the fimbriated end of the fallopian tubes. A woman must have at least one normal fallopian tube for this procedure. If fertilization occurs, the embryo(s) may travel through the fallopian tube to the uterus. Because GIFT requires a surgical procedure, laparoscopy, it is rarely performed at most ART centers. For this reason, IVF has become the treatment of choice.

Donor Oocytes

Using donor oocytes is an obvious extension of the IVF process, and, perhaps, one of the most exciting. It means that women without functioning ovaries who have a normal uterus can now conceive. Following the common model for donor sperm, oocyte donation can be made anonymously, or known donors can be selected. While there are potential concerns with the use of known donors, no documented problems can be found. Many programs in the United States require recipients to identify their own donor. The use of anonymous donors is increasing, with most large ART programs having an extensive list of available anonymous donors.

Oocyte donation starts with the removal of eggs (through oocyte retrieval methods previously discussed) from a donor after ovarian stimulation. Next, donor oocytes are fertilized with the recipient partner's sperm. The resulting embryo(s) are transferred to the uterus of the recipient by the IVF procedure. The challenge of this procedure is the synchronization of the donor and recipient's cycles; consequently, hormone therapy is required for the recipient.[7]

Screening of the donor varies from program to program. Current (2006) American Society for Reproductive Medicine guidelines request that standard preconception testing—psychological, genetic, and serological testing (RH, syphilis, HIV-1, hepatitis B and C, and CMV antibody)—be completed before initiation of oocyte donation.[8] As technology evolves, these recommendations may change.

To date, ART, with oocyte donation, is one of the most successful treatments performed in any infertility program. Pregnancy rates as high as 50% have been reported, though more commonly, 41% of the procedures are successful.[5] Many young gynecologic oncology patients have lost one or both ovaries to borderline, early stage epithelial ovarian tumors or germ cell tumors. Oocyte donation is a viable option for this patient population.

Surrogate Gestational Carrier

For a woman without a uterus but with intact ovaries, a surrogate gestational carrier (host uterus) provides the only opportunity for a biological child. In this procedure, the woman who desires pregnancy is stimulated with medication to produce oocytes. The eggs collected through oocyte retrieval are fertilized with her partner's sperm, and then the resulting embryo(s) is placed into the surrogate's uterus (ET). If synchronization of the cycles of the patient and surrogate is not possible, the resulting embryos may be frozen for later transfer to the gestational carrier. Currently, most couples are required to find their own carrier. The concept of gestational surrogacy introduces many social, ethical, and legal issues that will be clarified over time and with experience.[9]

Surrogate Mother

Surrogacy, or surrogate motherhood, is an alternative when a woman has neither a functioning uterus nor ovaries. In this procedure, the surrogate mother is inseminated with the sperm of the infertile woman's partner. The male donor must complete extensive testing similar to that described for the oocyte donor.

Insemination can be done either intracervically or as an intrauterine (IUI) procedure. Intracervical insemination is a simple process. The sperm of the infertile woman's partner are drawn into a syringe and, with a speculum in place, deposited into the fertile mucus found in the cervical os of the surrogate. With IUI, a speculum is placed in the vagina, the cervical os is identified, and using a very thin catheter, washed sperm are deposited directly into the uterine cavity of the surrogate. Both procedures need to be timed very carefully to coincide with ovulation.

The surrogate mother has a genetic link to the offspring, making legal implications challenging and worrisome. There is, however, a biblical precedent for surrogate mothering in Jacob's wife, Rachel. Laws regarding surrogacy need to become standardized to prevent the intended parents from disappointment and further expense. To date, few cases have gone to litigation and those that have, have favored the intended parents.[9]

Surrogate mother applicants, whether for gestational surrogacy or surrogate motherhood, undergo an extensive screening process. Most programs require that only women who have had successful, uncomplicated pregnancies with children of their own become candidates. Furthermore, it is desirable that candidates be motivated by factors other than money (e.g., the desire to help another or the view that surrogacy is a personally rewarding experience). After the initial interview, psychological testing is done on both potential candidates and their spouses. Intelligence, ability to understand treatment plans, reliability, self-esteem, coping mechanisms, support systems, and sensitivity are a few of the important screening criteria. Similar psychological screening is done on the infertile couple. When psychological and medical screening is complete on all parties, they are matched and introduced, usually with the guidance of a psychologist. Ongoing psychological counseling is important to the outcome.

Cryopreservation and Embryo Donation

The human embryo has been successfully frozen at many stages of development. Stimulation of the ovary with medications during an IVF or GIFT cycle usually produces more oocytes than can be safely transferred at one time. For this reason, cryopreservation can offer a woman additional attempts at pregnancy without the necessity of repeating ovulation induction or egg retrieval. Another advantage of frozen embryo transfer (FET) is that transfer can occur at the time in a natural ovulatory cycle when endometrial receptivity is highest. Cryopreserved embryo donation, where permitted by law, provides an opportunity for children in infertile couples.

The success rate of frozen embryos is approximately 10% less than that for fresh embryos; this is in part because only 75% of cryopreserved human embryos survive after thawing.[10] However, on average, fewer embryos are transferred in frozen cycles than in fresh cycles, a partial explanation for the lower success rates. Frozen embryos can be stored indefinitely. A nominal fee for embryo storage is not uncommon. Counseling is required regarding the future use of frozen embryos.

Like other aspects of ART, laws regarding human embryo freezing vary from state to state. Each program has well-defined legal contracts to protect both the patient and the medical community. Ownership and control of embryos must be decided before cryopreservation. Currently accepted practice in most states regarding legal ownership of embryos resulting from the fertilization of the wife's ova by the husband's sperm is that the embryos shall be considered joint property of both partners.[10]

One major disadvantage of cryopreservation of embyros is the time required from start to finish of the procedure, usually 2–5 weeks. For some cancer patients, this delay in starting cancer treatment is unacceptable and not practical due to the risk involved with delaying treatment for some forms of cancer.

Autotransplantation of Cryopreserved Ovarian Tissue

A process currently in clinical trials by researchers in both the United States and Great Britain is the freezing of human ovarian tissue. Research by Gosden and colleagues, using animal tissue, offers the possibility for a more desirable approach to preserving reproductive potential in the female cancer patient. Gosden removed ovaries from sheep and then froze thin slices of the cortical tissue, which contain thousands of oocytes.[11] At a later date, the tissue was thawed and replaced in the region of the residual ovarian site, near the fimbriated end of the fallopian tube. In view of the fact that this is an autograft, there was no risk for immunological graft rejection. These sheep have since gone on to have normal ovulatory cycles and,

more importantly, to bear and deliver normal offspring. Eggs in slices of human ovarian tissue survive cryopreservation and thawing like animal ovaries. Ovarian tissue has been successfully reimplanted in a small number of healthy women volunteers in the United States, where it has functioned normally for a few weeks. More research is imperative in this field. Female cancer patients have the potential to benefit greatly from this procedure because ovarian tissue could be frozen prior to cancer treatment in much the same way as sperm are frozen and later thawed for use.[12]

Current recommendations by the ASRM are that clinical trials be carried out according to the guidelines of each institutional review board. Approved, written consent forms must be carefully presented and clearly understood, before signing, when a woman is offered this research protocol. Some female cancer patients have already had ovarian tissue frozen, but, to date, few have had the tissue transferred back.[12] There are two reported live births in cancer patients from this procedure. The primary reason tissue has seldom been transferred is the concern about the presence in the cryopreserved tissue of microscopic metastatic disease and the possibility of tumor reimplantation. This is still considered to be an experimental procedure. Areas of research are focusing on these important issues, with the goal that many women with cancer will benefit in the near future.

Radical Vaginal Trachelectomy

Radical vaginal trachelectomy is a surgical procedure that has been practiced in Europe for years and is gaining popularity in the United States. This procedure removes the cancerous portion of the cervix, leaving the ovaries and uterus. The diseased portion of the cervix is removed directly through the vagina. With the rest of her reproductive system intact, the woman is usually able to have children. However, the future children must be delivered by cesarean section because the cervix will be unsuitable for natural delivery.[13]

This procedure could be recommended for young women of reproductive age who desire children and have *selected* stage Ia1, Ia2, or Ib1 of either squamous or adenocarcinoma lesions less than 3 cm in diameter with limited endocervical involvement. Patients are told that this is not standard procedure for cervical cancer; however, with more than 500 cases reported in the literature, risk of recurrence is unchanged to those with radical hysterectomy.[13]

Breast Cancer/Tamoxifen Stimulation

Breast cancer is the second most common malignancy in women of reproductive age, and of the 180,000 new cases in the United States each year, 15% occur in women during their reproductive years.[14] Many of these young women are treated with alkylating agents following mastectomy or lumpectomy. Alkylating agents can have adverse effects on ovarian function, and each course of chemotherapy will result in a significant loss of ovarian reserve. Even those women who do not immediately become menopausal following chemotherapy are likely to experience infertility as time passes and they await a disease-free interval. Most oncologists recommend that a

woman have a disease-free interval of at least 3 years before attempting pregnancy.[15]

As women become more aware of the adverse effects of breast cancer treatment on ovarian function, many more are seeking ART procedures to preserve fertility. Embryo cryopreservation is the recommended option and is a well-established clinical approach. However, to be able to store embryos, a woman must produce multiple oocytes during her IVF procedure, and it is clearly documented that women who have received chemotherapy have a difficult time producing multiple oocytes.[15] Breast cancer cells can be affected by estrogen, the most common drug used to stimulate the ovary to produce multiple follicles. Most oncologists discourage the use of estrogen-producing drugs in breast cancer patients.

Recent studies by Oktay and colleagues showed that the combination of low-dose FSH with tamoxifen (a chemotherapeutic agent that suppresses breast carcinogenesis) and letrozole (an aromatase inhibitor that suppresses estrogen production and was shown to be superior to tamoxifen in the treatment of advanced-stage postmenopausal breast cancer) results in high embryo yield.[15] Recurrence rates of cancer do not seem to be increased. The letrozole protocol may be preferred because it results in lower estrogen levels.

Legal and Ethical Issues

The advent of ART has called into question some of our culture's most fundamental assumptions, beliefs, and practices with respect to how children are conceived. The ethical aspects of reproductive technology have raised debates since 1978, when IVF was first introduced. Since 2003, the Vatican has formally denounced all ART as amoral.[16] As techniques such as embryo splitting to produce identical twins continue to grow more sophisticated, the debates will intensify.

Statutes, regulations, judicial decisions, and the constitutional protection of right to privacy to make procreative decisions can profoundly influence which infertility services are offered and in what manner.[17] The law shapes the standards by which healthcare professionals must practice, and it likewise influences the rights and responsibilities of both the infertile couple and society with respect to a resulting child.[17] To prevent misunderstandings, all parties must be fully informed about the legal situation in their jurisdiction. These disclosures should include legal uncertainties as well as already established law.

It is impossible to discuss all the ethical and legal ramifications of ART. In fact, laws are not well established and are changing rapidly, but ultimately, the use of ART lies with the individual or couple. Founded both in statutory and case law, the doctrine of informed consent protects the patient's decision making and right to control his or her own body.[17] Informed consent requires education. Options that exist must be presented in a clear and concise manner, a challenge for the healthcare team. We will see more complex problems with the application of new technologies; therefore, we must remain ever vigilant of the eventual ethical issues.

Adoption or Childfree Living

Two other options not often addressed by health providers are adoption and childfree living.

ART frequently overlooks these in the quest for family building.

In the United States, it is estimated that 2%–4% of the population is adopted. Approximately 50,000 adoptions of nonrelated, healthy children occur annually in the United States, with over 8000 adoptions of foreign children and 10,000 adoptions of children with special needs[18] taking place. There are many different types of adoption—open and closed, private and agency, domestic and international, and special-needs adoptions. Advising a couple to contact organizations such as RESOLVE, Adoption Resources, or the National Council for Adoption as soon as possible is extremely helpful. These organizations can inform couples of what is available, approximate costs, waiting times, risks and benefits, and what is legal in their state.

It is advisable to encourage couples to start pursuing adoption early in the infertility workup, even if they are not yet committed to adoption. By doing so, the couple can learn what the racial, religious, and age restrictions are in various agencies, which should prevent confusion or disappointment concerning these issues when they are ready to proceed.

The couple preparing for adoption due to cancer-related infertility has many feelings related to loss of genetic continuity and inability to experience pregnancy and birth. They need time to grieve these losses and encouragement to set realistic expectations for them. Advising them to spend time with people who respect them and to meet with both adoptive and nonadoptive families are also helpful interventions.

The possibility of childfree living should also be discussed early. Assurance by a health provider that this option is a viable one may remind the couple that they are valuable for more than just their reproductive potential. The nurse can suggest alternatives, such as volunteering for children's activities, returning to school, starting a business, or traveling. Open communication regarding what the couple's life values are and prioritizing these values will enhance their self-esteem. And, like couples who are considering adoption, using resources such as RESOLVE and spending time with families committed to childfree living can help the couple to resolve their grief. Hopefully, when a couple comes to terms with the loss of childbearing capabilities and completes the grieving process, they will begin to develop realistic expectations for the future.

The Nurse's Role

The nurse's role in caring for the infertile oncology patient is multifaceted. Adviser, communicator, educator, counselor, and provider of support are the primary roles. The nurse must have the ability to listen and respond with empathy, recognizing and respecting the unique pain of the infertile woman and her partner. There may be no words to comfort someone whose life's dreams have been shattered by a diagnosis of malignancy and infertility. Nurses who have positive self-esteem and can acknowledge their own life sufferings and who possess an excellent knowledge base are best prepared to provide coping strategies in these cases. Fertile Hope, a nonprofit organization founded by a young female cancer patient for women who desire reproductive information, support, and hope, is an excellent resource for female cancer patients (www.fertilehope.org).

Cancer patients suffer intense emotional upheaval. They must learn to recognize, cope with, and resolve feelings of denial, isolation, grief, anger, and depression.[19] Adequate time for verbalization of feelings and for grieving must be given. Reassurance that grief is normal and that it will take time for resolution must be reinforced frequently.

Women of reproductive age who have cancer should be referred to an appropriate assisted reproductive center as soon as the diagnosis is made to enable them to discuss their future reproductive options and maximize their future chance of pregnancy. This is an extremely important nursing intervention.

Widening the patient's support system to include family, friends, social and religious services, and organizations, such as RESOLVE, ASRM, Fertile Hope, Susan G. Komen Breast Cancer Foundation, or others, are important nursing strategies. Encouraging the couple to ask for support so that the systems may be beneficial in resolving grief and diffusing anger is an important nursing goal. **Table 12-2** provides a list of questions for the patient who is considering ART. This list is not all inclusive. Each couple will have their own set of questions and concerns. Referring a couple to a list of reading materials, such as that in **Table 12-3**, adds to the nurse's armamentarium.

In addition, the use of various Web sites, such as www.sart.org, www.asrm.org, www.fertilehope.org, and others, will provide important information and programs available throughout the United States and Canada.

Table 12-2 QUESTIONS THAT A NURSE SHOULD BE PREPARED TO ANSWER ABOUT ASSISTED REPRODUCTIVE TECHNOLOGIES (ART).

1. What are the risks and benefits of the procedure?
2. What does our state allow; what is allowed in neighboring states?
3. How many IVF or GIFT cycles does the program complete per year?
4. What is the pregnancy rate; what is the take-home baby rate?
5. What are the projected costs of the program?
6. How are the donors screened?
7. How long does it take to conceive; how many attempts must I consider?
8. What drugs will I receive, and what are potential side effects?
9. What is the time commitment for the various procedures?
10. How is the procedure done?
11. Will confidentiality be maintained?
12. What about medical insurance; who will be covered and who pays for it?
13. Should life insurance be purchased?
14. What is the incidence of miscarriage?
15. What is the risk of congenital anomalies?
16. What is the risk of HIV or other sexually transmitted diseases?
17. Should we tell the offspring, and if so, what?
18. What support systems are in place for us as a couple? As individuals?
19. After its birth, to whom does the child legally belong; must we adopt that child?
20. What is the chance a surrogate mother will refuse to relinquish a child?
21. What are the age limits of the program?
22. Are single women accepted into the program?

Table 12-3 BOOKS ABOUT INFERTILITY.

1. Taking Charge of Your Fertility
2. Dr. Richard Marr's Fertility Book
3. Conquering Infertility
4. Getting Pregnant Naturally
5. In-vitro Fertilization: The A.R.T. of Making Babies
6. The Infertility Diet: Get Pregnant and Prevent Miscarriage
7. Adopting After Infertility
8. Expecting Miracles
9. When Empty Arms Become a Heavy Burden
10. Infertility Sucks

Summary

In the process of developing a therapeutic relationship, nurses can assess a woman's desire to have a family, provide basic information regarding the effects of disease and possible effects of therapy, provide support, and promote hopefulness. As new treatment modalities evolve, it is essential that the nurse remain informed about how he or she can affect the patient's quality of life. It certainly seems appropriate to tackle infertility concerns just as aggressively as current treatment modalities aim for cure. The nurse can instill in the patient a realistic sense of hope that infertility issues related to the disease and therapies may be overcome and that it may indeed be possible to have the family she desires.

References

1. Patridge AH, Gelber S, Peppercorn J, et al. Web-based survey of fertility issues in young women with breast cancer. *Gynecol Oncol.* 2005;97:90–95.

2. Wenzel L, Dogan-Astes A, Habbal R, et al. Defining and measuring reproductive concerns of female cancer survivors. *J Natl Cancer Inst.* 2005;(monogr):91–93.

3. Kim SS. Fertility preservation in female cancer patients: current development and future directions. *Fertil Steril.* 2006;85(1).

4. Cousineau TM, Domar AD. Psychological impact of infertility in best practices and research in clinical obstetrics and gynaecology. 2007;21(2):293–308.

5. American Society for Reproductive Medicine. Assisted reproductive technology in the United States: 2006 results generated from the American Society for Reproductive Medicine/Society for Assisted Reproductive Technology Registry. Press release. http://www.asrm.org. Published 2008.

6. Marrs RP, Vargyas JM. Human in vitro fertilization: state of the art. In: Mishell Jr DR, Davajan V, eds. *Infertility, Contraception & Reproductive Endocrinology.* Oradell, NJ: Medical Economics Company; 1986:565.

7. Navot D, Rosenwaks Z. Ovum donation. In: Seibel MM, ed. *Infertility: A Comprehensive Text.* Norwalk, CT: Appleton & Lange; 1990:513.

8. American Society for Reproductive Medicine. Guidelines for gamate and embryo donation. *Fertil Steril.* 2006;86(suppl 4):S.38–S.50.

9. Batzofin M, Brisman M, Madsen P. Gestational surrogacy: consistent laws are necessary to provide effective treatment. *Fertil Steril.* 2005;(84)1: S355–S356.

10. Dudzinski DM. Ethical issues in fertility preservation for adolescent cancer survivors: oocyte and ovarian tissue cryopreservation. *J Pediatric Adolesc Gynecol.* 2004;17:97–102.

11. Gosden RG, Baird DT, Wade JC, et al. Restoration of fertility to oophorectomized sheep by ovarian autografts stored at -196 degrees C. *Hum Reprod.* 1994;4(9):597–603.

12. Kim SS. Fertility preservation and reproduction in cancer patients. *Fertil Steril.* 2005;83(6): 1–11.

13. Beiner M, Covens A. Surgery insight: radical vaginal trachelectomy as a method of fertility preservation for cervical cancer. *Natl Clinical Pract Oncol.* 2007; 46(6):353–361.

14. Jemal A, et al. Cancer statistics. *CA Cancer J Clin.* 2008;58:71–76.

15. Oktay K, Buyuk E, Libertella N, Akar M, Rozenwaks Z. Fertility preservation in breast cancer patients: a prospective controlled comparison of ovarian stimulation with tamoxifen and letrozole for embryo cryopreservation. *J Clin Oncol.* 2005;23(19):4347–4353.

16. Sheaj B. The moral status of invitro fertilization (IVF) biology and method. Jan/Feb 2003. *Catholic Insight.* 2006;14:18,37.

17. Patrizio P, Butts S, Caplan A. Ovarian tissue preservation and future fertility: emerging technologies and ethical considerations. *J Natl Cancer Inst Monogr.* 2005;107–110(34).

18. American Fertility Society. *Adoption: A Guide for Patients.* Birmingham, AL: American Fertility Society; 2007.

19. Lee S, Schover L, Patridge A, et al. American Society of Clinical Oncology recommendations on fertility preservation in cancer patients. *J of Clin Oncol.* 2006; 24(18):2917–2930.

Chapter 13

Menopause

Barbara C. Poniatowski, MS, RN-BC, AOCN®

Introduction

Menopause is a natural biological event in the reproductive cycle of the middle-aged woman. The average age for menopause is 51–52 years.[1–4] This phase of a woman's life, known as the climacteric, starts with the decline of ovarian activity and ends when ovarian functioning ceases.[5] During menopause, biological fertility and endocrine ovarian activity cease with a marked decline in estradiol levels and an elevation of gonadotropin in early follicular phase.[6] Menopause can be delineated into three phases. The premenopausal phase is defined as having menstruated within the last 3 months. A last menstrual period within 3 to 12 months defines the menopausal phase, with the absence of menstruation for at least 12 months defining the postmenopausal phase.[7,8] The transition from premenopausal to postmenopausal state may take 2–8 years.[7] Physical and environmental factors may affect the age of menopause. These factors include nutrition, smoking, reproductive history, and socioeconomic status.[6,7] Malnutrition, smoking, lower height and weight, null parity, never using oral contraceptives, race, and ethnicity contribute to an early menopause and a shorter premenopausal period.[4,6,7,9] Body weight increase is associated with later menopause.[4]

Women who experience menopause prior to the age of 40 are classified as having premature menopause. Premature menopause can be induced through surgical ablation (bilateral oophorectomy with or without the removal of the uterus), radiation, and chemotherapy. Women who have a family history of premature menopause, Sheehan syndrome, or XX chromosomes may also experience a premature menopause.[3,6,8,10,11]

Menopausal Symptom Experience

It is difficult to consider a woman's menopausal symptoms without reviewing the history of menopause for the last 2 centuries. Sociological events of the 19th and 20th centuries, including a change in the role of women, the focus on menopause as a disease, and society's perception of menopause, have defined the menopause experience.[12] The classification of menopause as a disease and a change in the woman's role from independent to submissive and dependent occurred simultaneously.[1,2,10] The classification of menopause as a disease created fear, isolation, and negativity that survived into the 21st century.[3,10,13,14] The Healthy Women's Study (HWS) explored the myths and realities of menopause with a survey of 541 women.[13] A majority of these women felt that menopause did not change a woman but that they themselves were likely to become depressed. A follow-up study revealed that a negative attitude and other life changes affected the woman's quality of life and health.[13] Hunter's[15] review of five large studies supported this contention that a negative view of menopause impacts a woman's menopausal symptoms and quality of life.

Researchers began to question the validity of menopause as a disease during the last 2 decades of the 20th century. Previous research had methodology flaws that included preselection, the use of retrospective data, poorly constructed data collection tools, the measurement of psychological morbidity, and failure to account for cultural impact.[2,16,17]

Identifying menopausal symptoms can be challenging. Kaufert, Gilbert, & Hassard[18] detailed a number of methodological issues they faced when trying to determine what menopausal symptoms a woman experiences. These issues include preparation of symptom lists, measuring psychological morbidity, minimizing the impact of cultural beliefs, and short longitudinal studies and follow-up.[4] Variables that affect a woman's experience during the menopause include cultural diversity, role changes, society's attitude, health beliefs, physical and emotional health, and attitude toward menopause.[4] Control of these variables in the design of a study can be problematic. Problems are evident when you compare the symptoms included in the Blatt Menopausal Index, the Greene Index, and the Neugarten and Kranes Checklist. These lists were developed from reported symptoms, from treatment-seeking women, from symptoms assigned by a physician, or from symptoms garnered from the literature.[16,17,19] The Melbourne Women's Midlife Health Study, a community-based cross-sectional study of 2001 women aged 45–55 years, found that women who do not seek help during menopause had different health behaviors and symptom reporting than women who do seek help.[19] This has been validated by the Massachusetts Women's Health Study (MWHS) report that health status at menopause reflected prior levels of health as well as previous healthcare practices.[17] A study by Maureen Broughton[3] explored a woman's interpretation of the menopause experience and found that menopause knowledge, culture, event timing, and internalization of the meaning of menopause influence the experience. Taechakraichana and colleagues[5] reported that the Study of Women's Health Across the Nation (SWAN) clearly demonstrated racial and ethnic differences for menopausal symptoms.

During the 1990s, researchers categorized menopausal symptoms into domains. Hildritch and colleagues[20] categorized the symptoms of menopause into five domains: vasomotor, physical, psychological, sexual, and global. Perez[21] listed symptoms in three domains: general, somatic, and psychobiological. A NIH Consensus Panel[4] indicated that hot flashes, night sweats, vaginal dryness, and sleep disturbance are symptoms that are strongly or moderately linked to menopause. The panel also concluded that evidence did not support a strong relationship between menopause and mood symptoms, cognitive disturbances, somatic symptoms, or urinary incontinence. While Sterns and Hayes[22] stated that 30% of women complain of symptoms that may last up to 5 years, with 20% continuing to have symptoms for 15 years, the NIH Conference[4] was unconvinced that enough data exists about the severity, frequency, and duration of symptoms to draw any conclusions.

Vasomotor Symptoms

Vasomotor disturbances include hot flashes, night sweats, nausea, chills that may lead to symptoms of insomnia, early morning awakening, mood disturbances, muscle aching, fatigue, and palpitations.[5,23,24] Symptoms may be preceded by an aura of palpitations and headache.[25] After the vasomotor instability, the woman may experience diaphoresis, coldness, tiredness, dizziness, or fainting.[5] Hot flashes at night interrupt REM and non-REM sleep patterns. Interruption of sleep may result in daytime dizziness, loss of ability to concentrate, and forgetfulness.[5] Vasomotor disturbance can translate to uncontrolled mood changes, irritability, depression, fear of being alone in public, loss of self-confidence, feeling tense, difficulty making decisions, anxiety, feeling unworthy, and loss of libido.[5]

It has been calculated that 55%–93% of menopausal women experience hot flashes and that one-third of the women find the hot flashes to be intolerable.[4,8,22,26,27] Approximately one-third of the women will seek treatment with a healthcare provider.

Factors that affect the incidence of hot flashes and the resulting sequelae include early progesterone hormone fluctuation, weight, negative attitudes, alcohol use, early menarche (before age 12), a lower level of education, caffeine intake, spicy foods, culture, environment, and early menopause (before age 47 years).[7,26–28]

The Seattle Midlife Women's Health Study established a relationship between hot flashes and low estrogen/hypothalmic levels. Hot flashes occur more frequently at night because the hypothalamic/pituitary axis peaks at night.[7] The intensity of the hot flash may vary with weight. Thinner women tend to experience more severe and more frequent flashes due to decreased amount of adipose tissue and reduced ability to transform androstenedione to estrone and estradiol.[29] Alcohol, caffeine, stress/anxiety, and a warm environmental temperature also trigger the hot flash.[29] Findings from the MWHS showed that women with a negative attitude toward menopause reported a high frequency of hot flashes.[17] However, in the same study, the vast majority of women (69%) did not report being bothered by hot flashes or night sweats. An earlier sample of 1746 women, age 40–66 years, concluded that less than half the women with hot flashes ever report moderate to severe symptoms.[24] However, this earlier study was based on Swedish women, and cultural differences could have been a mitigating factor in the findings. Cultural differences in hot flash reporting were seen by Lock[30] in a study of Japanese women and menopause. According to Lock, Japanese women do not report hot flashes as a symptom of menopause. This cross-sectional survey maintains that Japanese women associate menopause with gray hair, changes in eyesight, short-term memory loss, headaches, shoulder stiffness, dizziness, unspecified chest pain, and lassitude. Participants in the SWAN study of 14,906 women from a variety of cultures revealed that African American women and women with surgically induced menopause report greater vasomotor symptoms.[28,31]

The same study found that postmenopausal women had more vasomotor symptoms than premenopausal women. Rostom[32] communicated that vasomotor symptoms appeared to be more severe in women who had estrogen abruptly withdrawn, smoked, or whose mothers had severe hot flashes.

Urogenital Symptoms

Approximately 95% of menopausal women experience urogenital symptoms, such as frequent urination, urgency, leakage, vaginal dryness, or itching or burning in the vagina or vulva. For as many as 40% of women, these symptoms may be moderate to severe.[33] These symptoms begin to occur well before menses cease, and endogenous estrogen withdraw to the epithelium is credited with initiating the urogenital changes that occur in the bladder, urethra, vagina, vulva, and surrounding structures.[33,34] See **Table 13-1** for a list of the causes of urogenital atrophy and **Table 13-2** for the physical characteristics of urogential atrophy.

Dyspareunia and related sexual problems (i.e., decreased desire and responsiveness) are a direct consequence of urogenital pathophysiology. Ballinger[35] implies that sexual behavior is influenced by menopause. The sexual problems are in part caused by dyspareunia related to vaginal

Table 13-1 CAUSES OF UROGENITAL ATROPHY.

Cause	
Antiestrogen medications	Lupron
	Clomid
	Provera
	Synarel
	Nolvadex
	Danocrine
Postpartum breastfeeding	Absence of placental estrogen
	Antagonistic action of prolactin on estrogen
Premenopausal	Premature ovarian failure
Extraneous causes	Surgery (oophorectomy)
	Chemotherapy
	Radiation
	Menopause
Other milder forms	Heavy smoking (reduce estrogen absorption)
	Reduced sexual activity
	Inadequate systemic ERT

Source: Adapted from Carcio H. Urogenital atrophy. *Advance for Nurse Practitioners.* 2002;October.

Table 13-2 PHYSICAL CHARACTERISTICS OF UROGENITAL ATROPHY.

Urogenital Area	Characteristics
Labia	Less prominent, flattened, fusion of labia minora, lax and wrinkled, thinning cell layer, prominent sebaceous glands, positive sticky glove sign, easily traumatized, irritation due to continuous use of pad for urinary incontinence
Clitoris	Less prominent, retracts beneath the prepuce, slight atrophy
Subcutaneous fat	Diminished
Pubic hair	Thin, less coarse
Vaginal wall epithelium	Thin, friable, shiny, small ulcerations, patches of granulation tissue, petechial spots (resemble trichomoniasis), fissures, ecchymotic areas from exposed capillaries, loss of rugae, decreased vascularity (pale), less lubrication (dryness), loss of distensibility, elasticity, decreased discharge
Vagina	Introital stenosis (less than two fingers), shortened, shrinkage of fornices, less elasticity, possible cystocele, rectocele, or pelvic prolapse
Discharge	Variable, watery to thick and cloudy, may be serosanguineous from friable surfaces
Maturation index	Preponderance of parabasal cells
Cervix	Shrinks, flattens into vaginal wall, Os becomes tiny, squamo-columnar junction recedes up the cervical canal, atrophied crypts and ducts in canal
Uterus	Smaller, endometrium thins (less granular, atrophic), uterine stripe less than 4 mm, fibroids may shrink
Perineum	Minor laceration at posterior fourchette
Urethra	Caruncle (red, berry-type protrusion, atrophy, polys, prolapsed/eversion urethral mucosa)
Pelvic floor	Muscle tone diminishes, cystocele, rectocele
Ligaments and connective tissue	Lose strength and tone
Bladder mucosa and urethra	Decreased tone

Source: Adapted from Carcio H. Urogenital atrophy. *Advance for Nurse Practitioners.* 2002;October.

atrophy, vaginitis, and a general reduction in sexual responsiveness. Decrease in sexual interest is associated with hormone withdrawal, low social class, symptoms of depression, and poor marital relations.[7,16,35] Stone and Pearlstein[16] associated five changes in sexual functioning with menopause: diminished sexual responsiveness, dyspareunia, decreased sexual activity, decline in sexual desire, and a dysfunctional male partner. Symptoms of sexual dysfunction may last 5–15 years in 15%–30% of patients.[16] Vaginal atrophy and vaginitis that causes dyspareunia are related to loss of ovarian estrogen, causing the vagina to become friable and pale.[15,16] The loss of estrogen leads to vaginal mucosal thinning, decreased vaginal secretions, and secretions that lose acidity. Tissue is then more sensitive to trauma, inflammation, and infection resulting in dyspareunia.[10] Stearns and Hayes[22] associated the early loss of estrogen or premature menopause with worse symptoms of sexual dysfunction. Work by Freedman[34] suggests that decreases in estrogens, androgens, and progesterone affected the clitoral sensitivity, the vulvar blood flow, and the ability of the woman to achieve orgasm.

Psychological Symptoms

Ballinger[35] and Hunter[15] reviewed the psychiatric literature concerning menopause and found no major effect on a variety of psychiatric symptoms. Schmidt and Rubinow[36] suggest that an excess of somatic, mood, and behavioral symptoms do appear to be associated with surgically induced and natural menopause. These authors reference several studies that suggest an increase in a woman's vulnerability to mood disorders during the menopause stage of life.

Historically, researchers felt that depression triggered menopause.[10,17] In the HWS of 541 premenopausal women, age 41–50 years, women were asked if a woman would get depressed during menopause. Eighty percent responded affirmatively.[13] Fifty-five percent of the same women thought they themselves would get depressed. The MWHS found that the variables most associated with depression were lower education, marital status (higher rates in widowed, divorced, and separated women), physical health, and stress from worry about others. This study also reported that women who did not report psychological symptoms prior to menopause most likely had a college education, did not smoke, and exercised regularly.[17] Several authors suggest that mood changes are secondary to distressing physical and biological symptoms and that depression is caused by other significant life and role changes in the woman's life (i.e., empty nest syndrome, caring for aging parents, and such).[10,16,35] Soltes[37] lists mood swings, anxiety, depression, and irritability as commonly reported psychological changes during menopause. This investigator felt that hormonal changes, a diagnosis of cancer, and the aging process influence psychological changes. In addition, Soltes[37] noted that depression could also be related to serotonin levels that were not measured in most studies.

Schmidt and Rubinow[36] identified several factors to consider when trying to determine the presence of psychiatric illness in a menopausal woman. Some of these factors are confirmation of menopausal status, determination of relationship between somatic symptoms and psychiatric problems, and determination of the origin of the problem.

Telephone interviews by Bosworth and coinvestigators[38] explored the relationship between depression and menopausal symptoms. The conclusions pointed to an association between depressive symptoms and declines in estrogen related to biochemical changes in the brain. Interestingly, they also found that smoking increases the risk and that exercise decreases the risk for depressive symptoms. However, the study did not examine current depressive status, daily living conditions, chronic disease, or family problems.[38] Taechakraichana et al.[5] suggest that psychological symptoms, such as mood changes, irritability, depression, fear of being alone in public, feeling tense, and feeling unworthy, may be due to personality, premenopausal feelings, and family, social, and work environments. Shepherd and Bopp[7] relate mood changes to estrogen levels, life stresses, and society's negative view of aging women. A review of the literature by Freedman[34] cites a study by Majos et al. (1986) that highlights the association between high progestin levels and increased psychological symptoms, such as depression, anxiety, and irritability. Vanwesenbeeck and colleagues[39] propose that menopausal symptoms are related to negative attitude and negative health status prior to menopause.

Cognitively, a relationship between menopause and Alzheimer's disease was explored in a cohort of 2509 members from Leisure World Community. Alzheimer's disease was found in 138 of these women. The study concluded that there was an increase in the incidence of Alzheimer's disease due to estrogen deficiency.[40] A more recent study by Farrag and coresearchers[11] looked at the relationship between surgical menopause and cognitive function and concluded that estrogen deficiency is associated with a decline in neurocognitive functioning. The NIH Consensus Panel[4] concluded that evidence was insufficient to suggest a relationship between menopause and cognitive dysfunction.

Other Menopausal Symptoms

A variety of other acute symptoms have been identified and associated with menopause. These symptoms are joint pain, forgetfulness, muscle pain, tiredness, tiredness on awakening, restless leg, pins and needles, lack of energy, shortness of breath, dry eyes, skin changes (dry, flaking), wrinkles, waist thickening, increase in bra size, and muscle, breast, and body changes.[3,5,8,22]

Long-term effects of estrogen reduction include osteoporosis and coronary heart disease. These will be discussed in the following section about symptom management.

Symptom Management

The management of menopausal symptoms can be challenging because of symptom heterogeneity and a lack of consensus on the effectiveness of the therapeutic options. This section will focus on the use of pharmaceuticals, botanicals, herbs, and lifestyle changes for the prevention and treatment of menopausal symptoms.

Hormone Replacement Therapy—Cardiovascular Disease

Cardiovascular disease is the leading cause of death in American women.[41] The majority of these deaths are postmenopausal women.[27] Recent trials have suggested that hormone replacement therapy (HRT) cannot prevent cardiovascular events.

The Women's Health Initiative (WHI) stopped the estrogen/progestin arm of this clinical trial early. This randomized, double-blinded, placebo-controlled trial of 16,608 healthy postmenopausal women discovered evidence that estrogen plus progestin increased the risk for nonfatal myocardial infarctions but not coronary death. Additionally, there was increased risk for invasive breast cancer, stroke, deep vein thrombosis (DVT), and pulmonary emboli (PE).[42–44] However, about 40% of women in treatment groups were noncompliant, taking less than 80% of their medications at one point during the study. This suggests an even greater risk for HRT users. Methods of statistical analysis for primary and secondary endpoints continue to be questioned by some practitioners.[43] The estrogen replacement therapy (ERT) alone arm of the WHI continues. Three years of follow-up in the WHI suggest that women in the group who had taken HRT versus the placebo group no longer had an increased risk of cardiovascular disease.[45]

Previous studies—Heart and Estrogen/Progesterone Replacement Study (HERS), Postmenopausal Estrogen/Progestin Intervention Trial (PEPI), and the Nurses Health Study—also investigated the use of estrogen/progestin for prevention of cardiovascular events. The Nurses Health Study monitored 120,000 women, age 30–45 years, over a 20-year period. A potential for increased risk of cardiovascular heart disease was shown.[23,43] The HER trial of 2760 women demonstrated an increased risk for DVT, PE, and gallstone surgery.[23,46] HERS found coronary events to be more frequent in the first year of HRT use. HER investigators continued to follow the participants in the HER II study. At the conclusion of HER II, the investigators recommended against using HRT for reducing the risk of coronary heart disease in women with coronary heart disease.[43]

The PEPI trial of 875 women tested unopposed estrogen and three estrogen/progestin products against placebo. Drug effect on high-density lipoprotein (HDL), cholesterol levels, systolic blood pressure, serum insulin levels, and fibrinogen levels were endpoints. At the conclusion of the study, results showed an increase in HDL (all groups), no changes in insulin levels or blood pressure (between groups), and an increase in endometrial hyperplasia in the unopposed estrogen group. The investigators suggested that HRT had a cardioprotective effect because of increases in HDL and decreases in fibrinogen levels, unchanged blood pressure, and insulin levels. Many practitioners questioned the study results because of the study length and design.[43] The Progression of Coronary Artery Atherosclerosis study supported the beneficial effects of HRT on HDL but did not demonstrate a slowing of the progression of athersclerotic lesions.[23,43]

Recently, the US Preventive Services Task Force (USPSTF)[47] recommended against the routine use of estrogen/progesterone for prevention of chronic conditions (including coronary heart disease) in postmenopausal women. This task force was charged with reviewing the scientific evidence and preparing recommendations. The American College of Obstetrics and Gynecology, The North American Menopause Society (NAMS), and the American Heart Association have also recommended against the use of HRT for primary or secondary prevention of cardiovascular disease.[47]

A variety of alternatives have been suggested to prevent coronary heart disease (CHD) in the postmenopausal woman. Alternatives include drugs, lifestyle changes, dietary interventions, smoking cessation, and physical exercise. Suggested pharmaceuticals include statins to lower cholesterol, hypertensives to control blood pressure, and selective estrogen receptor modulators (SERMs) to reduce total cholesterol and increase HDL.[23,25,48] The Raloxifene Use for the Heart (RUTH) study of 10,101 women completed enrollment in August 2000. With a median follow-up of 5.56 years, it was reported that there was no significant difference between raloxifene and placebo for death from coronary cause, non-fatal myocardial infarction, or hospitalization for acute coronary syndrome. However, the study did show a reduction in risk for invasive breast cancer.[49] Statins may reduce new cardiovascular events by 30%.[23] The American College of Cardiology recommends statins rather than HRT for primary and secondary prevention of HRT.[23] Stress reduction, regular exercise, decreasing caffeine and alcohol, low fat/low cholesterol diet, and adequate sleep are lifestyle changes reported to help prevent CHD. Isoflavones (phytoestrogens) have estrogenic properties and have therefore garnered much interest as a substitute for HRT for management of menopausal symptoms. It appears that isoflavones with their SERM qualities do not affect endometrial cell proliferation, may slightly decrease serum triglyceride levels, reduce or do not affect platelet aggregation, and do not increase thrombosis.[44] In 1999 the US Food and Drug Administration (FDA) approved a health claim that soy protein can reduce cholesterol levels. The FDA set 25 g/day as the target soy intake goal for cholesterol reduction.[44] Further research is needed to support the claim that soy can decrease blood pressure and inhibit low-density cholesterol.[44] A meta-analysis of 38 studies revealed that an intake of 47 g/day of soy protein decreased total cholesterol, low-density lipoprotein, and triglycerides in individuals with moderate to severe hypercholesterolemia.[50] Conversely, a study of the effect of isoflavone supplementation on endothelial functioning using oral soy isoflavone for 2 weeks found no benefit to endothelial functioning in healthy menopausal women. Researchers concluded that soy supplements do not have the same effect as high-soy protein diets.[51]

Rigorous studies need to be designed to investigate isoflavones' affect on prevention of CHD.[52]

Hormone Replacement Therapy—Osteoporosis

Osteoporosis is defined by the National Institute of Health Consensus Panel in Osteoporosis Prevention, Diagnosis and Therapy as "a skeletal disorder characterized by compromised bone strength predisposing a person to an increased risk of fracture."[5,53] Twenty percent of white women older than age 50 years have osteoporosis, with an additional 35%–50% having low bone mass. African Americans have the lowest osteoporitic rates.[54] Bone mineral density (BMD) and bone quality is used to measure the risk of osteoporosis. Peripheral dual energy X-ray absorptiometry (pDEXA) or computed tomography technology measures BMD.[55] The portability and low cost of these devices has improved the accessibility of BMD testing.[56] BMD that is 2.5 standard deviations or more below the average for young healthy women is considered to be osteoporosis.[53]

Bone loss increases at the time of menopause by an average of 3% per year, with losses higher in the early postmenopausal years.[27,57] Estrogen therapy appears to decrease bone resorption and turnover.[54] The PEPI trial of 875 postmenopausal women showed an improvement in BMD for lumbar spine and hip.[23] Other studies have shown a reduction in bone loss and an increase in bone mass associated with HRT.[5,27]

NAMS's review of more than 50 randomized, placebo-controlled trials revealed that using ERT/HRT increases BMD in the spine and hip. The Study of Osteoporotic Fractures revealed a risk reduction of 34% for nonspine fracture in HRT or estrogen-alone users.[54] A secondary outcome of the study was the finding that HRT or ERT is more effective if started within 5 years of menopause and used longer than 10 years. Estrogen products are FDA indicated for prevention of osteoporosis but not for treatment of osteoporosis. FDA treatment indication was withheld because of lack of data from rigorous clinical trials.

NAMS[54] management recommendations for osteoporosis involve identification of risk factors and reduction of morbidity. The more osteoporitic risk factors—genetics, lifestyle, hormonal status, medication use (such as glucocorticoids), treatment with cytotoxic agents, calcium imbalances, GI diseases, hematological cancer, nutritional disorders, rheumatoid arthritis, and chronic renal disorders—the higher the risk. Pharmacological interventions are appropriate for women with DEXA scores greater than 2.5, women with DEXA scores of −2 to −2.5 and one additional risk factor, or postmenopausal women with osteoporitic fracture.[54] Interventions included ERT/HRT, bisphosphanates, SERMs, calcitonin, parathyroid hormone, tibolone, and statins. HRT was shown to improve BMD, prevent bone loss, and increase bone mass.[5,23] ERT/HRT preparations that might be used for prevention and treatment of osteoporosis are conjugated equine estrogens, esterified estrogens, estradiol tablets and transdermal patch, and estropipate.[58] In spite of good evidence that estrogen and progestin increase BMD and reduce the risk for fracture, the US Preventive Services Task Force recommended against routine use of estrogen and progestin for the prevention of chronic conditions in postmenopausal women. This task force believed that the harmful effects of HRT exceeded the prevention benefits. Likewise, the WHI recommendations against HRT use in CHD because of increased risk for CHD and breast cancer directly impacts the ability to utilize HRT for osteoporosis.[42]

Bisphosphanates decrease bone resorption (with no adverse effect on the breast or uterus), and increase BMD (hip and spine) and risk of vertebral and nonvertebral fracture.[23,27,53,54] The bisphosphanates, alendronate and risedronate, are indicated for the prevention and treatment of osteoporosis. Trials that have shown the benefit of bisphosphanates include the Fracture Intervention Trial (FIT).[23,27] SERMs decrease the risk of vertebral fractures with no effect on the endometrium or breast.[23,48,53] The Multiple Outcomes of Raloxifene Evaluation (MOORE) study supported the use of SERMs for prevention of fractures.[23,25,27,48] Calcitonin (intranasal or injectable) is used for treatment, but not prevention, of osteoporosis. The Prevent Recurrence of Osteoporitic Fracture (PROOF) study showed the effectiveness of nasal calcitonin in preventing further fractures.[23] The statins require trials to establish their effectiveness in fracture prevention.[23]

NAMS[54] recommends lifestyle changes that might aid in preventing and/or treating osteoporosis. These changes are dietary (increase fruits and vegetables, decrease fat, consume adequate protein), calcium and vitamin D supplements, magnesium, exercise, smoking cessation, alcohol avoidance, and falls prevention. Cook and Pennington[59] investigated the effect of the combination of herbs, vitamins, and minerals on BMD in early postmenopause with unsuccessful results. The combination of herbs, vitamins, and minerals was unsuccessful in protecting against bone loss with decreases in BMD in the spine, hip, and forearm. Conversely, vitamin C was found to have a beneficial effect on BMD with the greatest effect in women who were concomitantly using ERT and calcium supplements.[60] The recommendation for calcium supplements is 1200 mg per day for women over 51 years of age, 1000 mg per day for women aged

25–50 years, 1000 mg per day for postmenopausal women under 65 years of age who are taking ERT, and 1500 mg per day for all women over the age of 65. It is recommended that from age 51–70 years, women should consume 400 IU per day of vitamin D. For women over the age of 70 years, the intake of vitamin D supplement should be 600 IU per day.[54]

Hormone Replacement Therapy—Vasomotor and Urogenital Symptoms

ERT and HRT decrease hot flashes by 50%–100% and are the most consistent and effective treatment of hot flashes.[4,22] Hot flashes result from estrogen deficiencies and the hypothalamic response to the lowered estrogen levels.[7] HRT is approved for relief of menopausal symptoms, but many women choose not to take HRT or never seek to take HRT for a variety of reasons.[8] Hing and Brett[61] analyzed data from the National Ambulatory Medical Care Survey and the National Hospital Ambulatory Medical Care Survey for 2001–2003. Their analysis showed a significant decline (43.6% for HRT and 35% for estrogen alone) in prescriptions for hormone therapy (estrogen plus progestin) and estrogen during that period. Studies cited earlier in this chapter presented findings that HRT may have detrimental effects on the health of the postmenopausal woman (increased risk of CHD and breast cancer).

Unopposed estrogen places women at risk for endometrial cancer. The risk increases with dose and duration. Approximately 36% of women in the PEPI trial who were randomized to receive unopposed estrogen developed adenomatous or atypical hyperplastic endometrial tissue.[58] Estrogen and progestin increased the risk of CHD and breast cancer. Women in the WHI had a 15% increased risk for breast cancer with less than 5 years of estrogen and progestin use and a 53% increased risk with more than 5 years of use.[42] The risk for ovarian cancer associated with HRT use is not clear and requires further study.[58]

Estrogen and progestin agents available for symptom management include conjugated equine estrogens, esterified estrogens, estropipate and other estrogen sulfates, micronized 17 beta estradiol, ethinyl estradiol, transdermal estradiol patches, vaginal estrogenic preparations, medroxyprogesterone acetate, levonorgestrel, norethindrone, micronized progesterone, transvaginal progesterone, and 17-acetoxy progesterone.[58,62] ESTRING, Estrace, and Vagifem are estrogen creams that are available for management of urogenital symptoms. Systemic estrogen absorption from vaginal creams is of concern for breast cancer survivors. A small amount of systemic absorption is expected, and detrimental effects have been reported.[63,64] An early study by Nilsson and Heimer[65] found no significant increase in plasma estrogen in patients who received 1.2 mg per day of vaginal ESTRING.

For women who are not candidates for HRT (i.e., those with breast, ovarian, or endometrial cancer) or who choose not to take HRT, alternative therapies may be utilized for symptom management. Bioidentical HRT has been proposed as one alternative for systemic HRT. These customized preparations are compounded by the pharmacist and contain hormones identical to endogenous hormones—estradiol, estriol, estrone, progesterone, and testosterone. These products use plant-based bioidentical hormones extracted from plants such as soy and yams. There is a lack of efficacy and safety data for bioidentical products.[4] At question is the skill of the compounding pharmacist and the validity of the product bioavailability. Women who use the compounded hormones should consult a physician before using the products and have follow-up visits to measure hormone levels.[7] Triestrogen, bioestrogen, and estriol are examples of bioidentical HRT.

Psychological Symptom Management

Women who experience depression during menopause should have a thorough assessment to determine the physiological and/or psychological causes for the depression. Interventions to treat the depression might be either pharmacological or nonpharmacological. Nonpharmacological interventions could include psychotherapy, support groups, exploration of coping mechanisms, control of related symptoms (i.e., sleep disorders, irritability, and hot flashes), behavior modification, relaxation techniques, visual imagery, and exercise.[66] Serotonin reuptake inhibitors (SSRIs) or tricyclic antidepressants (TCAs) may be used for pharmacological treatment. SSRIs and TCAs have been reported to be very effective in treating major depression. These drugs are also recommended for the treatment of moderate to severe depression.[67] The SSRIs that may be prescribed are fluoxetine (Prozac), paroxetine (Paxil), sertraline (Zoloft), or trazodone (Desyrel). Nortriptyline (Pamelor), amitriptyline (Elavil), or desipramine (Norpramin) are the TCAs most often prescribed.[67]

Alternatives to HRT for Vasomotor and/or Urogenital Symptoms

Other drugs have reported efficacy in the management of menopausal symptoms. Venlafaxine acetate, clonidine, megestrol acetate, Bellergal-S, and gabapentin have purported to improve menopausal symptoms. The nonhormonal agent venlafaxine has been studied for control of hot flashes. Barton and colleagues'[64] continuation study of 102 postmenopausal women taking venlafaxine reported intermediate-term efficacy and good tolerability for treatment of hot flashes.

Clonidine's affect on hot flashes has been mixed. Some investigations have found that clonidine decreases hot flashes, while others found it inferior to conjugated equine estrogen.[27] Megesterol acetate controls hot flashes but increases weight gain, which may be unacceptable to many women.[23] Loprinzi et al.[68] treated hot flashes with megesterol acetate and demonstrated a reduction in the hot flashes. A randomized trial of 60 postmenopausal women comparing estrogen and gabapentin to placebo determined that gabapentin was as efficacious as estrogen in treating hot flashes.[69] It has been suggested that findings from this study need to be confirmed in a larger trial.

Alternative Therapies for Menopausal Symptoms

More than 40%–42% of Americans use some form of alternative medicine, and as many as 63%–83% of breast cancer patients use alternative medicine.[70] Mahady and colleagues[71] interviewed 500 women to determine their use of botanical dietary supplements. This racially and ethnically diverse group reported a 79% use of botanicals or dietary supplements, with 36.5% reporting daily use. In this study the most commonly used botanicals were soy, green tea, chamomile, gingko, ginseng, echinacea, and St. John's wort. Study participants admitted that they combined the botanicals with prescription drugs and over-the-counter medications. While isoflavones and phytoestrogens have received extensive scrutiny with mixed results, most studies do not provide enough information on long-term adverse effects.[4] Office visits to providers of alternative therapies numbered more than 628 million in 1997, compared to 385 million visits to primary care providers.[27] The cost of alternative therapy is estimated at $27 billion per year.[70] Safety and efficacy data for herbs as alternative therapy is sparse.[72] See **Table 13-3** for a list of herbs that are suggested as alternatives for treatment of menopausal symptoms.

Table 13-3 ALTERNATIVE THERAPIES/SYMPTOMS THEY CLAIM TO IMPROVE.

Herb/Alternative	Vasomotor Symptoms	Urogenital Symptoms	Other Symptom
Moisturizers		Yes	
Black cohosh	Yes		Fatigue
Dong quai	Yes	Yes	Insomnia
Ginseng	Yes		
Licorice root	Yes		
Evening primrose	Yes		
St. John's wort			Depression
Ginseng			General well-being
Gingko biloba			Improvement in sleep, mood, memory
Chamomile			Stabilize mood, sleep
Valerian root			Insomnia, anxiety
Balm	Under study		Improve sleep, memory
Wild yam		Yes	
Chaste berry	Yes		
Hops	Under study		Improve sleep, memory
Isoflavones	Yes		Improve sleep, memory
Gotu kola	Yes		
Witch hazel		Yes	
Sage	Yes		
Sarsaparilla			
Agrimony		Yes	
Chaste tree		Yes	

Source: Eichholz et al. 2002; Warren et al. 2002; Bratman and Girman 2003; Komesaroff et al. 2001.

Commission E of the German Federal Health Authority is an agency that regulates the safety and efficacy of herbs and phytomedicinals. Herbs are defined as crude drugs of vegetable origin that are utilized for treatment of disease or to attain or maintain health. Herbs include tinctures and extracts. Commission E considers the following herbs to be safe for menopausal symptoms: balm, black cohosh, chaste tree/chaste berry, ginkgo, ginseng, passion flower, St. John's wort, and valerian. The commission did not approve licorice root, agrimony, angelica, catnip, chamomile, damania, dandelion, dong quai, hop, sage, fenugreek, gotu kola, and sarsaparilla.[25] For a review of the side effects of herbs, please refer to an up-to-date herbal therapy reference text.

Two herbs not mentioned by Commission E are red clover and wild yam. Red clover, with its four estrogenic isoflavones, has no benefit for menopausal symptoms.[4,73] Wild yam extract or cream was found to have no effect on menopausal symptoms. After 3 months of treating 23 healthy women with wild yam cream, investigators found no statistical differences between the yam cream and placebo.[74]

Black cohosh is the most extensively studied of the herbal remedies. Remifemin is a commercially available black cohosh that has shown inconsistent results.[75] In some studies, the symptoms moderately decreased but showed no change in vaginal cytology or hormone concentrations.[75] Commission E recommends a 6-month limitation of the use of remifemin. Methodology flaws may account for the inconsistent results in black cohosh studies. Many studies lack placebo groups, have no randomization, are not double blinded, have small groups, or are inconsistent in dosing.[8] Randomized studies of 85 women stratified on tamoxifen use

were assigned to either black cohosh or placebo. At the completion of the 60-day study, black cohosh was not more efficacious than placebo.[76] The National Institutes of Health is currently conducting scientifically rigorous black cohosh studies. Bratman and Girman's[50] *Mosby's Handbook of Herbs and Supplements and Their Therapeutic Uses* rates the usefulness of drugs and herbs for menopause, with 4 having the strongest clinical evidence and 1 the weakest. Estriol is rated as a 4, with progesterone cream a 3. Soy received a rating of 3, with black cohosh receiving a 2. Red clover, ginseng, vitamin E, and dong quai rated a −1 or −2. The authors found no evidence to support the use of alfalfa, bioflavonoids, chaste berry, essential fatty acids, flax seed, gamma oryzanol, licorice, St. John's wort, or vitamin C for menopausal symptoms.

Taechakraichana et al.[5] have suggested that lifestyle changes could augment medications for the treatment of vasomotor symptoms. Lifestyle changes include dressing in layers; wearing woven cotton clothing; using loosely woven bedding; avoiding caffeine, alcohol, and spicy foods; sucking on ice; and a cool environment. Stearns and Hayes[22] recommend acupuncture, meditation, applied relaxation, biofeedback, and paced respirations to help in the management of hot flashes.

Conclusion

The Massachusetts Women's Health Study (MWHS) of 2570 women identified the average age of menopause as 50 with a range of 45–55 years.[9,10] In 2001, 42,635,000 women in the United States were older than age 50 years.[22] It is estimated that 6000 women reach menopause every day (two million a year).[77] These statistics emphasize why it is imperative that prevention and treatment of menopausal symptoms and associated long-term effects continue to receive investigator attention. The WHI has heightened interest in discovering safe and efficacious therapies for the prevention of CHD. The WHI findings directly impact decision making by women and their physicians for the prevention and treatment of osteoporosis and acute symptoms. As the numbers of women of menopausal and postmenopausal age continues to increase, it will become critical that we are able to offer these women short-term and long-term management of symptoms resulting from menopause. Interventions that are safe and cost effective with minimal side effects are necessary to minimize the effect that this large population of women has and will continue to have on our healthcare dollars. Safe, cost-effective interventions with minimal side effects are crucial to maintaining the quality of life of these women. Well-designed studies with valid instruments are critical to determining safe and efficacious interventions to treat menopausal symptoms.

Implications for Nursing

With the average woman's life span now at approximately 80 years, nursing will play a crucial role in assisting the menopausal and postmenopausal woman to live greater than one-third of her life as an active individual free of menopausal-associated chronic diseases. Nursing should be on the forefront of research that explores the safety and efficacy of alternative therapies and the impact of those drugs, herbs, and treatments on the woman's quality of life. Nurses need to educate women to make informed decisions about prevention and treatment of menopause sequelae. Consumer education about treatment risks and benefits is greatly needed. Nurses must be involved in supporting legislation that will regulate and standardize recommended alternative and complementary therapies. Nurses should be cognizant of the cost of alternative treatments and recognize that impact on healthcare dollars. Education is critical. Every nurse should have the same knowledge of alternative and complementary medicine that they have of pharmaceutical products and treatments. Like every area of healthcare, knowledge about the prevention and treatment of menopausal symptoms and long-term sequelae continues to explode. We must have the most up-to-date information or the ability to find that information if we are to assist our patients in making informed, competent decisions about their healthcare.

References

1. McPherson K. Menopause as a disease: the social constructs of a metaphor. *Adv Nurs Sci.* 1981;3:95–110.
2. McPherson K. Nurse researchers respond to the medicalization of menopause. *Ann NY Acad Sci.* 1990;591:180–184.
3. Boughtron M. Premature menopause: multiple disruptions between the woman's biological body experience and her lived body. *J Adv Nurs.* 2002;37(5):423–430.
4. National Institutes of Health (NIH) Conference. National Institutes of Health State-of-the Science Conference statement: management of menopause-related symptoms. *Ann Int Med.* 2005;142(12):1003–1013.
5. Taechakraichana N, Panyakhamlerd K, Limpaphayom K, Jaisamrarn U, Chaikittisilpa S. Climacteric: concept, consequence and care. *J Med Assoc Thai.* 2002;June:81–86.
6. Khaw, K. Epidemiology of menopause. *Br Med Bull.* 1992;48:249–261.
7. Shepherd J, Bopp J. Pharmacy-based care for perimenopausal and postmenopausal women. *J Am Pharm Assoc.* 2002;42(5):700–711.

8. Mahady G, Fabricant D, Chadwick L, Dietz B. Black cohosh: an alternative therapy for menopause? *Nutr Clin Care.* 2002;5(6):283–289.

9. McKinlay S, Brambilla D, Posner J. The normal menopause transition. *Maturitas.* 1992;14:103–115.

10. Quinn A. Menopause: plight or passage. *NAACOG Clin Issues Perinat Women Health Nurs.* 1991;2: 304–311.

11. Farrag A, Khedr E, Abdel-Aleem H, Rageh T. Effect of surgical menopause on cognitive functions. *Dement Geriatr Cogn Disord.* 2002;13:193–198.

12. Poniatowski B, Grimm P, Cohen G. Chemotherapy-induced menopause: a literature review. *Cancer Invest.* 2001;19(6):641–648.

13. Matthews K. Myths and realities of the menopause. *Psychosom Med.* 1992;54:1–9.

14. Estok P, O'Toole R. The meanings of menopause. *Healthc Women Int.* 1991;12:27–39.

15. Hunter M. Predictors of menopausal symptoms: psychosocial aspects. *Bailliere Clin Endocrinol Metab.* 1993;7:32–45.

16. Stone A, Pearlstein T. Evaluation and treatment of changes in mood, sleep, and sexual functioning associated with menopause. *Prim Care Mat Woman.* 1994;21:391–403.

17. Avis N, McKinlay, S. The Massachusetts Women's Health Study: an epidemiologic investigation of the menopause. *J Am Med Women Assoc.* 1995;50:45–59.

18. Kaufert P, Gilbert P, Hassard T. Researching the symptoms of menopause: an exercise in methodology. *Maturitas.* 1988;10:117–131.

19. Morse C, Smith A, Demerstein L. The treatment seeking woman at menopause. *Maturitas.* 1994;18: 161–173.

20. Hildritch J, Lewis J, Peter A, et al. Menopause-specific quality of life questionnaire: development and psychometric properties. *Climacteric.* 1996;24: 161–175.

21. Perez J. Development of the menopause symptom list: a factor analytic study of menopause associated symptoms. *Women Health.* 1997;25:53–69.

22. Stearns V, Hayes D. Approach to menopausal symptoms in women with breast cancer. *Curr Treat Options Oncol.* 2002;3:179–190.

23. Pinkerton J, Santen R. Use of alternatives to estrogen for treatment of menopause. *Minerva Endocrinol.* 2002;27:21–41.

24. Hagstad S, Janson P. The epidemiology of climacteric symptoms. *Acta Obstet Gynecol Scand.* 1986;134:59–65.

25. Warren M, Shortle B, Dominguez J. Use of alternative therapies in menopause. *Clin Obstet Gynecol.* 2002;16(3):411–448.

26. Schwingl P, Halka B, Harlow S. Risk factors for menopausal hot flashes. *Obstet Gynecol.* 1994;84: 29–34.

27. Eichholz A, Mahavni V, Sood A. Allopathic and complementary alternatives to hormone replacement therapy. *Expert Opin Pharmacother.* 2002;3(7): 951–955.

28. Women's Health Across the Nation. www.edc.gsph. pitt.edu/swan/. Accessed June 15, 2008.

29. Shaw C. The perimenopausal hot flash: epidemiology, physiology, and treatment. *Nurs Pract.* 1997;22: 55–56.

30. Lock M. Contested meanings of the menopause. *Med Cult.* 1991;337:1270–1272.

31. Avis N, Stellato R, Crawford S, et al. Is there a menopausal syndrome? Menopausal status and symptoms across racial/ethnic groups. *Soc Sci Med.* 2001;52:345–356.

32. Rostom A. The management of menopausal sequelae in patients with breast cancer. *Clin Oncol.* 2001;13:174–180.

33. Carcio H. Urogenital atrophy a new approach to vaginitis diagnosis. *Adv Nurs Pract.* 2002;October: 40–48.

34. Freedman M. Quality of life and menopause: the role of estrogen. *J Women Health.* 2002;11(8):703–718.

35. Ballinger C. Aspects of the menopause. *Br J Psychiatry J Med Sci.* 1990;156:773–787.

36. Schmidt P, Rubinow D. Menopause-related affective disorders: a justification for further study. *Am J Psychiatry.* 1991;148:844–852.

37. Soltes B. Therapeutic options for menopause in cancer survivors. *Oncl Nurse Updat.* 1997;4:1–12.

38. Bosworth H, Bastian L, Kuchibhatla M, et al. Depressive symptoms, menopausal status, and climacteric symptoms in women in midlife. *Psychosom Med.* 2001;63:603–608.

39. Vanwesenbeeck I, Vennix P, van de Wiel H. Menopausal symptoms: associations with menopausal status and psychosocial factors. *J Psychosom Obstet Gynecol.* 2001;22(3):149–158.

40. Paganini-Hill A, Henderson VW. Estrogen deficiency and risk of Alzheimer's disease. *Am J Psychiatry.* 1994;140:256–261.

41. Cardiovascular disease. www.cardiovascular-disease. org. Accessed June 15, 2008.

42. Writing Group for the Women's Health Initiative Investigators. Risks and benefits of estrogen plus progestin in healthy postmenopausal women. *JAMA.* 2002;288(3):321–369.

43. Biscup P. Risks and benefits of long-term hormone replacement therapy. *Am J Health Syst Pharm.* 2003;60:1419–1425.

44. Messina M. Soy foods and soybean isoflavones and menopausal health. *Nutr Clin Care.* 2002;5(6): 272–282.

45. Women's health initiative. www.whi.org. Accessed June 15, 2008.

46. Nair G, Klein K, Herrington D. Assessing the role of estrogen in the prevention of cardiovascular disease. *Fin Med Soc Duodecim Ann Med.* 2001;33:305–312.

47. US Preventive Services Task Force. Postmenopausal hormone replacement therapy for the primary prevention of chronic conditions: recommendations and rationale. *Am J Nurs.* 2003;103(6):83, 85, 86, 89–91.

48. Boyack M, Lookinland S, Chasson S. Efficacy of raloxifene for treatment of menopause: a systematic review. *J Am Acad Nurse Pract.* 2002;14(4):150–155.

49. Barrett-Connor E, Mosca L, Collins P, et al. Effects of raloxifene on cardiovascular events and breast cancer in post menopausal women. *NJM.* 2006;755(2): 125–137.

50. Bratman S, Girman A. *Mosby's Handbook of Herbs and Supplements and Their Therapeutic Uses.* St. Louis, MO: Mosby; 2003.

51. Hale G, Paul-Labrador M, Dwyer J, Merz C. Isoflavone supplementation and endothelial function in menopausal women. *Clin Endocrinol.* 2002;56: 693–701.

52. Eden J. Managing the menopause: phyto-oestrogens or hormone replacement therapy. *Fin Med Soc Duodecim Ann Med.* 2001;33:4–6.

53. Choo W, Loh F, Ng S. Osteoporosis in relation to menopause. *Ann Acad Med.* 2002;31(1):30–36.

54. The North American Menopause Society. Position statement management of postmenopausal osteoporosis. *Menopause.* 2002;9(2):84–101.

55. Pouilles J, Tremollieres F, Martinez S, Delsol M, Ribot C. Ability of peripheral DXA measurements of the forearm to predict low axial bone mineral density at menopause. *Osteoporos Int.* 2001;12:71–76.

56. Palumi C, Chiarenza M, Zizza G, et al. Role of DEXA and ultrasonometry in the evaluation of osteoporotic risk in postmenopausal women. *Maturitas.* 2002;42:113–117.

57. Ahlborg H, Johnell O, Nilsson B, Jeppsson S, Rannevik G, Karlsson M. Bone loss in relation to menopause: a prospective study during 16 years. *Bone.* 2001;28(3):327–331.

58. Wright L, Kalantaridou S, Calis K. Update on the benefits and risks of hormone replacement therapy. *Formulary.* 2002;37:78–80, 82, 86, 91–93.

59. Cook A, Pennington G. Phytoestrogen and multiple vitamin/mineral effects on bone mineral density in early postmenopausal women: a pilot study. *J Women Health Gend Med.* 2002;11(3):53–60.

60. Morton D, Barrett-Connor E, Schneider D. Vitamin C supplement use and bone mineral density in postmenopausal women. *J Bone Miner Res.* 2001;16(1):135–140.

61. Hing E, Brett K. Changes in US prescribing patterns of menopausal hormone therapy, 2001–2003. *Obstet Gynecol.* 2006;108(1):33–40.

62. Goolsby M. Management of menopause. *J Am Acad Nurse Pract.* 2001;13(4):147–150.

63. Barton D, LaVasseur B, Loprinzi C, Novotny P, Wilwerding B, Sloan J. Venlafaxine for the control of hot flashes: results of a longitudinal continuation study. *Oncol Nurs Forum.* 2002;29(1):33–39.

64. Barton D, Loprinzi C, Gostout B. Current management of menopausal symptoms in cancer patients. *Oncol.* 2002;16(1):67–79.

65. Nilsson K, Heimer G. Low-dose oestradiol in treatment of urogenital deficiency: a pharmacokinetic and pharmacodynamic study. *Maturitas.* 1992;15:121–127.

66. Dow K. *Pocket Guide to Breast Cancer.* 2nd ed. Sudbury, MA: Jones and Bartlett; 2002:260–262.

67. St. Marie B. Depression. In: Camp-Sorrell D, Hawkins R, eds. *Clinical Manual for the Oncology Advanced Practice Nurse.* Pittsburgh, PA: Oncology Press; 2000:927–930.

68. Loprinzi C, Michalak J, Quella S, et al. Megastrol acetate for the treatment of hot flashes. *N Engl J Med.* 1994;331:347–352.

69. Reddy S, Warner H, Guttuso T, et al. Gabapentin, estrogen and placebo for treating hot flashes, a randomized controlled trial. *Obstet Gynecol.* 2006;108(1):41–48.

70. DiGianni L, Garber J, Winer E. Complementary and alternative medicine use among women with breast cancer. *J Clin Oncol.* 2002;20(18):34s–38s.

71. Mahady G, Parrot J, Lee C, Yun G, Dan A. Botanical dietary supplement use in peri- and postmenopausal women. *Menopause.* 2003;10(1):65–72.

72. Amato P, Christophe S, Mellon P. Estrogenic activity of herbs commonly used as remedies for menopausal symptoms. *Menopause.* 2002;9(2):145–150.

73. Fugh-Berman A, Kronenberg F. Red clover (trifolium pratense) for menopausal women: current state of knowledge. *Menopause.* 2001;8(5):333–337.

74. Komesaroff P, Black C, Cable V, Sudhir K. Effects of wild yam extract on menopausal symptoms, lipids and sex hormones in healthy menopausal women. *Climacteric.* 2001;4:144–150.

75. McKenna D, Jones K, Humphrey S, Hughes K. Black cohosh: efficacy, safety, and use in clinical and preclinical applications. *Altern Ther.* 2001;7(3):93–100.

76. Jacobson J, Troxel A, Evans J, et al. Randomized trial of black cohash for the treatment of hot flashes among women with a history of breast cancer. *JCO.* 2001;19(10):739–745.

77. North American Menopause Society. www.northamericanmenopausesociety.org. Accessed June 15, 2008.

Chapter 14

The Sequelae of Cancer and its Treatment

Susan J. McIntyre, RN, MN, ANP-BC, AOCN®

Introduction

Today over 10 million Americans have either been cured of or are in remission from cancer. Sixty-five percent of cancer patients survive more than 5 years. Earlier diagnosis and increasingly efficacious treatment of cancer have led to increasing numbers of individuals living with cancer and the aftermath of its treatment. There were an estimated 1,444,920 new cases diagnosed in 2007, with about 559,650 expected cancer deaths.[1] Many cancer survivors are living normal lives, caring for their families, working, participating in sports, and contributing to their communities. Preventing or minimizing side effects has become increasingly important. The diagnosis of cancer continues to elicit fear; however, the occurrence no longer equates to mortality from the disease. As our society moves from perceiving cancer as a universally terminal illness to a chronic illness or even an illness with likelihood of cure, preservation of function and enhancing quality of life become critically important.

Conceptual Framework

Chronic illness (or the impact of its treatment) is permanent. It requires costly and frequent intervention(s) and results in significant changes of lifestyle, life goals, personal and professional role functions and opportunities, and recreational activities.[2] Managing chronic illness is not a two- or three-dimensional phenomenon; rather it is multidimensional, just as working with human beings is always multidimensional. Therefore, a definition offered by Lubkin and Larsen for chronic illness recognizes well the complexity of chronicity in the cancer patient because nobody exists in a vacuum:

> *Chronic illness is the irreversible presence, accumulation or latency of disease states or impairments that involve the total human environment for supportive care and self-care, maintenance of function and prevention of further disability.*[3]

Furthermore, it may not be the disease itself (having been controlled or cured), but the aftermath that compromises quality of life and forces adaptation on the patient's and her support system's part. Differences between treatment arms may be slight, but the impact they render on one's life in the aftermath may not be insignificant. In addition, in the last couple of decades, treatment strategies became increasingly complex and toxicities provided an equally complex picture. Therefore, the National Cancer Institute encouraged researchers to consider how treatment impacts one's life, and not simply in the form of reported toxic effects. As a result, measuring quality of life before, during, and after treatment emerged as an additional objective of many cancer clinical trials.

Quality of life is difficult to define and measure. Just as pain is subjective and when measured is defined according to what the patient says it is, quality of life has the same constraint on definition and is multidimensional. For the purpose of evaluating it within a clinical trial, it is considered to be "a pragmatic, day-to-day functional representation of a patient's physical, psychological, and social response to a disease and its treatment."[4] Quantifying the concept may be accomplished with A Quality of Life Questionnaires—FACT-BRM and FACT-O. These self-report questionnaires have questions that relate to the categories of a "Physical Well Being," a "Social/Family Well Being," an "Emotional Well Being," a "Functional Well Being," and "Additional Concerns." ONLY the individual suffering from cancer and its treatment can determine this important parameter.[5,6] Appearances may depict an individual with multiple health, financial, and social problems, but that individual may describe herself as enjoying high quality of life. Conversely, individuals with every outward appearance of

the constituents of high quality of life may describe themselves as lacking in all areas of contentment and happiness.

Systems Theory proposes that any system finding itself in a state of disequilibrium will attempt to reestablish balance. Whether nurses view their patients within the context of the traditional medical model or utilize one of the many conceptual models of nursing, their "patient system" (whether it is an individual or family or community) will always attempt to reestablish a state of equilibrium or balance. Our current healthcare system has fallen short of providing extended support to the chronically ill, including the cancer patient who has completed active treatment. Nurses must position themselves as the key entity to bridge this gap. Part of this role responsibility includes informing themselves and their patients about the possible sequelae of cancer and its treatment. Anticipating these possible consequences may lead to eventual preventative interventions, and if not, perhaps methods of symptom relief can be found that lessen the severity of experienced long-term side effects, resulting in significantly improved quality of life.[7,8]

Review of the Literature

The review of the literature is certainly not exhaustive. Clearly certain topics which may be considered long-term sequelae of the treatment of gynecologic malignancies have been omitted. These topics include long-term changes secondary to radiation therapy, as well as psychiatric disorders that a survivor may attribute to the trauma of the cancer experience. The reader is encouraged to read nursing and medical texts and periodicals devoted solely to these topics and those devoted to specific gynecologic disease sites for information regarding other long-term effects of gynecologic cancers and the respective treatments for information regarding these topic areas.

The reader may also note that for the topic areas included, there may be a wealth of medical citations, but no nursing citations, or the opposite may be true. For example, research exists (though it is not plentiful) in the area of cognitive dysfunction, in medical periodicals. Nursing studies in the area are almost nonexistent. This does not mean that nursing research should not be done on this topic. On the contrary; not only should nursing research be done, but this topic has numerous nursing implications for the nursing clinician and her/his patient population. In contrast, a dearth of literature exists in medical journals and texts on the topic of lymphedema. More has been done in this area in nursing. If one researches this topic in the gynecologic oncology arena, both medical and nursing professionals have their work cut out for them. The topic is infrequently discussed, let alone researched. Hopefully the topics discussed in this chapter will motivate the reader to do more reading on the long-term effects of female cancer and its treatment, and to dedicate considerable energy to researching possible ways for nurses to remedy these significant problems.

Cognitive Dysfunction

Cognitive function is a multidimensional concept that describes the domains resulting from healthy brain performance, specifically attention and concentration, executive function, information processing speed, language, visuospatial skill, psychomotor ability, learning, and memory.[9]

Attention enables an individual to triage relevant inputs, thoughts, or actions while ignoring other input that distracts or is irrelevant. The three types of attention include selective, sustained, and directed. Selective attention allows the individual to focus on specific objects, or stimuli, excluding other stimuli for brief periods of time. Sustained attention, or concentration or vigilance, allows the maintenance of attention toward a stimulus for more extended periods of time. Directed attention refers to one's ability to attend to two or more competing tasks simultaneously, or what many of us speak of when we say we are "multitasking." Attention is the basic building block of cognitive function and is needed for the expression of other cognitive domains. It acts as a mediator to integrate, direct, and influence memory, perception, and language.[10]

Executive function is a higher-order cognitive process that includes initiation, planning, hypothesis generation, flexibility, utilization of information, and self-perception. Executive function deficits manifest themselves by the inability to follow directions, decreased ability to handle personal finances, disorganized behavior or thinking, loss of motivation, and increased need for external structure. This adversely affects an individual's work habits and ability to plan for the future.

Information-processing speed simply refers to the brain's ability to process simple and complex information rapidly. It includes all aspects of the brain's processing of sensory, perceptual, and conceptual input, from storage and analysis to output.

Language includes verbal and written communication used to express thoughts. Processing language involves representing, comprehending, and communicating symbolic information in written and spoken form. Impairment in this area of cognitive function inhibits the ability to communicate with others and follow instructions without repetition and explanation.

Motor function relates to motor performance and includes speed, strength, and coordination. The cerebellum has a moderating role between the several areas of the central nervous system (CNS) that are needed for movement. Decreased motor function is manifested by gait changes, weakness, tremors, or dexterity problems.

Visuospatial skill is the ability to process and interpret visual information regarding the location of things in space. It is dependent on processes that start in the retina, where visual sensations begin. Communication between a number of locations in the brain allows for object recognition and other areas of brain communication support for spatial aspects of vision. Impaired visuospatial skill causes altered perceptions or inability to recognize familiar objects, possibly resulting in decreased ability to perform manual tasks.

Learning involves the process of acquiring new information or knowledge. Memory, in turn, involves the persistence of learning so that this information can be utilized later in time. Learning and memory, which results from repetition of newly acquired information, pertain to the ability to acquire, store, and utilize new information.

Short-term memory, often called working memory, refers to brief memory storage with a decay rate of a few seconds. Consolidation is the neuropsychological mechanism that enables us to store memories more permanently. Long-term memory, or semantic memory, allows us to learn, store, and recall acquired knowledge and facts.[10] (The reader is referred to this citation for additional information regarding the corresponding anatomical locations and interactions of these cognitive functions and anatomical components.)

Cognitive dysfunction or impairment has been reported in 17%–75% of patients who receive adjuvant chemotherapy. Incidence rates vary widely in the research studies and may be secondary to differences in the time since treatment, doses and regimens of drugs, menopausal status, and utilized testing methods. Areas of dysfunction identified include poor concentration, slowed mental and motor speed, impaired short-term memory (especially acquiring new information and recalling recently learned information), and impaired psychomotor functioning. Deficits are usually graded as mild to moderate in severity and are associated with both standard-dose and high-dose chemotherapy. Higher chemotherapy doses, however, are associated with more severe and persistent impairment. Dysfunction is frequently noted during chemotherapy but has been documented up to 10 years after treatment.[11]

Research focusing on gynecologic cancer patients receiving chemotherapy is limited.[12] Forty-one patients with advanced-stage ovarian cancer received one of two graduated doses and schedules of paclitaxel, gemcitabine, and carboplatin, for six cycles, with filgrastim support. In addition to determining response rates from this regimen, researchers longitudinally assessed impact on cognitive function. Psychomotor speed, cognitive flexibility, attention, and concentration were measured, as well as quality of life. In addition, patients were interviewed regarding their own perceptions of possible cognitive changes. Cognitive function was assessed before, during, and after chemotherapy. Researchers found a trend toward stable or improved psychomotor speed, cognitive flexibility, attention, and concentration during chemotherapy and 6 months after the completion of treatment. Although women classified as highly educated perceived themselves with compromised concentration and memory, objective measures did not support these perceptions. Other studies focusing on cognitive dysfunction in gynecologic oncology patients only measure patients' perceptions within the context of quality of life.[13]

Remaining studies that objectively evaluate cognitive function in chemotherapy patients primarily focus on patients with breast cancer. Sample sizes usually are small, and methodologies sometimes are flawed.[9,14] **Table 14-1** summarizes findings and limitations of some of the more recent studies of cognitive dysfunction in breast and ovarian cancer patients following treatment.[12–22]

A significant problem encountered by those doing longitudinal evaluation is attrition of the sample groups, which inevitably occurs in high-risk populations. This alone pleads the case for a well-designed cooperative group clinical trial in the gynecologic cancer population. Methodology needs attention: Pretreatment evaluation is a must to rule out preexisting impairment, and evaluation tools need fine tuning to reduce the time required for evaluation (eliminating test fatigue in the study subjects) and to simplify data collection.

What actually causes cognitive dysfunction in the chemotherapy patient is not clearly understood. Higher doses of chemotherapy result in more severe cognitive impairment.[15] More recently, comparisons of PET scans and MRI scans have documented structural changes in the brains of those who have received chemotherapy.[23,24,17] This leaves little doubt that chemotherapy impacts cognitive function. Speculation exists regarding how this happens because many agents are believed to be unable to permeate the blood brain barrier because of limited solubility or high molecular weight. Many agents are severe irritants and may cause tissue necrosis, thereby damaging blood vessels and in turn allowing crossover. This potentially results in direct damage to brain tissue or brain transmitters. In addition, chemotherapeutic agents may disturb the normal physiology of the brain by direct injury to neurons from an uncontrolled inflammatory response initiated by cytokines. (The cytokines are proteins that are released by immune cells in the body, which are activated in response to inflammation, stress, or direct injury to neurons.) Proinflammatory cytokines augment the immune system's response to facilitate efficient resolution of injury. The brain, in turn, interprets the increased levels of proinflammatory cytokines as signals of sickness. Not only does this trigger all resources in defense against infection and tissue injury, but it also initiates the behavior response known as "sickness behavior." Sickness behavior results in weakness, decreased physical activity, and anorexia, as well as decreased concentration, listlessness, and decreased ability to learn. Others suggest that cytokines may enter the central nervous system through passive diffusion, active transport, or by stimulating prostaglandins to signal the brain to induce cytokine synthesis in the brain.[14,10]

Other explanations for how this happens include anemia and hormonal changes. Acute oxygen deprivation may lead to damage to the frontal and temporal lobes, the hippocampus, the basal ganglia, and the cerebellum. This insufficiency of brain oxygenation leads to impaired alertness, attention and concentration, memory, motor function, and mental flexibility.

Table 14-1 REVIEW OF COGNITIVE DYSFUNCTION STUDIES IN CANCER PATIENTS WHO HAVE RECEIVED CHEMOTHERAPY.

Author(s)/ Publication	Sample (size and type)	Comparison Group	Measuring Tools of Cognitive Function	Areas of Cognitive Dysfunction	Major Findings	Limitations
Ahles, et al. *J Clin Oncol.* 2002;20(2). Dartmouth-Hitchcock Medical Center[16]	35 breast cancer patients and 36 lymphoma patients; all patients received tx 5 years ago	Patients who had received local treatment only (surgery)	See note below	Psychomotor functioning (seen in patients 10 years or more after receiving chemotherapy)	Low correlation between higher number of chemotherapy cycles and lower neuropsychological performance	1. Small sample size—cannot draw conclusions about different agents or regimens 2. Lack of pretreatment assessment
Brezden, et al. *J Clin Oncol.* 2000;18(14). University of Toronto[17]	31 breast cancer patients on adjuvant chemotherapy; 40 breast cancer patients who received chemotherapy 2 years ago	36 healthy controls	1. High sensitivity cognitive screen 2. Profile of mood state (POMS)	(Trends only) Impairment in: 1. Domains of memory and language in patients in treatment 2. Language and visual-motor skills in patients who completed tx more than 1 year ago	No difference between the three groups in POMS scores Statistically significant difference in cognitive function in the actively treated group and the control group	1. Small sample size 2. Control group was much younger and tended not to be menopausal (as was the case in the treatment groups)

Chan, et al. *Gynecol Oncol.* 2003;88(1). Hong Kong[13]	17 ovarian cancer patients on neoadjuvant platinum/taxol (only 12 patients completed the study)	Historical	European Organization for Research and treatment of cancer QOL questionnaire	Not able to identify—tool used was global in its measurement	(Not statistically significant) Initially decreased role functioning and cognitive functioning at 3 months after completing chemotherapy	1. Small sample size 2. Comparison was based on historical control
Tchen, et al. *J Clin Oncol.* 2003;22(15). University of Toronto[18]	110 breast cancer patients receiving various adjuvant chemotherapy treatments	100 patients selected "matched" (by age) controls	1. High sensitivity cognitive screen 2. Attention span 3. Reaction time	(Trends only) Language, attention span, concentration, self-regulation, and planning in treatment group	16% moderate to severe impairment in the patient group 4% found impaired in the control group	1. Small sample size 2. Patients selected their own controls
Mar Fan, et al. *J Clin Oncol.* 2005;23(31). University of Toronto[19]	91 breast cancer patients at 1 year after treatment; 83 breast cancer patients at 2 years after treatment	81 controls (patient selected)	High sensitivity cognitive screen	Not specifically discussed	16% of patients who were 1 year post-treatment had moderate to severe impairment; 4% of patients who were 2 years	1. No baseline measurements were done 2. Patients selected their own controls

(continues)

Table 14-1 REVIEW OF COGNITIVE DYSFUNCTION STUDIES IN CANCER PATIENTS WHO HAVE RECEIVED CHEMOTHERAPY continued.

Author(s)/Publication	Sample (size and type)	Comparison Group	Measuring Tools of Cognitive Function	Areas of Cognitive Dysfunction	Major Findings	Limitations
					posttreatment had moderate to severe impairment	
Kreukels, et al. *Clin Breast Cancer.* 2006;7(1). Netherlands Cancer Institute[15]	12 breast cancer patients received high-dose chemotherapy, 17 received conventional doses	23 breast cancer patients needing no further therapy	Reaction time Amplitudes and latencies of P-3 (a portion of event-related potentials; see note below)	Electrophysiologic alterations were seen in patients who received high-dose therapy	Amplitude of P-3 was significantly decreased in patients on high-dose therapy; no difference in reaction times between the groups	1. Small sample size 2. Complexity of tasks was too difficult to perform for all three groups of patients at the time they performed the tasks
Wefel, et al. *Cancer.* 2004;100(11). MD Anderson Cancer Center[21]	18 breast cancer patients	None—patients served as their own controls	See above and list of the tests used below	Domains of attention, learning, and processing speed	33% had impairment before treatment; Long-term finding: 50% of those patients who showed decline	1. Small sample size 2. No true control group

Schagen, et al. *Ann Oncol.* 2002;13: 1387–1397. Netherlands Cancer Institute[22]	Breast cancer patients: 23 on standard dose treatment; 31 on another standard dose treatment; 22 on high-dose treatment	27 breast cancer patients who received no chemotherapy	Self-report, perception questions (regarding health, QOL, depression, anxiety, and see below)	None: findings of this study suggest cognitive dysfunction after chemotherapy may be transient	showed improvement with time 4 years after therapy completion there were no differences found between the groups 1. Small sample size 2. Significant number of patients were lost to follow-up 3. Survival rates were different for the groups, making comparisons and conclusions difficult over time
Hensley, et al. *Gynecol Oncol.* 2006;102(2). Memorial Sloan Kettering Cancer Center[12]	27 patients with stage III or IV ovarian cancer	Patients served as their own controls with baseline tests done before chemotherapy was started	Self-perceptions were reported and see below	Patients perceived dysfunction, however scores did not reflect this; even perceptions of cognitive function returned to baseline at 6 months	No decrease in cognitive function 1. Small sample size 2. No long-term measurements were done 3. Possibility exists that the domains affected were not measured

Explanation of the cognitive tests used in some of the studies summarized in Table 14-1:

Ahles, et al. (2002):

Wechsler Adult Intelligence Scale
Boston Naming Test
Wechsler Memory Scale
Gordon Diagnostic System—Motor Functioning
Spielberger State-Anxiety Inventory
Center for Epidemiological Study—Depression

Wide Range Achievement Test
California Verbal Leaning Test
Continuous Performance Test
Squire Memory Self-Rating Questionnaire
Fatigue Symptom Inventory

Kreukels, et al. (2006):

Amplitudes and latencies of P3, which is an electrophysiologic index of information processing that presents a task with different conditions related to input, central, and output processing of information.
Reaction time, which measures *the efficiency of procesing* that is involved in each of the *stages* of the performed task.

Wefel, et al. (both citations) (2004):

Wechsler Adult Intelligence Test
Nonverbal Selective Reminding Test
MMPI

Verbal Selective Reminding Test
Multilingual Aphasia Exam
Quality of Life Inventory

Schagen et al. (2002):

Rey Auditory Verbal Learning Test
Digit Span of the Wechsler Adult Intelligence Scale
Trailmaking A and B
D2 Test
Fepsy Finger Tapping Task
Fepsy Binary Choice Test
Dutch Adult Reading Test

Complex Figure Test: Copy and Recall*
Digit Symbol of the Wechsler Adult Intelligence Scale
Word Fluency Subtest from the Dutch Aphasia Society Test
Stroop Test
Fepsy Visual Reaction Test
Fepsy Visual Search Test

*To reduce the risk of practice effect, Form II of the Complex Figure Test was used in the second assessment.

Hensley, et al. (2006):

FACT-O for QOL
Trailmaking A and B (for cognitive flexibility and psychomotor speed)
Wechsler Adult Intelligence Test
Scale—R Digit Span Subtest (attention and concentration)

Myelosuppressive chemotherapy agents cause anemia, and its incidence depends upon the dose intensity and cumulative courses of treatment. The most optimum hematocrit level for optimizing cognitive function is not known. Again, there is speculation that decreased concentration occurs with the hemoglobin level less than eight or a hematocrit level less than 25%.[10]

Hormones are chemical substances capable of acting on cells located at a distance. Acetylcholine may be involved in memory consolidation. Estrogen increases the level of an enzyme required for acetylcholine synthesis. There are multiple estrogen receptor sites throughout the brain, especially in locales involved in attention, memory, and learning. Chemotherapy and radiation are known to induce menopause, and many gynecologic oncology patients face surgically induced menopause. These modalities induce a more rapid drop in estrogen than natural menopause induces. It is not known if an accelerated drop in estrogen results in more cognitive impairment than a more gradual drop.[10]

Chemotherapy-induced cognitive impairment occurs in varying degrees. Oncology nurses need to be informed about this potential side effect of chemotherapy. Valid and reliable tools for assessing cognitive impairment and grading its impact do not yet exist. Knowing of its existence is not enough. Several factors impact the likelihood of the problem occurring. These factors fall into one of three different categories: 1) disease-related factors; 2) patient-related factors, and 3) specific chemotherapy-related factors. Although mechanisms of action are not clearly understood, nurses must ensure that patients and caregivers are aware of the possibility of cognitive impairment so that informed decision making can occur. Risk of impaired cognition can be minimized by monitoring for signs and symptoms of anemia and other aggravating conditions, such as anxiety or depression, and intervening appropriately.[11]

The *Cancer Care Information Series* offers suggestions to improve concentration. This resource is available via an 800 phone number or their Web site (see Resource List). In recent years, numerous articles have appeared in newspapers and on the Internet regarding keeping your brain limber and healthy. Whether or not these suggestions would help reduce chemotherapy-induced cognitive impairment is unknown. Nevertheless, these exercises offer possibilities for study and may impact a patient's quality of life if they perceive themselves as still cognitively capable. Other suggestions entertain the possible benefits of antidepressants, exogenous hormones, physical activity, and behavioral strategies.[25,26,19] Many of these techniques remain untested.

Peripheral Neuropathy

The peripheral nervous system consists of three major functional parts—autonomic, motor, and sensory nerves—and includes the cranial nerves. Peripheral neuropathy (PN) is inflammation, injury, or degeneration of the peripheral nerve fibers. It may occur as a part of the disease process of cancer; it may result from chemotherapy treatment, or, like cognitive dysfunction, it may be present before treatment commences.[20,21,25,27–29] Symptoms of the neuropathy will depend upon the specific injury and whether the dysfunction involves the sensory, motor, autonomic, and/or cranial nerves. Symptoms may range from paresthesias to severe, disabling sensorimotor pain and resulting muscle weakness.[27] This discussion is limited to chemotherapy-induced PN. Other cancer-related sources of PN include paraneoplastic syndrome, compression of the spinal nerves, radiation therapy, and surgery.

PN is primarily induced by the vinca alkaloids, the platinols, and the taxanes. Half of all individuals who receive vincristine will develop paresthesias of the hands and feet; between 20% and 90% of those receiving cisplatin (dose dependent) and about 60% of those receiving paclitaxel will experience PN.[30,31] The sensory nerves sense touch, pain, temperature, position (proprioception), and vibration. The motor nerves are responsible for voluntary movements, muscle tone, and coordination, and the autonomic nerves control intestinal motility, blood pressure, and involuntary muscles. There are two types of peripheral nerve fibers. Small fiber nerves are unmyelinated and sense pain and temperature. For the most part, they are composed of microtubules, which act as a transport mechanism for proteins. Large fiber nerves are myelinated and sense position and vibration, along with serving in motor control. They are composed primarily of neurofilaments that serve as the framework of the axon. Both the small and the large fibers connect with their respective tracts or columns in the spinal cord and serve as a relay system to the sensory areas of the brain. Most chemotherapy drugs usually affect one type of nerve over another: platinols affect the large fibers to varying degrees, taxanes and vinca alkaloids affect small fibers, and all agents capable of causing PN can lead to the loss of deep tendon reflexes (DTRs). Because the platinol agents primarily affect the large fibers, sensory, motor, and autonomic neuropathies may all be observed. Sensory neuropathies may include loss of the sense of position and vibration and what is known as Lhermitte sign.

Lhermitte sign is described as a lightening-like sensation that starts in the neck and radiates down the back and legs when the neck is flexed. Foot and wrist drop are examples of motor dysfunction seen with cisplatin toxicity, which is usually seen after moderate to severe sensory loss occurs. Orthostatic hypotension is an example of the rare autonomic dysfunction that may occur with these agents. With the platinol agents, PN usually occurs later in the treatment period and may not happen until a regimen of chemotherapy is completed. Increased cumulative doses and prolonged infusions increase the likelihood of platinol-induced PN.[32]

Taxanes are plant-derived compounds that cause microtubular aggregation, and their use has brought greater attention to the problem of peripheral neuropathy. The risk of taxane-induced PN depends upon the agent used, its administration schedule, cumulative dose, and if the taxane is combined with another neurotoxic agent.[33-35] Arthralgia/myalgia, as well as sensory and motor neurotoxicity incidence and severity, are reported as less in docetaxel than in paclitaxel and therefore may suggest its substitution in place of paclitaxel if a presenting patient is at especially high risk of PN development.[36,37] Vinca alkaloids are usually limited to the treatment of germ cell tumors and stromal tumors in the field of women's cancers. Although PN has been reported with vindesine and vinblastine, neurotoxic potential is highest with vincristine. As many as 57% of patients receiving vincristine may encounter paresthesias in the feet and hands, and up to 34% may experience motor weakness manifested by foot drop. It affects large fibers, although its strongest effect is on the small fiber nerves. Symptomatically, this is seen as loss of pain and temperature sensation with myalgias and distal paresthesias seen even earlier. Vincristine may also impact the autonomic system, resulting in intestinal dysmotility, orthostatic hypotension, urinary retention, and abnormal pulse responses.[32] Comprehensive assessment of PN should include three major components prior to the initiation of potentially neurotoxic chemotherapy and upon treatment completion. Assessment may also include interval and follow-up evaluations if PN is considered one of the dose-limiting toxicities of a new treatment regimen. One of the three major components is a thorough medical history. Preexisting conditions that lead to PN's presence at baseline or an increased likelihood of it occurring from neurotoxic chemotherapeutic agents include diabetes, herpes zoster, alcohol abuse, atherosclerotic heart disease, HIV infection, vitamin B deficiency, Charcot-Marie-Tooth disease, and various prescription drugs.[29] Knowing the patient's vocation and avocations may lead to different chemotherapeutic combination selections. Physical assessment for the presence of PN should include evaluating the cranial nerves, assessing cerebellar function and proprioception, and testing sensory function the deep tendon reflexes.[29,38,39]

Few instruments exist for purposes of measuring the patient's subjective experience with PN. Improved control of other chemotherapy-related toxicities has brought the problem of PN to the forefront, especially in the arena of quality of life. Many quality of life indexes include items addressing PN in their questionnaires, while others have led to the development of instruments measuring the subjective experience and its impact on one's functional status.[31] Future research needs to address the fine-tuning of preexisting instruments, thereby developing measuring tools that are practical for use in the clinical setting but global enough to build upon our knowledge base of PN.[31,37–39]

Preventative options for PN include pre- and postmedicating with pharmaceutical and nutritional agents as well chemotherapeutic regimen modifications. Amofostine, a cytoprotective agent approved to reduce renal toxicity associated with Cisplatin, has had mixed results in reducing neuropathy. Not only does it add to the expense of chemotherapy, but it has its own set of unpleasant side effects, which must be prevented for it to be *patient acceptable*.[40,41] Glutamine is a nonessential amino acid that serves as a fuel source for small intestine enterocytes and a precursor of neurotransmitters. Patients are given 10 grams/day for 3–4 days starting the day after treatment. Like amifostine, glutamine has had mixed success in reducing taxane-induced dysesthesias and numbness in the fingers and toes.[27,41,42,43,46,47] One reliable preventative method exists: to administer nonneurotoxic chemotherapeutic agents. Unfortunately, for ovarian cancer, the most active drugs for the disease are the platinums and the taxanes. Carboplatin has been shown to be equally as effective as cisplatin in combination with Taxol. With the reemergence of intraperitoneal cisplatin as the standard of care for patients with optimally debulked stage III disease, this may become a less attractive option. Vitamin E supplementation was shown to be safe and effective in protecting against cisplastin-induced peripheral neuropathy, but a small sample size necessitates further study to validate this finding.[44] For patients with preexisting conditions lending higher risk to PN development and those whose professions and avocations in which PN will impair their dexterity and balance, docetaxel has been substituted for paclitaxel.[37,45,46]

Analgesics are used for symptom control of PN, although they do not prevent it and they do not affect the underlying cause. Antidepressants and anticonvulsants have been heavily relied upon to relieve the pain resulting from most PN. Their use in chemotherapy-induced PN originated in their success in relieving pain secondary to diabetes- and herpes-associated PN. In addition to borrowing from these knowledge bases, Smith, Whedon, and Bookbinder developed a three-level algorithm that mirrored the World Health Organization's analgesic ladder.[47] Mild analgesic agents that usually can be purchased over the counter (OTC) are grouped in level one. These include extended-relief acetaminophen and nonsteroidal antiinflammatory drugs (NSAIDS). Level two consists of anticonvulsants and antidepressants, and opioids are grouped in level three. Many of these agents successfully relieve the discomfort; however, they too have unpleasant side effects that make their use unacceptable for some individuals.

In addition, the oral route may not be a viable option for others. For example, Gabapentin is a calcium-channel blocker that inhibits the release of excitatory neurotransmitters. It is not effective in treating acute pain or pain without an objective nerve injury. Common side effects of Gabapentin include drowsiness, gastrointestinal disturbance, and cognitive impairment in the elderly.[48] Collaboration between pharmacists and podiatrists, as well as the emergence of compounding pharmacies, has resulted in the formation of several topicals that make it possible to get good pain relief with less drowsiness (see **Table 14-2**). If agents are totally ineffective, they are eliminated as an option; if agents are partially effective at their maximum dose, they are used in combination with other medications in another category.[47]

Nonpharmaceutical methods for pain relief include hydrotherapy, water exercise, gentle massage, hot and cold applications, acupuncture, and TENS. Nurses can assist patients in

Table 14-2 ALGORITHM FOR PHARMACOLOGIC INTERVENTIONS FOR PERIPHERAL NEUROPATHY.

Level I
Extended relief acetaminophen*(recommended dose: 1300 mg three times a day)   NSAIDs*(recommended dose: 800 mg three times a day)   * Both medications are contraindicated in patients with impaired liver or renal function and those with duodenal ulcers.

Level II	
Tricyclic *Antidepressants*	
Amitriptyline	Start with 10–25 mg and titrate up to 50–150 mg.
Clomipramine	Given at bedtime, used to treat burning, shooting, or
Desipramine	tingling pain. Side effects include dizziness, dry mouth,
Doxepin	drowsiness, weakness, weight gain, and constipation.
Imipramine	
Nortriptyline	

Table 14-2 ALGORITHM FOR PHARMACOLOGIC INTERVENTIONS FOR PERIPHERAL NEUROPATHY *continued.*

Anticonvulsants	
Carbamazepine	Start with 200 mg and titrate up to 600–1200 mg.
Phenytoin	Start with 300 mg and titrate up to effective dose.
Valproic acid	Start with 10–15 mg/kg/day in 1–3 doses and titrate up to 750–2000 mg.
Gabapentin	Start with 300 mg/day and titrate up to as high as 3600 mg in three divided daily doses.
Pregabalin (Lyrica)	Start at 50 mg three times a day and increase up to 300 mg tid.

Level III

Opioids	Doses are determined by patient tolerance and titrated to
Morphine	analgesia.
Hydromorphone	

Oxycodone
Fentanyl
Methadone

Topical Applications or Local Anesthetics

Lidocaine 5% patches (May use up to three patches at a time.)

NeuroGel
Ketoprofen 5%
Amitriptyline 2%
Carbamazepine 2%
Gabaclon
Gabapentin 6%
Clonidine 0.2%

NeuroGel 2
Ketamine 10%
Gabapentin 6%
Baclofen 2%
Amitriptyline 2%
Clonidine 0.1%

Lyrica Gel

Morphine Gel

Source: Based on information from Almadrones et al., 2002; Smith et al., 2002; Marrs & Newton, 2003; Wilkes, 2004; Armstrong et al., 2005; Wamboldt & Kapustin, 2006.

trying these approaches, as well as referring patients for physical and occupational therapy. In addition, nurses need to discuss safety issues inside and outside of the home.

Urinary Tract Dysfunction

Urinary tract dysfunction is a common problem for women past the age of menopause. Fifteen to 30 percent of women over 60 years old who are not institutionalized report having at least occasional urinary incontinence. Estrogen protects the lining of the urethra and normal function of the urinary tract. Lack of estrogen due to natural menopause or menopause induced by surgery, chemotherapy, or radiation may hasten the onset of urinary tract dysfunction.[49] Treatment infusions may hasten or decrease the woman's ability to avoid incontinence. Many chemotherapy regimens require additional intravenous fluids that increase urinary output. Drugs that cause decreased alertness and mobility, such as diphenhydramine, prochlorperazine, lorazepam, and metoclopramide, as well as narcotic pain relievers and antidepressants, may decrease the sensation of bladder fullness. The chemotherapeutic drugs such as cisplatin, vinca alkaloids, and taxanes can cause or exacerbate neuropathy.[49,50,53] Urinary tract function is dependent on both the central nervous system and the peripheral nervous system. Bathroom facilities may be inaccessible because of poor proximity, occupation by others, or inability to move independently. Peripheral neuropathy may alter the bladder sensation, resulting in frequency, urgency, and incontinence.[29,51]

Frequent urinary tract infections, common in women with a gynecologic malignancy, may be due to the disease or to one or more of its treatments.[52] Radiation treatment to the pelvis may disrupt the normal smooth lining of the bladder, hampering its ability to destroy and expel bacteria. Radiation cystitis exhibits many symptoms of bladder infection, including dysuria, urinary urgency, and hematuria.[51] Long-term use of low-dose prophylactic antibiotic therapy may be necessary to prevent recurrent urinary tract infections. Agents may need periodic rotations. Attention should be given to cost and tendency for organism resistance, as well as to culture and sensitivity results, when selecting the appropriate antibiotic.

Radiation cystitis (irritating pain in the bladder secondary to radiation damage) exhibits many symptoms of bladder infection, including dysuria, urinary urgency, and hematuria. Adequate hydration reduces symptom severity if one avoids bladder irritants, such as caffeinated and carbonated beverages and citric and cranberry juices. Phenazopyridine hydrochloride is a topical analgesic excreted via the kidney, and it may be used to relieve bladder inflammation symptoms manifested as painful bladder spasms, dysuria, frequency, and urgency. (Remember to inform the patient that her urine will turn orange-red and it may stain clothing.) Oxybutynin chloride relaxes the smooth muscle of the bladder, relieving symptoms of frequency and urgency. Other effective agents for this purpose of relieving bladder spasms include flavoxate hydrochloride and hyoscyamine sulfate.[52]

Urinary tract obstruction is often seen with advanced cervical cancer and possibly other pelvic tumors if the tumor impinges on the ureter(s) or, less commonly, the bladder. Obstruction may lead to kidney dysfunction, often detected by an increase in the serum creatinine. Nephrostomy tubes are used to relieve the kidneys by diverting the urine, or stents may be placed to ensure patency of the ureters to drain the affected kidney. An obstructed urinary tract is highly susceptible to infection, which may be the symptom of obstruction. Even after a nephrostomy tube or stent is placed, the patient is vulnerable to infection because of the presence of a foreign body in the urinary tract. Prophylactic antibiotics may be prescribed in this case.[53]

Renal dysfunction in women with gynecologic cancer is most commonly caused by urinary tract obstruction. It may also be caused by nephrotoxic drugs, such as cisplatin. Underlying chronic illnesses, however, like diabetes, hypertension, and cardiac disease, may increase susceptibility to renal dysfunction. Patients should be encouraged to maintain adequate hydration and electrolyte balance and to avoid nephrotoxic drugs as much as possible. Amifostine (Ethyol) may be used if a nephrotoxic drug, such as cisplatin, is the chosen drug for treatment. Amifostine provides protection against cisplatin-induced nephrotoxicity. It may be used to decrease anticipated nephrotoxicity, as well as to prevent cumulative renal toxicity. Amifostine is dosed at 940 mg/m^2 after prehydration and is given IV push over 15 minutes or less to minimize toxicity. Toxicity is immediate with nausea, vomiting, and/or hypotension. Premedication with antiemetics, positioning the patient in a flat position, and infusing the drug over 3 to 5 minutes can minimize toxicity. Many patients tolerate the drug without side effects when these precautions are taken.[40,41,44]

Thromboembolic Events

Thromboembolic events (TE) have been discussed within the context of cancer for over a century.[54] Cancer-associated coagulation may occur in more that 90% of patients, and TE may be responsible for as many as 200,000 deaths among hospitalized patients in the United States each year.[55] Two recent gynecologic oncology studies documented the problem in 16% of a selected group of their patients.[54,56,59]

Virchow's triad, or the three factors involved in the pathogenesis of venous thrombosis, include damage to the vessel wall, venous stasis, and hypercoagulability.[56] Cancer cells may activate the clotting system directly (by stimulating thrombin production) and indirectly (by stimulating mononuclear cells to produce procoagulant materials). Tumors may damage the endothelium by direct vessel invasion and by secreting vascular permeability factors, which accounts for the accumulation of extravascular fibrinogen around tumors. Cancer treatments including chemotherapy, radiation, and surgery are also responsible for direct injury to the vessel wall.[54]

Venous stasis may result in TE by preventing activated coagulation factors from being diluted and cleared by normal blood flow. Stasis results in hypoxic damage to endothelial cells, resulting in prothrombotic changes. Venous stasis results from immobility in debilitated postoperative patients or from obstruction from extrinsic vascular compression from bulky tumor masses.

Hypercoagulability has been documented in cancer of the ovary. In this situation, a cascade of events occur:

> *a hematocrit-independent hyperviscosity syndrome with elevated platelet count with the concurrence of increased coagulation activation, reduced red blood cells deformability, dehydration due to malignant ascites, and activation of the host inflammatory response, may alter the rheologic properties of blood and contribute to reduced blood flow.*[54]

Patient risk factors (some of which have been previously mentioned) that predispose cancer patients to TE include: advanced age (greater than 60 years), obesity (BMI greater than 25), previous thrombosis, smoking, varicose veins, comorbidities, treatment with erythropoietin, and higher staged malignancies, as well as bulky tumors.[54,57,60]

Signs or symptoms of TE include unilateral swelling of an affected extremity, positive Homans sign, and shortness of breath or chest pain, indicating a possible pulmonary embolus.[58] Diagnosis of TE is usually confirmed with Doppler ultrasound of the affected limb, and if swelling of the limb is accompanied by chest pain or shortness of breath, chest X-ray, with or without spiral CT, is used to confirm pulmonary embolus.[56]

Treatment of TE must be aggressive. One usually begins with unfractionated heparin or low molecular weight heparin (LMWH) with rapid conversion to warfarin for chronic anticoagulation. Warfarin's half life of 2 to 3 days makes dose titration to maintain an International Normalized Ratio (INR) between 2 and 3 slow and tedious.[58] During the initial anticoagulation interval, INR levels must be followed closely. Patient education should address vitamin K: Patients should understand that it offsets the effect of warfarin and they should know which foods are rich sources of vitamin K. Other medications and medical disorders often offset the action of warfarin. Antibiotics upset the delicate balance of bacteria in the lower gastrointestinal tract, which produce one of three forms of vitamin K.[59] Liver dysfunction may affect the warfarin dose required for target anticoagulation.[49,58,61] Other medications, such as aspirin and most NSAIDs, potentiate the effect of anticoagulants. Patients need to be reminded of those effects as well.

For the patient who has a dangerously high INR, the effect of the warfarin may persist for 2 to 5 days after discontinuing the drug. Although vitamin K reverses dangerously high anticoagulation, fresh frozen plasma is often used to more moderately decrease the anticoagulation effect. This reduces the risk of thrombosis due to total reversal of the anticoagulation.[55,58,61]

Lymphedema

Lymphedema is persistent swelling resulting from an abnormal accumulation of protein-rich fluid in an affected anatomical location. Primary lymphedema is a birth defect in which an individual suffers a deficit of lymph channels. Primary lymphedema generally shows an autosomal dominant pattern of inheritance with incomplete penetrance and variable expression and age of onset.[60] Secondary lymphedema results from tumor or trauma (infection, surgery, or radiation), causing obstruction of the lymphatic system. For the woman with a gynecologic malignancy, swelling in the abdomen, pelvis, perineum, and lower extremities develops from absence or obstruction of the pelvic or inguinal lymph nodes. Breast cancer patients suffer from swelling of the arm on the affected side, but also the trunk (especially the chest region), axilla, and scapular regions. Treated and untreated, secondary lymphedema extensively impacts quality of life of women who survive breast or gynecologic cancer. Physically, it potentially results in cellulitis, lymphangitis, open draining wounds, impaired mobility, and even life-threatening septicemia and lymphangiosarcoma. The disease disfigurement and management compromises self-esteem, body image, occupational capabilities, and interpersonal and family relationships.[60–67,70]

The incidence of secondary lymphedema is difficult to establish for both populations: those women with a history of breast cancer and those with a previous gynecologic malignancy. Incidence rates vary from 10% to nearly 68% in the breast cancer population.[64,68,71] In the gynecologic cancer population, incidence rates vary from 2.5% to 47%.[62,63,69,66,72] With one exception, all figures originated from retrospective studies. In the one prospective study, no statistically significant differences were found regarding age, race, body mass index, cancer stage, surgical procedure, or having received versus not having received radiation therapy, between those with or without lymphedema.[68] Others claim that the extent of treatment (sampling a higher number of lymph nodes, administering radiation therapy to a wider field) and obesity impact risk, while age and involvement of dominant limb versus nondominant limb have minimal impact.[65] Multiple studies show lower incidence rates of lymphedema after sentinel lymph node biopsy versus auxiliary lymph node dissection.[70] Studies with the longest follow-up generally report the highest incidence. Limited sample sizes, retrospective versus prospective methodology, and variability in defining and measuring lymphedema explain the broad range of reported statistics.[61]

The water displacement or volumetric measurement (the gold standard) is generally considered to be the most accurate method of assessment and evaluation of lymphedema and demonstrates interrater reliability. The extremity is submerged in a tank of water, and water displacement is measured to determine the volume of the limb. Affected and unaffected limbs are easily compared without complicated equations. These comparisons allow the practitioner to document treatment progress. The volumetric method utilizes cumbersome equipment that requires lengthy set up and cleaning after each use. Consequently, its use is usually limited to specialty and research settings.[60,61,71,64,74]

Circumferential measurements are usually taken with a tape measure, making this method more conducive to the clinical setting. The limb is measured at specific points, and these points are measured at each assessment, with data recorded in table format.

A third method uses circumferential measurements, taken at 10 centimeter intervals, and applies the numbers to the formula for a truncated cone. Calculations are made on the unaffected limb for comparative purposes to determine the percentage of edema change. The method is quite cumbersome and allows for a high potential of calculation errors. Software would eliminate the chance of error; however, data entry would likely not occur until after the patient visit, diminishing the patient's immediate feedback.

The comparative circumferential measurement method (CCMM), developed by an occupational therapist, obtains measurements at specifically defined points, and additional points are included if a significant amount of edema is encountered in an area not generally covered by the specific measurement points. The unaffected limb is measured at the same points. Differences at each point are added together, rendering one calculated score upon which to base all future reassessments. No special equipment is required other than a tape measure. Measurements and calculations are easily performed in the clinical setting and recorded on a simple documentation form. This allows provision of feedback to patients and other caregivers.[60]

A newer measurement method is bioelectric impedance analysis, which uses electrical current to measure extracellular fluid in the extremities. Preliminary findings appear hopeful; however, for some settings the purchase of special equipment may present an impediment.[60] Another method estimates limb volume by infrared perometry and utilizes equipment marketed for fitting custom-made compression garments. Infrared perometry currently is being evaluated.[61]

Ideally, measurements would be done before treatment initiation. This major methodology flaw is unfortunately almost universal in the clinical setting. Consequently, statistics cannot truly reflect an accurate incidence rate of the problem.[60,61,64,68,71,72,74,75]

Lymphedema occurs when the amount of arteriovenous fluid diffusing into the interstitial tissue to nourish the cells overrides the lymphatic system's ability to transport the fluid rich in larger protein molecules out and back into the venous system. The accumulation of interstitial macromolecules leads to increased oncotic pressure in the tissues, which, in turn, pulls more fluid into the tissue. Protein accumulation triggers recruitment of neutrophils, macrophages, and fibroblasts into the edematous limb. A state of chronic low-grade inflammation ensues, which leads to the deposit of disorganized collagen fibers.

This fibrosis further undermines transport capability, again increasing lymph stasis. The stagnant, protein-rich fluid provides an excellent culture medium for bacteria leading to a local or regional infection (cellulitis or lymphangitis) which, left untreated, may progress to systemic sepsis.[61,70,73]

Early identification of lymphedema and initiation of therapy usually translates to more successful results. Nurses have provided patients with a handful of well known prevention principles for many years. No data exist, however, upon which to base these principles (see **Table 14-3**).[61,64,70,73] Future research needs to address possible predisposing variables, as well as testing these long-accepted principles of prevention.

Several schools of therapy exist for lymphedema.[71] All, however, unanimously agree that a multimodality program achieves the best therapeutic result. These programs, commonly termed "Comprehensive Decongestive Physiotherapy," (or similarly named programs), consist of four major components:

- Meticulous skin care: Prevents skin breaks and infections and maintains optimum moisture
- Exercise: Approached wearing a compression garment without extreme exertion or excessive weight bearing
- Manual lymphatic drainage (MLD): A light massage technique to facilitate lymphatic mobilization back into the central circulation
- Bandaging and compression garments: Implemented once the first three (particularly MLD) achieve maximum limb-size reduction

(See references 61, 70, 71, 73, & 74 for more detailed descriptions and explanations.)

A good program also includes a nutrition component, emphasizing sufficient fluid and protein intake and optimum weight management.

External compression therapy is the mainstay of lymphedema management. Manual lymphatic drainage is followed by compression bandaging and garments. Bandaging consists of short, nonelastic bands that exert high external

---

Table 14-3 PREVENTION PRINCIPLES FOR PATIENTS WHO HAVE UNDERGONE
LYMPH NODE DISSECTION.

---

1. Avoid punctures and cuts (injury). Practice meticulous skin, nail, and cuticle care.
2. Avoid injections, blood pressure monitoring, phlebotomy, and intravenous infusions in the affected limb.
3. Avoid constricting garments and jewelry. If possible, wear padded bra straps.
4. Avoid heat and sun exposure, hot tubs, steam baths, and saunas.
5. Avoid vigorous exercise and strenuous exertion by the affected limb. Consider vigorous aerobic arm exercise only when compression garments support the limb.

Source: Based on information in Petrek and Disa, 2005.

pressure against the inner working musculature and low external pressure when the muscle is at rest. Long elastic (Ace) bandages run the risk of creating a tourniquet effect, thereby completely collapsing the lymphatic vessel. Improved patient wear compliance of compression garments may be achieved by carefully reviewing their benefits (see **Table 14-4**).

Diuretic therapy is generally contraindicated. Diuretics temporarily decrease the fluid in interstitial tissue; however, the high protein macromolecules remain. Consequently, fluid rapidly reaccumulates and edema reappears. Benzopyrones have shown conflicting results and may induce liver dysfunction.[61,70,73] Surgical reanastomosis of lymphatic vessels to venous vessels remains an unknown and may result in infection, fibrosis, and scarring.[71] One study achieved good long-term results in a small group of women who had intractable lower extremity lymphedema after radical hysterectomy and staging laparotomy for cervical cancer. Physiotherapy was recommended to continue to achieve the best results.[73] Sentinel lymph node identification, as an option for patients with pelvic malignancies, as it is for those with breast cancer, is being explored.[74,75,78]

Osteoporosis

Osteoporosis is a "skeletal disorder characterized by compromised bone strength, predisposing a person to an increased risk of fracture."[76] An estimated 44 million Americans have or are at risk of developing osteoporosis or osteopenia. This represents 55% of all individuals age 55 years or older. Although it is considered to be non-gender specific, of the 10 million Americans with osteoporosis, 8 million are women.[77] In 2000, the direct and indirect costs of osteoporosis-related fractures were $7.5 billion a year in the United States. Of those suffering hip fractures related to decreased bone mineral density, one-third require long-term care, and only one-third return to their prefracture functional level. Furthermore, the mortality rate in the 5 years following fracture in these individuals is 12%–20% higher than in those of similar age and gender who have not suffered a fracture.[78,79,82]

Normal bone turnover in the skeleton depends upon balance between bone resorption and bone formation (otherwise referred to as skeletal remodeling). Osteoclasts remove or resorb old bone, and osteoblasts are the bone-forming cells. Osteoblasts produce collagen, alkaline

---

Table 14-4 Benefits of wearing compression garments.

1. Compression garments improve lymphatic flow and reduce accumulated protein.
2. Compression garments improve venous and lymphatic return.
3. Compression provides counter pressure against the muscle pump and helps mobilize protein in the tissue of fibrotic limbs.
4. The garments properly shape and reduce the size of the limb.
5. Compression garments help protect the limb from potential trauma.
6. Compression garments are essential to maintaining edema reduction.
7. Compression garments are essential to maintaining skin integrity and skin suppleness, and to compensating for the elastic insufficiency of the skin after volume reduction.

Source: Based on information from Petrek and Disa.

phosphatase, and other proteins and secrete them into the bone matrix (or resorption cavity). Normally the activities of the osteoclasts and osteoblasts are tightly coupled during adulthood. With advancing age, however, the rate of bone resorption vastly exceeds the rate of bone formation. This is thought to be partially due to lifespan shortening of the osteoblasts and lifespan lengthening of the osteoclasts. Estrogens act directly and indirectly to limit bone resorption and maintain bone density. With the fall of estrogen levels, there is an increase in osteoclast formation and survival.[77,80,81,83,84]

The loss of estrogen, rather than aging, is the major determinant of postmenopausal bone loss. Women treated for endometrial and ovarian cancer abruptly enter menopause as a result of the surgical portion of their treatment (removal of the ovaries in addition to hysterectomy and bilateral salpingectomy with the staging procedures). The ovaries may or may not be removed in early invasive cancer of the cervix, and for those with advanced cervical disease, radiation therapy will likely ablate ovarian function unless surgical ovarian transposition occurs during the surgical staging procedure.[82]

Data suggest that ovarian failure secondary to adjuvant chemotherapy for breast cancer results in rapid falls in estrogen levels similar to what occurs after surgically induced menopause (rather than the more gradual decrease that occurs over several years with natural menopause). Ovarian failure secondary to chemotherapy results in rapid (within 1 year of treatment) bone loss in breast cancer patients treated with cyclophosphamide in the adjuvant setting. The resulting ovarian failure is dependent upon the cumulative dose of chemotherapy given and the age of the woman receiving treatment. Those over age 40 years and those receiving higher doses of chemotherapy were at greater risk of becoming menopausal.[83–85,88]

Significant bone loss can occur in breast cancer patients treated with selective estrogen-receptor modulators (SERMs) and aromatase inhibitors (AIs).

Although tamoxifen (a SERM) has been shown to prevent bone loss in postmenopausal women, tamoxifen and raloxifene (which is used to prevent and treat osteoporosis in postmenopausal women) were shown to result in bone loss in the hip and spine in premenopausal women.[84] Hence, the impact of SERMs on bone density in premenopausal women requires further investigation. Aromatase inhibitors may accelerate bone loss in postmenopausal women, due to their profound suppression of circulating and tissue estrogen levels.[81] Bone fracture rates differ among the various clinical trials with specific treatment arms and defined patient populations. Nevertheless, all AIs appear to result in loss of bone density of about 4%–5% in the first 2 years of treatment.[86–88,91]

With the exception of most women with a history of breast cancer and some women with a history of a gynecologic malignancy, hormone replacement therapy was frequently recommended as a means to prevent osteopenia and osteoporosis before the results of the Women's Health Initiative Study were published a few years ago. However, before this, despite the undesirable consequences of menopause, only one in six of the 36 million women age 50 years or older took hormone replacement therapy.[78,81,84] This sorry statistic coincides today with the low percentage of women who are at high risk of developing reduced bone density who do not get screened. Furthermore, although bone loss is known to be accelerated 2 years before menopause through the first 5 years after menopause, the National Osteoporosis Foundation and World Health Organization do not recommend dexa scan screening in the general population until age 65 years.

Bisphosphonates (risedronate, clodronate, alendronate, pamidronate, and zoledronic acid) not only increase bone mineral density but reduce the likelihood of vertebral and non-vertebral fractures. They are approved both for the prevention and treatment of osteoporosis. Clinical trials are now taking place to determine whether bone loss is more severe in women who have had ovarian ablative treatment, receive either tamoxifen or anastrozole, and receive or do not receive zoledronic acid.[81] A Gynecologic Oncology Group study is evaluating whether or not zoledronic acid can reduce bone loss in women who have prophylactic bilateral oophorectomy to reduce their risk of ovarian cancer.[89]

Fatigue

Cancer-related fatigue (CRF) is a distressing, persistent, subjective sense of tiredness or exhaustion related to cancer or cancer treatment that is not proportional to recent activity and interferes with usual functioning.[90] Other definitions of the concept are simpler: *a sensation of tiredness*, and, therefore support approaching fatigue research as a self-perceived state. Regardless of one's accepted definition or study approach, the knowledge base of CRF during treatment and after treatment has mushroomed over the last 25 years. Depending upon the patient population, its incidence is between 75% and 100% during the active treatment phase.[91,92,95] The incidence of CRF long after treatment completion (2.5 to 5–10 years) can be up to one-third of the studied sample.[91,93,95,96]

CRF may result from the nature of the malignancy itself, the treatment approach, and preexisting patient variables. As treatment becomes more complex (combined modalities) and dosing schedules become more intense, fatigue also becomes more common and more intense.[96] Biotherapy as a solitary modality results in a high incidence of CRF. If combined with conventional chemotherapy or a second biotherapeutic agent, it becomes a certain sequelae in the cancer experience.[97]

CRF presents a tremendous clinical challenge for the following reasons: (1) CRF is a multidimensional phenomenon with potential to be physical, mental, or affective in expression, which leads to the second reason for its challenging nature; (2) it has multiple correlates, that is, it may correlate and coexist with depression, anxiety, anemia, quality of life, cognitive dysfunction, and perceived social support;[91,94,98,101] 3) the etiology or cause may be multifactorial.

Fatigue may result from the malignancy itself and, in fact, may be one of the patient's presenting symptoms. Fatigue induced by radiation therapy usually ensues after the first or second week of therapy and may continue up to a year after its completion.[99] Chemotherapy-induced fatigue starts a few days after drug delivery and may last until the next treatment course is administered. Fatigue will be intensified if these two modalities are combined with one another or combined together or alone with surgery or biotherapy.[100]

Preexisting patient variables include the following:

- Activity level, including decreased activity and deconditioned state
- Anemia
- Comorbidities
- Emotional distress, including depression and anxiety
- Nutritional deficits
- Pain
- Sleep disturbance[90]

A patient may present with anemia before treatment initiation. Anemia may also be treatment induced. Hemoglobin levels lower than 12g/dL have been shown to correlate with lower quality of life and more fatigue. In addition, anemia has been associated with decreased survival. Strong clinical evidence supports the use of epoetin alfa, and its use has been shown to increase hemoglobin levels and decrease the need to transfuse.[90,101,104] However, advisories have recently warned that using erythropoiesis-stimulating agents for cancer-associated anemia may increase the incidence of venous thrombosis and possibly stimulate tumor cell growth. Furthermore, raising hemoglobin levels has not yet been shown to improve the prognosis of anemic cancer patients.[102–104]

Preexisting psychological factors complicate clinical management of fatigue. Cancer patients at the highest risk for depression (frequently related to the stress of having a malignancy) have suboptimal pain control, preexisting mood disorders, advanced disease, or are in poor physical condition. In one group of cancer survivors, those suffering from fatigue were more likely to suffer higher levels of clinical depression. Research shows that fatigue and depression correlate with one another; this is not to be confused with a causal relationship. Although antidepressants may relieve depression, they rarely relieve fatigue.[100]

Many factors may contribute to long-term cancer-related fatigue, several of which are amenable to medical or nursing management. Consequently, thorough assessment is mandatory for the cancer survivor presenting with fatigue. Ruling out disease recurrence/progression is foremost in focused history taking and follow-up physical exam completion. When this and a comprehensive review of systems is completed, in-depth fatigue assessment focuses on onset, pattern, duration, whether or not change occurs over time, and aggravating or alleviating factors. Determining how much fatigue interferes with daily activities must not be neglected in the assessment process. Nutritional deficits may contribute to fatigue, especially if weight or caloric intake has changed. Electrolyte imbalances should not be overlooked, and inadequate fluid intake can be detrimental to energy levels. One must also consider whether fatigue is secondary to decreased physical activity or decreased physical fitness. Comorbidities that may compromise energy levels include infections and pulmonary, renal, hepatic, and neurologic dysfunction. Endocrine dysfunctions that may increase fatigue include hypothyroidism, hypogonadism, and adrenal insufficiency. Nail stresses that clinical assessment must be rapid and universally applicable, and recommends using published guidelines to thoroughly evaluate fatigue.[90,91,94] Most contributing factors are amenable to interventions, and thorough assessment, in turn, guides appropriate management.

Just as cancer-related fatigue is multidimensional and has multiple correlates, its management must be approached with an interdisciplinary team.

Information regarding expected patterns of fatigue for various treatment modalities must be provided at the initiation of therapy. Support groups focusing on information provision are helpful, as is keeping a daily symptom diary. Although energy conservation and distraction techniques have not been tested in any formal studies, patients may find this advice helpful. In fact, setting activity priorities may facilitate survivors to find meaning in their experience with fatigue.[105] Nonpharmacologic techniques that lend themselves to the enlistment of assistance from other disciplines include:

- Initiation of an exercise program: physical therapy or rehabilitative medicine can provide a plan of approach so that injuries are less likely to occur.[90,106,109]
- Stress management, relaxation, attention-restoring therapy, and support groups: therapists and experts in complementary care techniques can assist with devising a personal or family plan for this area. They may also help families return to some semblance of normalcy and intervene with sleep disorders.[90]
- Implementation of a healthy diet: assistance should be provided by a registered dietician who is familiar with cancer and treatment modalities.

In light of the recent warnings regarding epoetin alfa, cancer survivors who have completed active treatment should be evaluated for deficiencies and receive iron, folic acid, and vitamin B_{12} if indicated.[100,107,110] A recent warning from the United States Food and Drug Administration raised concerns about the potential adverse effects of erythopoiesis-stimulating agents (ESAs) in anemic cancer patients who are receiving chemotherapy. Survival has been found to be poorer in some patients, and the need for transfusion was not reduced in other cancer patients when ESAs augmented therapy.[102]

Research is limited in the area of pharmaceutical intervention for fatigue relief. Classes of medications that may potentially be useful include psychostimulants, selective serotonin-reuptake inhibitors, and low-dose corticosteroids. Although double-blinded randomized studies have not been conducted with methylphenidate, it has been helpful for outpatients with advanced cancer and melanoma patients on interferon who utilized it with an exercise program.[108–110]

Discussion and Future Needs

Accruing adequately sized samples is a ubiquitous problem in clinical research. Clinical studies of the long-term effects of cancer and cancer treatment have not evaded this problem. With a few exceptions, the cited research here had sample sizes that did not allow for comparisons that would allow for statistically significant results. Trends can be visualized, lending the clinician some hunches regarding the sequelae of oncologic interventions. This allows the nurse who is involved in patient care to at least inform the patient regarding what has been observed and hopefully to provide some reassurance as well as anticipatory nursing intervention.

Medical and surgical oncology has found a solution to the problem of small samples. Cooperative groups emerged in the early 1970s, making it possible to accrue clinical data more rapidly, improve survival and remission rates, and keep up with technology as well. The nursing profession needs to follow suit. The cooperative groups lend themselves nicely to this purpose. Nevertheless, we have not seen a great deal of nursing research generated by cooperative groups. Simply evaluating the incidence of the clinical problems establishes a list of priorities or needs in patient care. Pharmaceutical research has not developed perfect antineoplastics; therefore nurses and their patients continue to search for solutions to the problem of peripheral neuropathy. Nurses can be key people in the search for a worthy solution to this clinical problem. These potential solutions could be piloted in the environment of a cooperative group, much as phase I and II studies are piloted.

The majority of studied populations in the reviewed literature were breast cancer survivors. This is partly because it is easier to accrue samples of breast cancer patients than it is to accrue samples of ovarian cancer survivors, especially if one considers where some of these studies were conducted: in the department of (neuro) psychology versus the department of medical oncology. Nevertheless, studies of cognitive dysfunction, fatigue, lymphedema, and osteoporosis need to be done on the gynecologic oncology patient population as well. This allows findings to become more applicable to other groups and adds to the validity of the research.

Nursing Implications

On July 15, 2005, a three-day invitational conference occurred in Philadelphia. The conference was entitled *The State of the Science on Nursing Approaches to Managing Late and Long-Term Sequelae of Cancer and Cancer Treatment*. Goals of the symposium were to develop research priorities and recommendations for clinical care, education, and policy related to nursing care for survivors of cancer who complete initial treatment during adulthood and continue to live with the potential or actual sequelae of their cancer, its treatment, or both.[111] Symposium participants established numerous barriers to optimal care for cancer survivors and strategies to overcome them. At the top of their list was the knowledge deficit that exists among their own profession.

Nurses need to actively teach each other. As this committee of conference attendees established priorities; clinicians who function in collaborative roles with physicians in the outpatient setting need to do likewise. This applies to those working as case managers in the outpatient setting as well. As the Oncology Nursing Society holds trainer workshops for those interested in teaching nurses about chemotherapy and radiation therapy, similar strategies need to occur among nurses whose role it is to teach patients.

Health care needs to move from being illness-based to a wellness orientation. Such was the motivation behind training nurses to become nurse practitioners: to help our population live healthier lives by practicing good health promotion. Health maintenance protocols were developed for various population groups, taking into consideration gender, culture, and age. Similarly, these nursing committees could develop health promotion protocols with the plan to present survivors with this protocol soon after they complete active treatment. Sharing this perception of a healthy future cannot help but reduce a survivor's anxiety as she makes the transition out of active treatment.

Support groups play an important role in this endeavor. Peer support improves motivation to eat healthier and exercise regularly. Exercise in itself improves fatigue, cognition, lymphedema (if not approached too vigorously), and osteoporosis. Research shows that aerobic exercise decreases fatigue and depression and enhances one's level of alertness. No data exist regarding whether weight training benefits fatigue or cognition, although we do know that it benefits bone density and mood states in the elderly. This would be a relatively easy study to implement in the clinical setting, collaboratively with a physical therapist or personal trainer.

Oncology rehabilitation clinics have emerged to assist the patient cope with the transition from the active treatment phase to the follow-up phase. A team of nurses could easily implement this concept.

The general public and third-party players need to realize the benefits of such programs. Cancer is not our nation's number one health problem, but the cancer survivor population recently grew to 10 million. Nurses need to help our survivors become healthier people.

Conclusion

Cancer leaves one not unscathed. The research on the long-term physical impact of cancer treatment, specifically radiation therapy, surgery, and chemotherapy on the different tissues and organ systems, is not discussed here. Nor is the incredible psychological impact cancer and cancer treatment has on the female cancer survivor. These topics are usually well covered in the medical textbooks of gynecologic oncology and medical oncology. Nevertheless, one gets a glimpse of how treatment and the disease may impact a survivor over a long period of time. Just as our healthcare system does not serve those with chronic illnesses well, concerns of cancer survivorship are not well addressed. This area provides rich opportunities for advanced practice nurses and oncology nurse clinicians, much as their professional counterparts could function in internal medicine with the problems chronic illnesses present outside the acute care setting.

References

1. American Cancer Society. Cancer facts and figures. http://www.cancer.org. Published 2007. Accessed July 13, 2008.

2. Pitzele SK. *We Are Not Alone: Learning to Live with Chronic Illness*. New York, NY: Workman; 1986.

3. Lubkin IM, Larsen PD. *Chronic Illness: Impact and Interventions*. Sudbury, MA: Jones and Bartlett; 2006.

4. Schipper H. Guidelines and caveats for QOL measurement in clinical practice and research. *Oncol.* 1990;4(5):51–57.

5. Johnson J. *Intimacy: Living As a Woman after Cancer*. Toronto, ON: NC Press Limited; 1987.

6. Pazdur R, Coia LR, Hoskins WJ, Wagman LD. *Cancer Management: A Multidisciplinary Approach*. 9th ed. Melville, NY: PRR; 2006.

7. Carnevali DL, Reiner AC. *The Cancer Experience: Nursing Diagnosis and Management*. Philadelphia, PA: JB Lippincott; 1990.

8. Fitzpatrick JJ, Whall AL. *Conceptual Models of Nursing*. 4th ed. Upper Saddle River, NJ: Pearson, Prentice Hall; 2005.

9. Jansen CE, Miaskowski C, Dodd M, Dowling G. Chemotherapy-induced cognitive impairment in women with breast cancer: a critique of the literature. *Oncol Nurs Forum*. 2005;32(2):329–342.

10. Jansen C, Miaskowski C, Dodd M, Dowling G, Kramer J. Potential mechanisms for chemotherapy-induced impairments in cognitive function. *Oncol Nurs Forum*. 2005;32(6):1151–1161.

11. O'Shaughnessy J. Chemotherapy-related cognitive dysfunction in breast cancer. *Semin Oncol Nurs*. 2003;19(4)(suppl 2):17–24.

12. Hensley ML, Correa DD, Thaler H, Wilton A, Venkatraman E. PhaseI/II study of weekly paclitaxel plus carboplatin and gemcitabine as first-line treatment of advanced-stage ovarian cancer: pathologic complete response and longitudinal assessment of impact on cognitive functioning. *Gynecol Oncol*. 2006;102(2):270–277.

13. Chan YM, Ng TY, Ngan HY, Wong LC. Quality of life in women treated with neoadjuvant chemotherapy for advanced ovarian cancer: a prospective longitudinal study. *Gynecol Oncol*. 2003;88(1):9–16.

14. Matsuda T, Takayama T, Tashir M, Nakamura Y, Ohashi Y, Shimozuma K. Mild cognitive impairment after adjuvant chemotherapy in breast cancer patients—evaluation of appropriate research design and methodology to measure symptoms. *Breast cancer*. 2005;12(4):279–287.

15. Kreukels BP, Schage SB, Ridderinkhof KR, et al. Effects of high-dose and conventional-dose adjuvant chemotherapy on long-term cognitive sequelae in patients with breast cancer: an electrophysiologic study. *Clin Breast Cancer*. 2006;7(1):67–78.

16. Ahles TA, Saykin AJ, Furstenberg CT, et al. Neuropsychologic impact of standard-dose systemic chemotherapy in long-term survivors of breast cancer and lymphoma. *J Clin Oncol*. 2002;20(2):485–493.

17. Brezden CB, Phillips KA, Abdolell M, Bunston R, Tannock IF. Cognitive function in breast cancer patients receiving adjuvant chemotherapy. *J Clin Oncol*. 2000;18(14):2695–2701.

18. Tchen N, Juffs HG, Downie FP, et al. Cognitive function, fatigue, and menopausal symptoms in women receiving adjuvant chemotherapy for breast cancer. *J Clin Oncol*. 2003;21(22):4175–4183.

19. Mar Fan HG, Houede-Tchen N, Yi QL, et al. Fatigue, menopausal symptoms, and cognitive function in women after adjuvant chemotherapy for breast cancer: 1– and 2–year follow-up of a prospective controlled study. *J Clin Oncol*. 2005;23(31):8025–8032.

20. Wefel JS, Lenzi R, Theriault R, Buzdar AU, Cruickshank S, Meyers CA. 'Chemobrain' in breast carcinoma? A prologue. *Cancer*. 2004;101(3):466–475.

21. Wefel JS, Lenzi R, Theriault RL, Davis RN, Meyers CA. The cognitive sequelae of standard-dose adjuvant chemotherapy in women with breast carcinoma: results of a prospective, randomized, longitudinal trial. *Cancer*. 2004;100(11):2292–2299.

22. Schagen SB, Muller MJ, Booger W, et al. Late effects of adjuvant chemotherapy on cognitive function: a follow-up study in breast cancer patients. *Ann Oncol*. 2002;13:1387–1397.

23. Inagaki M, Yoshikawa E, Matsuoka Y, et al. Smaller regional volumes of brain gray and white matter demonstrated in breast cancer survivors exposed to adjuvant chemotherapy. *Cancer*. 2007;109(1):146–156.

24. Silverman DH, Dy CJ, Castellon SA, et al. Altered frontocortical, cerebellar, and basal ganglia activity in adjuvant-treated breast cancer survivors 5–10 years after chemotherapy. *Breast Cancer Res Treat*. 2007;103(3):303–311.

25. Barton D, Loprinzi C. Novel approaches to preventing chemotherapy-induced cognitive dysfunction

in breast cancer: the art of the possible. *Clin Breast Cancer*. 2002;3(3)(suppl):S121–S127.

26. Ganz PA. Cognitive dysfunction following adjuvant treatment of breast cancer: a new dose-limiting toxic effect? *J Natl Cancer Inst*. 1998;90(3):182–183.

27. Wilkes GM. Peripheral neuropathy. In: Yarbro CH, Frogge MH, Goodman M, eds. *Cancer Symptom Management*. 3rd ed. Sudbury, MA: Jones and Bartlett; 2004.

28. Ivanaj A, Pautier P, Rixe O, Duvillard P, Dubard T. Peripheral neuropathy in association with an ovarian dysgerminoma. *Gynecol Oncol*. 2003;89(1): 168–170.

29. Marrs J, Newton S. Updating your peripheral neuropathy "know how." *Clin J Oncol Nurs*. 2003;7(3):299–303.

30. Weiss RB. Miscellaneous toxicity: neurotoxicity. In: Devita VT, Hellman S, Rosenberg SA, eds. *Cancer: Principles and Practice of Oncology*. 8th ed. Philadelphia, PA: Lippincott Williams & Wilkins; 2008.

31. Almadrones L, McGuire DB, Walczak JR, Floria CM, Chunqiao T. Psychometric evaluation of two scales assessing functional status and peripheral neuropathy associated with chemotherapy for ovarian cancer: a gynecologic oncology group study. *Oncol Nurs Forum*. 2004;31(3):615–623.

32. Armstrong T, Almadrones L, Gilbert MR. Chemotherapy-induced peripheral neuropathy. *Oncol Nurs Forum*. 2005;32(2):305–311.

33. Almadrones L, Armstrong T, Gilbert M, Schwartz R. *Chemotherapy-Induced Neurotoxicity: Current Trends in Management; A Multidisciplinary Approach*. Philadelphia, PA: Phillips Group Oncology Communications; 2002.

34. Sehouli J, Stengel D, Mustea A, et al. Weekly paclitaxel and carboplatin, (PC-W) for patients with primary advanced ovarian cancer: results of a multicenter phase II study of the NOGGO. *Cancer Chemother Pharmacol*. 2008;61(2):243–250.

35. Augusto C, Pietro M, Cinzia M, et al. Peripheral neuropathy due to paclitaxel: study of the temporal relationships between the therapeutic schedule and the clinical quantitative score (QST) and comparison with neurophysiological findings. *J Neurooncol*. 2008;86(1):89–99.

36. Vasey PA. Survival and longer-term toxicity results of the SCOTROC study: docetaxel-carboplatin (DC) vs. paclitaxel-carboplatin (PC) in epithelial ovarian cancer (EOC) [abstract 804]. *Proc Am Soc Clin Oncol*. 2002;21:202a.

37. Rose PG, Smrekar M. Improvement of paclitaxel-induced neuropathy by substitution of docetaxel for paclitaxel. *Gyneocol Oncol*. 2003;91(2):423–425.

38. Berg D. *Advanced Clinical Skills and Physical Diagnosis*. 2nd ed. Malden, MA: Blackwell Science; 2004.

39. Seidel HM, Ball JW, Dains JE, Benedict GW, eds. *Mosby's Guide to Physical Examination*. 6th ed. St. Louis, MO: Mosby; 2006.

40. DeVos FY, Bos AM, Schaapveld M, et al. A randomized phase II study of paclitaxel with carboplatin +/- amifostine as first line treatment in advanced ovarian carcinoma. *Gynecol Oncol*. 2005;97(1):60–67.

41. Yalcin S, Nurlu G, Orhan B, et al. Protective effect of amifostine against cisplatin-induced motor neuropathy in rats. *Med Oncol*. 2003;20:175–180.

42. Jacobson SD, Loprinzi CL, Sloan JA, et al. Glutamine for preventing paclitaxel-associated myalgias and arthralgias: unfortunately a "no go" [abstract 1460]. *Proc Am Soc Clin Oncol*. 2002;21:366a.

43. Vahdat L, Papadopoulos K, Lange D, et al. Reduction of paclitaxel-induced peripheral neuropathy with glutamine. *Clin Cancer Res*. 2001;7:1192–1197.

44. Argyriou AA, Chroni E, Koutras A, et al. A randomized controlled trial evaluating the efficacy and safety of vitamin E supplementation for protection against cisplatin-induced peripheral neuropathy: final results. *Support Care Cancer*. 2006;14(11):1134–1140.

45. Josephs-Cowan C. Peripheral neuropathy in the ovarian cancer patient. *J Gynecol Oncol Nurs*. 2006;16(1): 6–11.

46. Armstrong DK, Bundy B, Wenzel L, et al. Intraperitoneal cisplatin and paclitaxel in ovarian cancer. *N Engl J Med*. 2006;354(1):34–43.

47. Smith EL, Whedon MB, Bookbinder M. Quality improvement of painful peripheral neuropathy. *Semin Oncol Nurs*. 2002;18(1):36–43.

48. Wamboldt C, Kapustin J. Evidence-based treatment of diabetic peripheral neuropathy. *J Nurs Pract*. 2006;2(6):370–378.

49. Stenchever MA, Droegemueller W, Herbst AL, Mishell DR Jr. *Comprehensive Gynecology*. 5th ed. Philadelphia, PA: Elsevier Science; 2006.

50. Page R. Common toxicities of chemotherapy. In: Pazdur R, Coia LR, Hoskins WJ, Wagman LD, eds. *Cancer Management: A Multidisciplinary Approach*. 9th ed. Melville, NY: PRR; 2006.

51. Bent AE, Cundiff GW, Swift SE. *Ostegard's Urogynecology and Pelvic Floor Dysfunction*. 6th ed. Philadelphia, PA: Lippincott Williams & Wilkins; 2007.

52. Itano JK, Taoka KN. *Core Curriculum for Oncology Nursing.* 4th ed. Philadelphia, PA: Elsevier Science; 2005.

53. Mutch DG, Grigsby PW, Markman M, Rubin S. Management of late effects of treatment. In: Hoskins WJ, Perez CA, Young RC, Barakat RR, eds. *Principles and Practice of Gynecologic Oncology.* 4th ed. Philadelphia, PA: Lippincott Williams & Wilkins; 2004.

54. Tateo S, Mereu L, Salamano S, et al. Ovarian cancer and venous thromboembolic risk. *Gynecol Oncol.* 2005;99(1):119–125.

55. Burke JJ, Osborne JL, Senkowski CK. Perioperative and critical care. In: Hoskins WJ, Perez CA, Young RC, Barakat RR, eds. *Principles and Practice of Gynecologic Oncology.* 4th ed. Philadelphia, PA: Lippincott Williams & Wilkins; 2004.

56. Jacobson GM, Kamath RS, Smith RS, Goodheart MJ. Thromboembolic events in patients treated with definitive chemotherapy and radiation therapy for invasive cervical cancer. *Gynecol Oncol.* 2004;96(2):470–474.

57. Wun T, Law L, Harvey D, et al. Increased incidence of symptomatic venous thrombosis in patients with cervical carcinoma treated with concurrent chemotherapy, radiation, and erythropoietin. *Cancer.* 2003;98:1514–1520.

58. Yarbro CH, Frogge MH, Goodman M. *Cancer Symptom Management.* 3rd ed. Sudbury, MA: Jones and Bartlett; 2004.

59. Busch F. *The New Nutrition: From Antioxidants to Zucchini.* New York, NY: John Wiley & Sons; 2000:105–106, 239, 283.

60. Brown, J. A clinically useful method for evaluating lymphedema. *Clin J Oncol Nurs.* 2004;8(1):35–38.

61. Armer J. Lymphedema. In: Hassey Dow K, ed. *Contemporary Issues in Breast Cancer: A Nursing Perspective.* 2nd ed. Sudbury, MA: Jones and Bartlett; 2004: 209–229.

62. Ryan M, Stainton C, Jaconelli C, Watts S, MacKenzie P, Mansberg T. The experience of lower limb lymphedema for women after treatment for gynecologic cancer. *Oncol Nurs Forum.* 2003;30(3):417–423.

63. Ryan M, Stainton MC, Slayton EK, Jaconelli C, Watts S, MacKenzie P. Aetiology and prevalence of lower limb lymphoedema following treatment for gynaecological cancer. *Aust N Z J Obstet Gynaecol.* 2003;43:148–151.

64. Radina ME, Armer JM, Culbertson SD, Dusold JM. Post-breast cancer lymphedema: understanding

women's knowledge of their condition. *Oncol Nurs Forum.* 2004;31(1):97–104.

65. McWayne J, Heiney SP. Psychologic and social sequelae of secondary lymphedema: a review. *Cancer.* 2005;104(3):457–466.

66. Brennan MF, Singer S, Maki RG, O'Sullivan B. Sarcomas of the soft tissues and bone. In: DeVita VT, Hellman S, Rosenberg SA, eds. *Cancer: Principles & Practice of Oncology.* 7th ed. Philadelphia, PA: Lippincott Williams & Wilkins; 2005:1583.

67. Aasi SZ, Leffell DJ. Cancer of the skin. In: DeVita VT, Hellman S, Rosenberg SA, eds. *Cancer: Principles & Practice of Oncology.* 7th ed. Philadelphia, PA: Lippincott Williams & Wilkins; 2005:1740.

68. Francis WP, Abghari P, Du W, Rymal C, Suna M, Kosir MA. Improving surgical outcomes: standardizing the reporting of incidence and severity of acute lymphedema after sentinel lymph node biopsy and axillary lymph node dissection. *Am J Surg.* 2006;192:636–639.

69. Abu-Rustum NR, Alektiar K, Iasonos A, et al. The incidence of symptomatic lower-extremity lymphedema following treatment of uterine corpus malignancies: a 12-year experience at Memorial Sloan-Kettering Cancer Center. *Gynecol Oncol.* 2006;103(3):714–718.

70. Petrek JA, Disa JJ. Rehabilitation after treatment for cancer of the breast. In: DeVita VT, Hellman S, Rosenberg SA, eds. *Cancer: Principles & Practice of Oncology.* 7th ed. Philadelphia, PA: Lippincott Williams & Wilkins; 2004:1483–1486.

71. Kalinowski B. Lymphedema. In: Yarbro CH, Frogge MH, Goodman M, eds. *Cancer Symptom Management.* 3rd ed. Sudbury, MA: Jones and Bartlett; 2004: 461–490.

72. Gerber LH, Vargo MM, Smith RG. Rehabilitation of the cancer patient. In: DeVita VT, Hellman S, Rosenberg SA, eds. *Cancer: Principles & Practice of Oncology.* 7th ed. Philadelphia, PA: Lippincott Williams & Wilkins; 2004.

73. Matsubara S, Sakuda H, Nakaema M, Kuniyoshi Y. Long-term results of microscopic lymphatic vessel-isolated vein anastomosis for secondary lymphedema of the lower extremities. *Surg Today.* 2006;36: 859–864.

74. Rob L, Strnad P, Robova H, et al. Study of lymphatic mapping and sentinel node identification in early stage cervical cancer. *Gynecol Oncol.* 2005;98(2): 281–288.

75. DiStefano AB, Acquaviva G, Garozzo G, et al. Lymph node mapping and sentinel node detection in patients with cervical carcinoma: a 2-year experience. *Gynecol Oncol.* 2005;99(3):671–679.

76. NIH Consensus Development Panel on Osteoporosis Prevention, Diagnosis and Therapy. Osteoporosis prevention, diagnosis, and therapy. *JAMA.* 2001;285(6):785–795.

77. Wright WL, Edwards WL, Recker RR, Ross RR. *Osteoporosis 2006: Latest in Diagnostic and Treatment Options to Improve Outcomes and Patient Adherence.* Ft. Myers, FL: Dowden Health Media; 2006:3–15.

78. Podczaski ES, Satyaswaroop PG, Mortel R. Hormonal interactions in gynecologic malignancies. In: Hoskins WJ, Perez CA, Young RC, Barakat RR, eds. *Principles and Practice of Gynecologic Oncology.* 4th ed. Philadelphia, PA: Lippincott Williams & Wilkins; 2004:213.

79. Guise TA. Bone loss and fracture risk associated with cancer therapy. *Oncologist.* 2006;11(10):1121–1131.

80. Lane NE. Epidemiology, etiology, and diagnosis of osteoporosis. *Am J Obstet Gynecol.* 2006;194(2)(suppl):S3–S11.

81. Van Poznak C. Clinical management of osteoporosis in women with a history of breast carcinoma. *Cancer.* 2005;104(3):443–456.

82. Lamb MA. Invasive cancer of the cervix. In: Moore-Higgs GJ, ed. *Women and Cancer: A Gynecologic Oncology Nursing Perspective.* 2nd ed. Sudbury, MA: Jones and Bartlett; 2000:82–112.

83. Fornier MN, Modi S, Hudis CA. (2002). Incidence of amenorrhea in breast cancer patients <40 years of age after paclitaxel-based adjuvant chemotherapy. Presented at: San Antonio Breast Cancer Symposia; 2002; San Antonio, TX.

84. Ganz PA, Greendale GA, Petersen L, Kahn B, Bower JE. Breast cancer in younger women: reproductive and late health effects of treatment. *J Clin Oncol.* 2003;21:4184–4193.

85. Ramaswamy B, Shapiro CL. Osteopenia and osteoporosis in women with breast cancer. *Semin Oncol.* 2003;30:763–775.

86. Coleman RE, Banks LM, Girgis SI, et al. on behalf of the IES Group. Skeletal effects of exemestane in the Intergroup Exemestane Study (IES). Two year bone mineral density and bone biomarker data. Presented at: 28th Annual San Antonio Breast Cancer Symposia; 2005; San Antonio, TX.

87. Coleman RE. (2006). Effect of anastrozole on bone mineral density: 5-year results from the 'Arimidex, Tamoxifen', alone or in combination (ATAC) trial. *J Clin Oncol.* 2006;24(18)(suppl), abstract 511.

88. Perez EA, Josse RG, Pritchard KI, et al. Effect of letrozole versus placebo on bone mineral density in women with primary breast cancer completing 5 or more years of adjuvant tamoxifen: a companion study to NCIC CTG MA 17. *J Clin Oncol.* 2006;24:3629–3635.

89. Gynecologic Oncology Group (www.gog.org). Information regarding protocol. http://ovarian-cancer.gog199.cancer.gov/gog215/.

90. National comprehensive cancer network. NCCN clinical practice guidelines in oncology: cancer-related fatigue. www.nccn.org. Published 2007.

91. Nail LM. Fatigue in patients with cancer. *Oncol Nurs Forum.* 2002;29(3):537–546.

92. Braun IM, Greenberg DB, Pirl WF. Evidenced-based report on the occurrence of fatigue in long-term cancer survivors. *J Natl Comp Cancer Network.* 2008;6(4):347–354.

93. Ahlberg K, Ekman T, Gaston-Johansson F, Mock V. Assessment and management of cancer-related fatigue in adults. *Lancet.* 2003;362:640–650.

94. Bower JE, Ganz PA, Desmond KA, et al. Fatigue in long-term breast carcinoma survivors. *Cancer.* 2006;106(4):751–758.

95. Holzner B, Kemmler G, Meraner V, et al. Fatigue in ovarian carcinoma patients: a neglected issue? *Cancer.* 2003;97(6):1564–1572.

96. Sura W, Murphy SO, Gonzales I. Level of fatigue in women receiving dose dense versus standard chemotherapy for breast cancer: a pilot study. *Oncol Nurs Forum.* 2006;33(5):1015–1021.

97. Porock D, Beshears B, Hinton P, Anderson C. Nutritional, functional, and emotional characteristics related to fatigue in patients during and after biochemotherapy. *Oncol Nurs Forum.* 2005;32(3):661–667.

98. Schwartz AL. *Pocket Guide to Managing Cancer Fatigue.* Sudbury, MA: Jones and Bartlett; 2004.

99. Bruner DW, Haas ML, Gosselin-Acomb TK. *Manual for Radiation Oncology Nursing Practice and Education.* 3rd ed. Pittsburgh, PA: Oncology Nursing Press; 2005.

100. Fu MR, McDaniel RW, Rhodes VA. Fatigue. In: Yarbro CH, Frogge MH, Goodman M, eds. *Cancer*

Nursing: Principles and Practice. 6th ed. Sudbury, MA: Jones and Bartlett; 2005:741–760.

101. Littlewood TJ, Bajetta E, Nortier JWR, Vercammen E, Rapoport B. Effects of epoetin alfa on hematologic parameters and quality of life in cancer patients receiving nonplatinum chemotherapy: results of a randomized, double-blind, placebo-controlled trial. *J Clin Oncol.* 2001;19(11)2865–2874.

102. Lappin TR, Maxwell AP, Johnston PG. Warning flags for erythropoiesis-stimulating agents and cancer-associated anemia. *Oncologist.* 2007;12(4):362–365.

103. Lavey RS, Liu PY, Greer BE, et al. Recombinant human erythropoietin as an adjunct to radiation therapy and cisplatin for stage IIB-IVA carcinoma of the cervix: a southwest oncology group study. *Gynecol Oncol.* 2004;95(1):145–151.

104. Lin A, Ryu J, Harvey D, Sieracki B, Scudder S, Wun T. Low-dose warfarin does not decrease the rate of thrombosis in patients with cervix and vulvo-vaginal cancer treated with chemotherapy, radiation and erythropoietin. *Gynecol Oncol.* 2006;102(1):98–102.

105. Thompson P. The relationship of fatigue and meaning in life in breast cancer survivors. *Oncol Nurs Forum.* 2007;34(3):653–660.

106. Stricker CT, Drake D, Hoyer KA, Mock V. Evidence-based practice for fatigue management in adults with cancer: exercise as an intervention. *Oncol Nurs Forum.* 2004;31(5):963–974.

107. Mock V, Olsen M. Current management of fatigue and anemia in patients with cancer. *Semin Oncol Nurs.* 2003;19(4)(suppl 2):36–41.

108. Bruera E, Driver L, Barnes EA, et al. Patient-controlled methylphenidate for the management of fatigue in patients with advanced cancer: a preliminary report. *J Clin Oncol.* 2003;21(11): 4439–4443.

109. Schwartz AL. Interferon-induces fatigue in patients with melanoma: a pilot study of exercise and methylphenidate. *Oncol Nurs Forum.* 2002;29(7)(online exclusive):E85–E90.

110. Wagner LI, Cella D. Fatigue and cancer: causes, prevalence and treatment approaches. *Br J Cancer.* 2004;91:822–828.

111. Houldin A, Curtiss C, Haylock PJ. Executive summary of the state of the science on nursing approaches to managing late and long-term sequelae of cancer and cancer treatment. *Am J Nurs.* 2006;106(3):6–11.

Resources

General Cancer Information and Support

The Chemotherapy Foundation
www.chemotherapyfoundation.org
212-213-9292

Dedicated to the control, cure, and prevention of cancer through innovative laboratory and clinical research and to the education of patients and physicians through symposia and educational literature.

Cycle of Hope
www.cycleofhope.org

Designed to help support early cancer detection, to reduce fear associated with treatment, to encourage a team approach, and to foster hope in patients and their families fighting the disease.

Gynecologic Cancer Foundation (GCF)
www.thegcf.org
800-444-4441

Ensures public awareness of gynecologic cancer prevention, early diagnosis, and proper treatment, as well as supports research and training related to gynecologic cancers.

National Cancer Institute
www.cancer.gov
800-4-CANCER

Free resources and educational materials on all cancer types.

National Coalition for Cancer Survivorship
www.canceradvocacy.org
877-NCCS-YES

Nationwide network of organizations and individuals serving all people with cancer.

National Comprehensive Cancer Network
www.nccn.com
888-909-6226

Dedicated to providing state-of-the-art care to patients, advancing research on prevention, and enhancing the effectiveness of cancer care delivery.

Building Mental Fitness

Belluck,P., As mind ages, what next? Brain calisthenics. *New York Times.* Dec. 29, 2006, 16:51:07.

Tannen, S., Mental fitness—exercises for the brain. http://www.bellydoc.com/articles/article7.htm

Ten steps to stay sharp as you age: http://www.palm-beachpost.com/health/content/shared-auto/healthnews/agng/600476.html

http://www.webmd.com/cancer/news/20070605/genius-pill-relieves-chemobrain

www.cancercare.org/pdf/fact_sheets/fs_chemobrain_cognitive.pdf

Cervical Cancer

Alliance for Cervical Cancer Prevention (ACCP)
www.alliance-cxca.org
Engender Health: 212-561-8000

Improving women's health and saving lives through cervical cancer prevention programs in developing countries.

CancerConsultants.com
www.cancerconsultants.com

Dedicated to providing comprehensive information on the prevention and treatment of cervical cancer, daily news, and clinical trials listings for cervical cancer patients and their families.

National Cervical Cancer Coalition
www.nccc-online.org
818-909-3849 or 800-685-5531

Dedicated to serving women with, or at risk for, cervical cancer and HPV disease.

National Cervical Cancer Public Education Campaign
www.cervicalcancercampaign.org
312-578-1439

In partnership with the Gynecologic Cancer Foundation (GCF), provides women and their doctors with information about what causes cervical cancer and the best ways of preventing it or detecting it.

Chemotherapy Side Effect-effect Information

CancerConsultants.com
www.cancerconsultants.com

Provides comprehensive treatment and side effect information.
www.ByMySide.com
www.ByMySide.com

An Amgen site that provides information on helping to protect against infection, treating anemia, and managing other side effects of chemotherapy. Includes tips for managing all aspects of your life as you go through the chemotherapy experience. Also includes Voices of Experience Support Network.

Lymphedema

Lymphatic Research Foundation.
www.lymphaticresearch.org
http//: www.lymphaticresearch.org/lymphedema.html

Lymphology Association of North America.
www.clt-lana.org/

National Lymphedema Network
www.lymphnet.org
800-541-3259

Works to standardize quality treatment for lymphedema patients nationwide.

Ovarian Cancer
Cancer Connection
www.ovarian-news.org
806-355-2565

The only international ovarian cancer organization that provides multiple matches for women seeking to contact other ovarian cancer fighters with similar circumstances. Publishes a free monthly newsletter that provides support, treatment information, and coping tips.

FORCE
www.facingourrisk.org
954-255-8732

A support and information site for women at risk of hereditary breast and ovarian cancer due to family history or BRCA genetic status.

National Ovarian Cancer Coalition
www.ovarian.org
888-OVARIAN

Promotes awareness and provides education and referrals for people affected by ovarian cancer.

Ovarian Cancer National Alliance
www.ovariancancer.org
202-331-1332

Promotes public policy, research, and awareness of ovarian cancer diagnosis and its treatment.

Ovarian Cancer Research Fund (OCRF)
www.ocrf.org
800-873-9569

Dedicated to finding an early diagnostic tool and a cure for ovarian cancer. Offers information and support to patients and their loved ones, and provides outreach programs to raise public awareness.

Share
www.sharecancersupport.org
866-891-2392

Providing support and a 24-hour hotline for women with breast and ovarian cancer.

Peripheral Neuropathy

Almadrones LA, Arcot R. Patient guide to peripheral neuropathy. *Oncol Nurs Forum.* 1999; nursing forum, 26:1359–1362.

This article provides nurses with practical tips for patients for use in the home and addresses safety needs. A patient education tool accompanies the article, which may be reproduced.

Donovan MA, Latov N. Explaining peripheral neuropathy. The Neuropathy Association, Inc., The Lincoln Building, 60 East 42 St., Suite 942, NY, NY, 1997. www.neuropathy.org

National Institutes of Health ClinicalTrials.gov http://clinicaltrials.gov/search/term=Peripheral+Neuropathy. http://clinicaltrials.gov/search/term=Peripheral+Neuropathy.

NCCTG: *Clinical Trial N00034.* http://ncctg.edu/n9741_index.html

Pace B. Neuropathy. (JAMA patientPatient page.) *JAMA.* 2000;284(17):2276.

This is a patient education tool that may be reproduced for noncommercial use by healthcare professionals to share with patients. It accompanies Apfel et al.'s article, "Efficacy and safety of recombinant human nerve growth factor in patients with diabetic polyneuropathy: a randomized controlled trial."

Chapter 15

The Impact of Gynecologic Cancer on the Family

Suzanne Lockwood, PhD, RN, OCN®, CHPN

The diagnosis and treatment of cancer is often a source of considerable physical and psychological stress for patients and their families. Gynecologic cancer affects the woman and her immediate and extended family, as well as her social network. Complicating the issue, besides the increasing incidence of cancer, is the fact that because of advanced and improved treatments, cancer patients are living longer. Cancer has become yet another one of the many chronic diseases that health care and society must address. Studies indicate that family and friends most often provide the physical and emotional support needed in the face of a devastating chronic illness.[1]

The event of cancer recurrence often means that individuals are faced with a disease that cannot be cured and must be endured over time. This reality requires patients and their families to undergo a change in personal perspective and often a change in the world that they live in. Living with or having a family member with cancer is a coping challenge and an emotional strain that healthcare professionals must be aware of. Although treatments have become increasingly effective for gynecologic cancers, the initial diagnosis still involves a threat of loss of life for many patients.

Even in cases where prognosis for survival is high, there may be a threat of loss to some significant aspect of physical functioning or damage to personal appearance. There is limited nursing research on the impact of the diagnosis of gynecologic cancer on women and their families, but the experience of gynecologic cancer for a patient and her family can mirror that of many other cancers.

A New Responsibility

Each family or social network is as unique as the gynecologic patient and her cancer. Reactions to the diagnosis and treatment of gynecologic cancer can have different manifestations that require different responses by the healthcare team. To further complicate the management of gynecological cancer, the needs of the family, caregivers, and patient will also change over time based on the stage of disease and family role involvement.

Families are being called upon to be strong, supportive, and flexible at a time when their loved one is battling and perhaps succumbing to probably the most feared diagnosis: cancer. The demand on families is not new, although the caregiver role has changed dramatically. Families are increasingly replacing skilled healthcare workers in the delivery of unfamiliar, complex care despite other obligations and responsibilities.[2] The length of time for family caregiving responsibilities has expanded from days and weeks to months and years as patients live longer. These new roles must be taken on in addition to their usual roles.

Family members become primary caregivers in the home, providing services that the nurse formerly provided in the hospital. Many families feel unprepared to take on this role. There is mounting evidence that changes in family roles and the burden placed on family caregivers may have negative effects on the quality of life for both the cancer patient and her caregivers, particularly during the advanced stages.[3] Family members are assuming physical caregiving responsibilities. "Standing by" and watching the patient's condition deteriorate has been reported to be the hardest task.[4] There is also mounting evidence of an increased vulnerability to symptoms of illness and the actual occurrence of illness in family members who are also caregivers to a loved one with cancer.

The burden of a cancer diagnosis and its treatment on family members has appeared in the cancer literature since the early 1980s. McCorkle and Pasacreta conducted a comprehensive review of the impact of interventions on cancer caregivers for the *Annual Review of Nursing Research*.[3] Findings indicated that family members felt inadequately prepared to provide care for their sick relatives in the home and identified a large number of informational and skill deficits. There is also evidence that cancer and its treatment have extensive psychological consequences for the entire family.[5]

The impact of gynecologic cancer on families is shaped by a number of factors, including the specific type of cancer and the implications of the diagnosis for the woman and her family, the meaning of the cancer experience to them, the social impact of physical changes, the timing of the cancer in the woman's and the family's lives, and the costs of the cancer to her family.[6] Women often play a central role in the day-to-day management of family life, the nurturing of children, and the care of extended family members; her ability to perform these roles is limited by gynecologic cancer, and thus the impact on the whole family can be overwhelming.

Caregivers

There is a difference between caring about someone (emotional) and caring for someone (the work).[7] Some individuals are able to manage and balance both aspects of caring, but others may be so devastated that they are barely able to manage one aspect. In some situations, caregivers may consciously or unconsciously decide that they can be responsible for one type of caring. The problem occurs when there is not a group or person willing to take on the other.

Families, or more generally, caregivers, are a patient's most important resource in adapting to cancer. Family is the "unit" of care; it is a "we" experience for most women. Family members provide most of the support, yet they are unprepared for the new role of caregiver and decision maker. Family as caregiver is a long-term commitment performed 24 hours per day, 7 days per week—a type of care very different than that provided by healthcare providers, and it thus imposes a different set of stressors or demands.[8] The psychosocial stressors for significant others may include emotional isolation, role reversal, and differences in communication styles between patient and family members. Caring responsibilities restrict social lives, and the sense of loneliness and isolation are recurrent themes in the literature.

Common concerns supported by empirical evidence include concerns and needs related to comfort for the patient, information about the disease and treatment, maintenance of household functioning, psychological and spiritual support, access to legal or financial advice, and availability of respite care.[7] Caregivers of family members with cancer report fatigue, poor health, and insufficient time for themselves, other family members, and friends.[9] Families can be partners in nursing efforts to meet the needs of the person with cancer; they can provide valuable unpaid informal assistance and serve as an extra set of ears and eyes.

Family, friends, and other members of a patient's social network play a significant role in how the patient adapts to cancer.[10] Social support protects people from harmful effects of stress and improves well-being and levels of adjustment. Oberst, Gass, and Ward reported that caregivers spend a majority of their time providing transportation, offering emotional support, and maintaining the household.[11] Although their research studied females with a variety of chronic diseases, breast cancer being one, Primomo, Yates, and Woods reported that the greater the woman's perception of affection and affirmation from her family and friends, the greater her self-reported quality of life, and her illness demands were lower.[12] Caregiving provides an opportunity for family members to find meaning and gain control over what is frequently seen as a very disruptive and out-of-control experience.

Identification of the patient's social network or caregivers is imperative. Steginga and Dunn reported that women's social supports were the most important factor in determining how they coped with gynecologic cancer.[13] The impact of gynecologic cancer on family and caregivers can be held in check to a certain degree, but discovering in the beginning who the patient's caregivers will be and the degree of involvement that the woman desires from each person can make all the difference. Inclusion of family or the patient's identified support system in discussions and planning must be considered. If individuals are best supported by their own social network, supporting and enhancing that network is appropriate for healthcare professionals.

Information Sharing

One of the most important concerns for family caregivers is the need for information.[14] Informational interventions are critical to helping caregivers cope with the patient's illness. Providing information about the physical aspects of the illness and treatment is expected. There is, however, a need for caregivers to be informed about what to expect from themselves and the patient regarding the emotional aspects of the illness. Identifications of who the recipient of information will be must be done early on.

Based on the literature review, information needs of family and/or caregivers can be categorized in the following way:

1. Understanding the condition
2. Improving coping skills
3. Dealing with family issues
4. Communicating effectively

5. Accessing community resources
6. Dealing with emotions
7. Long-term planning[15,16]

Addressing each category can be time consuming, but it is important that healthcare providers identify and prioritize these needs. It will be necessary to share information in small doses, and likely necessary to repeat it. The family's readiness and receptivity and the patient's current condition must also be considered; educators must evaluate their "ability to hear." Determining how each person learns can facilitate comprehension but may require a variety of teaching methodologies.

The times when information appears to be in greatest need includes the time of diagnosis, during hospitalization, at surgery, when a new treatment plan is implemented, and when recurrence occurs.[17] Focused programming and printed material addressing each of these categories and time periods in the cancer experience can be very helpful to family and caregivers.

In a comparative study of reactions to cancer, it was found that the period of greatest stress was immediately after the diagnosis had been communicated.[15] If the woman agrees, family members or other identified caregivers should be present when information is shared. Having another set of ears or eyes can be extremely helpful when the patient is trying to recall what the healthcare providers said. An additional area requiring assessment and sensitivity by the healthcare provider are the cultural or religious beliefs of the gynecologic cancer patient and her family or support system. The cultural burden of cancer in certain societies sometimes makes it impossible to inform the patient of the diagnosis and can tremendously

influence the treatment decisions that are made. Religious beliefs about the cause and purpose of illness, rationale and acceptance of medical treatments, and death must also be determined early on.

Nurses play an important role in ensuring that patients and families receive information and understand the goals, advantages, and disadvantages of treatment options and potential immediate and long-term outcomes of their choices. It is important to remember that every family member is unique and has varying informational needs. The type of information given is important. Printed materials provide the family and the patient with information that can be referred back to at a time that is convenient and when they are more ready to learn. Multimedia formats for information sharing can be useful, but it is important that the educator not assume that those being educated have access to the equipment or technology required for use.

Lalos studied endometrial and cervical cancer patients and their spouses and focused on how information about the diagnosis was shared.[18] The way of being informed provoked intense reactions for both. The aim should be to steer a course between blunt facts that might prove to be untrue and raising unrealistic hopes.[19]

Attention must be given to the needs of both the patient and her partner. Understanding details about the disease helps caregivers cope. Professionals can assume a lot about the patient's and caregivers' knowledge; it is imperative that questions be asked and that assumptions not be made. It is necessary to check and recheck the patient's and caregivers' understanding and satisfaction with the explanation that was given and realize that information needs will and do change over time, requiring repetition of information.

The Trajectory of Cancer

The diagnosis of cancer has also been described as a "roller coaster" of emotions. Oncology literature has largely addressed the needs of family caregivers as they experience a loved one's newly diagnosed cancer during two periods: treatment or at the end of life.

There is limited empirical evidence to support the magnitude of stress that cancer patients and their families experience with the initial discussions or mention of gynecologic cancer prior to surgery or a confirmed diagnosis. The initial cancer diagnosis imposes fear of the future of imminent death.[20] Other associated emotions include surprise, shock, disbelief, anger, denial, depression, and uncertainty.[9,15] Anecdotally, healthcare professionals who work in the gynecologic cancer arena are well aware of the impact that even the slightest suggestion of cancer can have on the woman and her family. Consequently, it behooves the nurse and other healthcare professionals to keep the family and patient informed about preoperative workups and radiological evidence as they communicate or demonstrate by their questions or other avenues for communication that exist within the healthcare setting.

The time of surgery has been described as a crisis situation for the entire family.[6,16] During the course of surgery, discovery that the cancer is more advanced than expected or that the intended procedures cannot be completed can be overwhelming. Many families will self-report being prepared for the worst, but when the worst becomes reality, reactions can run a wide spectrum. Surgery for advanced disease may lead to awareness in patients and families that the disease is progressing and patients are approaching the end of life.

Sources of help for women and their families who experience cancer consider the crisis over when the patients are home and beginning to resume normal activities. This reduction in the outside social network can increase the burden for the family and consequently impact the adjustment and even acceptance of the gynecologic cancer patient regarding her illness, treatment, and rehabilitation. Unlike some other chronic disease patients, women with gynecological cancer are faced with uncertainty and fear of recurrence. Recurrent disease extends the cancer experience for the patient and her family, reinforcing the insecurity about the future.[21]

Culturally, there may be factors that must be considered in relationship to adjustment to the cancer and understanding the requirements and possibilities for treatment and progression. A belief that the cancer is "punishment for a past mistake" is just one example. Others might see the cancer as a "gift," viewing the experience as a "wake-up call," an opportunity for communicating love, resolving old disagreements, and spending quality time together.

Cancer recurrence poses individual and family hardships, such as uncertainty, grief, and feelings of injustice, fear, and anger. The demand on caregivers escalates as treatment regimens progress and increase. Each new protocol provides a new set of circumstances for caregivers to adjust to. A fairly new concept to cancer nursing is rehabilitation. This is particularly important when the gynecologic cancer becomes a chronic disease. Issues new to this stage can include the importance of care continuity and home care needs. While a multidisciplinary approach should be used throughout the cancer experience, it is imperative in the rehabilitative stage.

The speed with which cancer progresses may influence a family's response to the illness, stretching their coping skills. Family exhaustion, conflict, and guilt are common when the family's and the patient's expectation of the cancer trajectory is different than what they experience. Underlying and complicating the cancer experience is a duty or commitment to care. Whether it is felt or real, it has an impact on the family and their adjustment to coping with the cancer. In the past when family members died in the healthcare facility, the home remained a separate place. With the increasing use of hospice and access to the resources for providing care at home, the place where many persons die has changed, bringing yet another set of issues.

Grbich confirmed that healthcare providers do not recognize the emotional needs of caregivers as the cancer patient approaches death, particularly when response to treatment does not occur. At the end of a cancer patient's life, it is not uncommon for caregivers to be left on their own.[9] Issues of "waiting" for the woman's death can frequently lead to feelings of guilt.

During the terminal stages, spouses are concerned about the patient's activity restrictions and have fears for the future. They worry about the patient's comfort, their emotional response to disease, the patient's death, their own physical illnesses and restrictions on their activities, as well as a feeling of helplessness. Some evidence reports concerns by family and caregivers that use of respite care

suggests that they are not "living up to their responsibility," resulting in guilt and a sense of failure.[15]

Illness and Treatment Impact

Recognition of both the physical and the nonphysical needs of the gynecologic cancer patient and her family members and caregivers is essential in promoting optimal care.

Chemotherapy and its side effects, particularly fatigue, nausea, vomiting, pain, anorexia, and low blood counts, are significant concerns for caregivers.[22] The medical team can assist the family or caregivers, in addition to the patient, by controlling treatment side effects and providing information on signs and symptoms to be monitored.

Timely administration of medications and teaching family members how to apply lotions, give injections, or change dressings makes them feel useful. In addition, caregiver training can save time for the healthcare provider. Pain management cannot be overstated for the patient's and the family's quality or life and their psychological adjustment to the cancer process.

As more women survive gynecologic cancer, they are faced with sometimes devastating chronic problems related to body image and functioning. Gynecologic cancer can have a significant impact on the social aspects of life for the woman and her family. It may alter the nature of, or isolate women from, social relationships that provide them energy, support, and encouragement; these relationships are needed more during their cancer treatment than in routine circumstances.

Issues of pain, surgical menopause, peripheral neuropathy, nausea, and alopecia can be the most devastating and sometimes most difficult for caregivers to manage. Caring for a loved one who is in pain poses many physical and psychological burdens for a family, including mood disturbance and disruption of relationships.[23] Nausea, like pain, can be managed; however, it requires adjustments. Caregivers must recognize and accept complaints of nausea and become somewhat creative in management. As a society that places extraordinary value on food and the "comfort" it can provide, it is very difficult for caregivers to accept that the woman does not want to eat or suddenly has a dislike for foods that are familiar. Because both are without obvious visible evidence, both pain and nausea can be ignored or given less attention. The medical management of both can be frustrating given the individuality of the nausea and pain symptoms. The process of identifying which combination of drugs works best for the woman without causing additional symptoms can be lengthy.

Explaining the surgical menopause associated with removal of the ovaries is a continual process.[24] Remaining sensitive to the complaints of hot flashes, dryness, and moodiness is important not only for healthcare providers but also for caregivers. The emotions associated with menopause, a condition of "old age," must be recognized and attended to. Explaining to the woman and her caregivers what might occur and giving them options for treating the symptoms will be helpful.

For the woman, the loss of hair can be one of the most devastating and emotionally charged aspects of treatment. The impact on families is just as overwhelming. The woman can easily avoid "seeing" the hair loss, particularly on her head, but for caregivers it is constant and cannot be ignored. Not reacting to seeing the bald head of the woman can be a challenge in itself. This serves as a constant reminder, even if the woman is symptom or disease free, that cancer and the chance of recurrence is now a part of their family.

Age at Diagnosis

The age of the woman when she is diagnosed with gynecologic cancer is also important. When gynecologic cancer happens in a young woman, issues for her and her family relate to starting careers, less-than-optimal finances, and caring for young children. Worries about life-threatening illness, body-changing surgery, threats to sexuality and sexual relationships, and side effects of treatment are common with gynecologic cancer patients.

Young, newly married couples who are trying to create their own families and separate from their families of origin may experience conflicts as the diagnosis pushes them back to intimacy with their parents and siblings.[6] During periods of life transitions, such as childbirth, career changes, and retirement, patients and their families may have a more intense response to the diagnosis and treatment.

Schaefer, Ladd, Lammers, and Echenberg looked specifically at the experience of living with ovarian cancer during the childbearing years.[24] Their analysis supported the struggle associated with the diagnosis and treatment for ovarian cancer, fear of recurrence, and inability to bear children. The women in their study stated that "they were different," and listening to their concerns and loss was incredibly important for their healing.[24] Of particular importance was the loss of choice related to deciding whether they wanted to have children. Offering choices to preserve this option, if possible, should be given, and couples or even single women should be referred to counseling or an infertility specialist prior to surgery. The impact on the spouse in the relationship to loss of childbearing has not been studied.

Coping

Family needs are dynamic throughout the cancer trajectory, and because the family is often the patient's resource for adapting to cancer, the coping mechanisms adopted by caregivers will affect the patient's own ability to cope.[25] The isolative and stressful nature of caregiving, increased stress, and a reported need for medication to help them cope with the burden associated with caregiving can also occur.[11] Hardwick and Lawson cite four main factors that influence the ability to cope when a family must deal with a chronic illness. They include:

1. Characteristics of the illness
2. Perceived threat to the family
3. Financial and social support
4. Previous experience with similar situations [25]

Finding meaning in the experience is important in the adjustment of the woman and her family. This may involve major shifts in how they view their family, life, values, and relationships. Understanding and coming to terms with the consequences of the cancer and finding sources of hope can also be the focus as the patient and caregivers come to terms with a life-changing diagnosis.

Issues of guilt about past events can lead to a variety of reactions. It is important to allow families the time and place to have these discussions. Try to keep the family focused on the present and what they can do to facilitate the medical plan of treatment and the significant changes that can occur. Help caregivers or family by encouraging conversation. Suppression of fears and feelings of anger are common. The healthcare provider should try to stimulate conversation, providing a safe outlet for an honest dialogue about concerns. It can be helpful to rely on common problems or issues that healthcare professionals have experienced in their practice.

Even the most cohesive families can encounter tremendous stress during the cancer event.[26] The experience can cause patients and caregivers to have different perceptions and reactions than they normally would have to varying sources of stress and physical symptoms.[27] In addition, these same reactions and concerns can contribute to family disagreements about treatment.

It is important to identify what activities are important to the family and what their priorities are.[28] Knowledge and planning to allow continued participation in these activities can assist families in adjusting to whichever stage of the disease the woman is in. Strategies used by families to cope with the stress and emotional strain of caregiving frequently include taking time for themselves, maintaining a sense of humor, and focusing on the present.[6]

Chambers, Ryan, and Connors identified ways of coping and adapting to a life-changing event such as cancer.[15] One method is to take a "time out," allowing for an opportunity to let off steam and a chance to get away from the situation. Another method is acceptance or deciding that "you just get on with it." Relaxation or "having a cup of tea" was also described as an intentional decision to think positive thoughts.

Zacharias, Gilg, and Foxall reported that the most frequently used coping strategy for spouses of gynecologic cancer patients was an attempt to escape the emotional distress by just "longing" and verbalizing a desire for the illness to go away.[5] Patients might also try to look for the positive aspects of the illness experience. Dodd, Dibble, and Thomas found that families used direct action for coping with cancer.[29] Taking a nap, orchestrating child care, seeking social support, and seeking information are some of the examples from their research. Family coping methods can also include talking and playing together, reassigning responsibilities, seeking outside help, and trying to keep a routine.[30]

Traditional Female Roles

Being a mother with a life-threatening illness adds yet another dimension to the gynecologic cancer experience. The frequently reported complaint of having no energy to do anything can have an impact on traditionally familiar roles and those that society has ascribed to women.

Fitch, Bunston, and Elliot conducted interviews with women living with cancer who had children age 18 years or younger living at home. Thirteen percent of these women had a diagnosis of gynecologic cancer, with the majority having breast cancer (46%).[30] Women in their study reported being reluctant to ask for help because it would mean failure. Many found they had to ask for help before they would receive it; others needed to be told what to do rather than just "jumping in."[30] Feeling a need to care for herself, yet knowing that she is responsible for the care of the household/family, is tremendous. Physical effects (nausea, fatigue) and hospital

visits (separation) were particularly disruptive to mothering roles.[30]

A change in appearance, even if it is only in the eye of the woman, may result in her not be willing to go out to social gatherings, to church, or to her usual activities. The family of the woman with gynecological cancer may also curtail her activities. Fatigue may limit her ability and willingness to see friends and demand the immediate attention of family time and energy, having a social impact on all of them.[6] Loss of sleep, a reduced appetite, treatment demands, time demands, and transportation issues each influence a woman's ability to maintain traditional roles. Hopelessness and uncertainty complicate the situation even further.

The role of mother is a significant caretaker role that requires balancing her own needs and those of her family. Loss of control over herself and her household has been repeatedly reported to be of particular concern for women who have not worked outside the home. Even with increased opportunities for outpatient treatment and cancer management, the woman or someone else has to organize child care. Trying to keep their children's lives normal—letting them be children but needing them to understand the situation—is essential.

Northouse has done much of the sentinel research on the impact of cancer on families. In a 1995 literature review, the impact of cancer on spouses was found to be significant for increased incidence of psychosomatic concerns, increased feelings of anxiety and depression, and high levels of distress similar to the wife diagnosed with cancer.[31] Spouses have a higher level of anxiety than most patients during initial hospitalization.[32] Husbands become more protective and seem to attempt to maintain a strong façade.[33]

Spouses rate cancer in their partners as a significant stressor and report a number of adverse effects of the disease on their marital relationship and daily functioning in the family.[34] Shifting roles can be overwhelming, not only for spouses but also for the woman with a gynecologic cancer. Anger and depression have been reported in husbands as the caregiver's role increases.[5,18]

Children and the Impact of Parental Cancer

The physical and psychological adjustment of children of cancer patients is even less well understood. Data on young adult, adolescent, and preadolescent children of cancer patients suggest that the degree of psychological distress is influenced by their age and sex and whether their mother or father is ill. While there is little empirical evidence on the effect of gynecologic cancer specifically on children, it can be inferred from other published reports that because the parent with cancer is the mother, the impact can be great.

Communication and parental coping with the disease and subsequent treatment can positively impact a child's adjustment to the gynecologic cancer diagnosis. An attempt to protect children from the knowledge and experience of cancer is impossible. Fears of worrying or frightening the children are not uncommon. However, children are often aware that something is going on, and their imagined fantasies are frequently more frightening than the reality.[21]

Younger children tend to be frightened by the parent's pain and loss of hair and weight, while adolescents want to alleviate some of these symptoms for their parent. Emotions associated with a parent having cancer range from a felt sense of helplessness to even avoiding contact and distancing because the cancer experience is so overwhelming. Anxiety and depression symptoms were higher for adolescents and young adults than for young children. The highest levels of anxiety, distress, and depression were found for adolescent girls whose mothers were sick.[34] Children of all ages may have adjustment problems, particularly when the mother is the patient; however, most of what is published is in relationship to adolescent girls.

Fitch, Bunston, and Elliot found that relationships with daughters became more distanced, with daughters frequently exhibiting anger, while relationships with sons became closer, with increased expressions of affection.[30] Older adolescent daughters are often concerned about heredity and whether or not this could happen to them.[6]

Adolescence is a time when parents and children typically have difficulty in their relationship as the adolescent attempts to separate, but cancer often requires that they become more emotionally involved. Increased demands to help around the house conflict with the adolescent's need to be more independent.[35] From doing more household chores and providing care to younger siblings to having to provide nursing care, girls take on this responsibility much more easily than boys.

Strategies for dealing with a mother's illness have been identified based on the empirical evidence that the reaction of children to a parent's diagnosis of cancer is dependent on their age. Younger children attempt to anticipate their mother's needs and want to help with chores or cooperate with other family members. Older children are more likely to express thoughts and feelings openly. Strategies used by all age groups involved avoiding the illness, maintaining normalcy, and spending more time together as a family.[16]

Economic Impacts

The necessity for most families has become that every adult must maintain employment outside the home. The need to then alter arrangements and lifestyle because of gynecologic cancer causes an immeasurable strain on financial resources. Cancer's economic impact on the family can be substantial, not only for those who are uninsured or underinsured, but even for those who have adequate insurance and experience the cost of cancer due to gaps in coverage or out-of-pocket or deductible expenses. Caring for the family member at home can have economic effects as family members deal with activities of daily living, living arrangements, and resort to functioning in what is basically a survival mode.

Family life changes result when severe disease- or treatment-related morbidity interferes with the patient's ability to function or work. Many people with cancer belong to double-income or single-parent households that are dependent on the finances and insurance by employment.[31,36] Treatments such as chemotherapy are significant expenses that are not always covered by insurance and thus can cause family stress. Quality of life costs related to reduced work effort, decreased productivity in the home, loss of promotion opportunities at work, and other factors have not been well studied but have been reported in various other venues.

Nursing Implications

In an effort to reduce or avoid crisis situations, healthcare professionals have a responsibility to assess family resources, promote self-care, and aid in gathering resources for patients and their caregivers. In addition to dealing with specific side effects, such as fatigue, low blood counts, and nausea and vomiting, families noted concurrent problems, such as work and finances, that can be intensified by a diagnosis and treatment of cancer.

In most situations, family members act as advocates for ensuring quality of care for those loved ones and can have a significant impact on treatment decisions and psychological well-being.[26] It is imperative that, early on, nurses and healthcare providers identify who the woman wants information to be shared with. Family disagreements about treatment decisions can result in a variety of problems. Integration of family in care planning can facilitate family communication and overall satisfaction and adjustment to the cancer experience.

As hospital stays shorten and the proportion of patients treated on an outpatient basis increases, nurses find themselves with less time to determine areas of concern or stress for families. Nurses need to assess a wide spectrum of potential family problems on a repeated basis. Some family problems tend to persist over a 6-month period of chemotherapy, while others are resolved more quickly.[22]

Family-based assessments are needed to determine how families adapt to the cancer and its treatment (see **Table 15-1**). Providing information or assistance that is specific to the patient's and caregivers' identified areas of need can provide the necessary assistance to everyone who is affected by the gynecological cancer diagnosis.

Table 15-1 Key starting questions.

Quick Family Assessment

1. Who does this woman consider to be her family, and are these the people most involved with her illness right now?
2. What is the most pressing/upsetting/distressing issue for the family right now? Is it the same for all immediate family members or does it differ from person to person? What are they doing right now to deal with the issue? With their distress? Are their strategies working?
3. Does this family have or know about resources it needs to deal with this issue and others? Do they know how to access the resources, and are there any barriers to doing this?

Source: Lowdermilk & Germino, 2000.

Table 15-2 Timing of information on gynecologic cancer for caregivers.

Phase of Illness	Information Needed
Diagnostic phase	• Explanation of procedures to be done, including preparation if needed • When to expect results • What emotions can be expected while awaiting diagnosis • Discuss familial risks if appropriate and available testing if recommended
Hospital phase	• Explanation of type of surgery planned • When to expect pathology report • Postoperative expectations/limitations
Treatment phase	• Explanation of type and length of treatment planned (radiation, chemotherapy) • Potential side effects and how to minimize • Effects on normal activities • Information on support groups
Adaptation phase	• Timing of follow-up tests and examinations if needed • Common concerns about follow up • Availability of support groups
Recurrent phase	• Explanation of type of treatment planned • Potential effects • Common feelings regarding recurrence • Ways to keep up hope • Support group availability • Community resources

Source: Lowdermilk & Germino, 2000.

It is important to reassess caregivers and patients at different intervals, particularly during times of transition and the beginning of new treatments, at recurrence, and when terminal care is considered (see **Table 15-2**).

Lev and McCorkle found that loss and grief could lead to positive and negative outcomes for family and caregivers.[4] It is important to provide interventions for family and/or caregivers that can positively influence their physical health as well as their recovery from the cancer experience and loss of a loved one.

Support Interventions

The sources of support available to cancer patients are many and varied, ranging from one-on-one interactions to myriad formal support groups and networks. Sources of support for family caregivers are more limited. Spouses in particular report little support from health professionals, which is often due to limited contact with physicians and nurses in hospital and outpatient settings. Increased referral of family members and caregivers to mental health professionals during the various phases of the patient's illness should be part of the plan of care.

The need to promote and maintain communication among family members is critical. Families may initially believe that they do not need any support or outside professional assistance with the care of their loved one; however, as the cancer persists, treatments change or increase, and the caregivers begin to experience a drain on physical and nonphysical resources, support may be needed. Sometimes they will deny the need or even avoid it due to issues of guilt or other feelings. The long-term nature of cancer care and the opportunity

for relationship development gives healthcare providers in this arena a unique opportunity to observe change and to develop relationships that allow for honesty and openness. It is because of this that healthcare providers must work within an interdisciplinary team. Early exposure to the team will facilitate the early access of families and caregivers to services that are available to them based on the setting, their insurance, and other community-based services.

Resources

Resources in the form of support groups, social workers, and others can be easily found within a healthcare setting. The issue for many, particularly early on, is where to go for more information that they can access as needed and sporadically or in "small doses." Books, other publications, groups, and Internet resources abound; however, guidance of patients and caregivers toward reliable resources is imperative. Access to the Internet, although it seems to be the norm, is not always available in rural areas of the country and world, nor can everyone afford it; traditional use of phones and printed material or booklets remains invaluable.

A survey was conducted with callers to Cancer Information Services (CIS) of the National Cancer Institute (NCI) to determine the usefulness and impact of the information received.[37] The survey results indicated that the CIS information exchange was beneficial to callers in a variety of ways. Nearly all respondents reported that all or most of the information they received over the telephone and through the mail was new to them. Survey results indicated that the CIS had a positive impact on callers' needs for assistance in coping with cancer, stating that the information they received made it easier to adjust to the illness, made them feel more knowledgeable about living with cancer, reassured them about the situation, and helped them find support in the community. The information gained was also disseminated to others by a substantial proportion of both patients and significant others.

As cancer patients and their families or caregivers attempt to deal with the diagnosis of cancer, a list of resources can be very helpful. The following is a list of resources that are of particular use for gynecologic cancer patients. The books cited are good general references, particularly for women. Due to the reality of publishing, the Internet sites, unlike the books, are updated frequently and provide access to information on the latest in treatments and research. The organizations, as a general rule, are excellent sources for printed materials, and many provide opportunities for individuals to ask questions and receive answers from others who are experiencing the same cancer.

Books (most available on www.amazon.com)

Anderson G. *Cancer: 50 Essential Things to Do*. Revised And Updated Edition. Plume Publishers; 1999.

Babcock E. *When Life Becomes Precious: The Essential Guide for Patients, Loved Ones, and Friends of Those Facing Serious Illnesses*. Bantam; 1997.

Baider L, Cooper CL, De-Nour AK, eds. *Cancer and the Family*. John Wiley & Sons; 2000.

Blachman L. *Another Morning: Voices of Truth and Hope from Mothers with Cancer*. Seal Press; 2006.

Brown PN. *Facing Cancer Together: How to Help Your Friend or Loved One*. Augsburg Fortress Publishers; 1999.

Gilbar O, Ben-Zur H. *Cancer and the Family Caregiver: Distress and Coping*. Charles C. Thomas Pub Ltd.; 2002.

Gould E. *Secrets of Cancer Survivors: A Book of Hope for Cancer Patients, Their Families and Friends*. ReadHowYouWant; 2008.

Harpham WS. *Diagnosis: Cancer: Your Guide to the First Months of Healthy Survivorship*. Norton, W.W. & Company, Inc.; 2003.

Harpham WS. *When a Parent Has Cancer*. HarperCollins Publishers; 2004.

Hartmann LC, Loprinzi CL, eds. *Mayo Clinic: Guide to Women's Cancers*. Kensington Publishing Corporation; 2005.

Heiney SP, Hermann JF, Bruss KV, Fincannon JL. *Cancer in the Family*. American Cancer Society; 2001.

Holland J, Lewis S. *The Human Side of Cancer: Living with Hope, Coping with Uncertainty*. Harper Paperbacks; 2001.

Hope L. *Help Me Live: 20 Things People with Cancer Want You to Know*. Celestial Arts; 2005.

Kalick R. *Cancer Etiquette: What to Say, What to Do When Someone You Know or Love Has Cancer*. Lion Books Publisher; 2005.

Kayser K. *Helping Couples Cope with Women's Cancers: An Evidence-Based Approach for Practitioners*. Springer Science & Business Media; 2008.

Levine M. *Surviving Cancer*. Broadway Publishers; 2001.

McCartney RA. *Understanding and Dealing with Cancer: A Book for Patients and Their Families*. Booklocker.com: 2001. (Limited availability)

McGinn KA, Haylock PJ. *Women's Cancers: How to Prevent Them, How to Treat Them, How to Beat Them*. Alameda, CA: Hunter House Books; 2003.

McKay J, Hirano N. *The Chemotherapy & Radiation Therapy Survival Guide*. 2nd ed. New Harbinger Publications; 1998.

Montz FJ, Bristow RE. *A Guide to Survivorship for Women with Ovarian Cancer*. Johns Hopkins University Press; 2005.

Moore K, Schmais L. *Living Well With Cancer: A Nurse Tells You Everything You Need to Know About Managing the Side Effects of Your Treatment*. New York, NY: Penguin Putnam; 2005.

Rose S, Hara R. *100 Questions & Answers About Caring for Family or Friends with Cancer*. Jones and Bartlett Publishers: 2004.

Rosenbaum E, Rosenbaum I. *Everyone's Guide to Cancer Supportive Care: A Comprehensive handbook for Patients and Their Families*. Andrews McMeel Publishing: 2005.

Russell N. *Can I Still Kiss You? Answering Your Children's Questions About Cancer*. Health Communications Incorporated; 2001.

Stern TA, Sekeres MA. *Facing Cancer: A Complete Guide for People with Cancer, Their Families, and Caregivers*. McGraw-Hill Professional; 2003.

Organizations

American Cancer Society	www.cancer.org	800-ACS-2345
CancerCare, Inc.	www.cancercare.org	800-813-HOPE
Cancer.com	www.cancer.com	888-227-5624
Centers for Disease Control and Prevention	www.cdc.gov/cancer	888-842-6355
Conversations! The International Newsletter for Those Fighting Ovarian Cancer	www.ovarian-news.org	806-355-2565
Eyes on the Prize.org	www.eyesontheprize.org	
Gilda Radner Familial Ovarian Cancer Registry	www.ovariancancer.com	800-682-7462
Gildas Club Worldwide	www.gildasclub.org	888-GILDA-4-U
National Cancer Institute Cancer Information Service	http://cis.nci.nih.gov	800-4 CANCER
National Cervical Cancer Coalition	www.nccc-online.org	800-685-5531
National Coalition for Cancer Survivorship	www.canceradvocacy.org	888-650-9127
Ovarian Cancer Canda	www.ovariancanada.org	877-413-7970
National Ovarian Cancer Coalition	www.ovarian.org	888-OVARIAN
WomensHealth.gov	www.4woman.gov	800-994-WOMAN
Ovarian Cancer National Alliance	www.ovariancancer.org	866-399-6262
Ovarian Cancer Research Fund, Inc.	www.OCRF.org	800-873-9569
Ovarian Plus International	www.Monitor.net/Ovarian	703-644-3162
Patient Advocate Foundation	www.PatientAdvocate.org	800-532-5274
SHARE: Self-help for Women with Breast or Ovarian Cancer	www.sharecancersupport.org	866-891-2392
Society of Gynecologic Oncologists	www.SGO.org	312-235-4060
The Wellness Community	www.thewellnesscommunity.org	888-793-WELL
Women's Cancer Network	www.wcn.org	312-578-1439

Conclusion

Cancer stands as a symbol of the unknown and dangerous, of chaos and anxiety, of suffering and pain, of guilt and shame. Gynecologic cancer, because of its impact on conventional roles within families, can be extraordinarily consuming. Given the advances in the diagnosis and treatment of gynecological cancer, it has also become a disease that impacts families and caregivers like any other chronic disease. Issues related to the disruption of household routines, balancing of work outside the home with care and treatment, and having to provide emotional support to the woman can be overwhelming.

The ability to adjust to gynecologic cancer is linked to the coping ability of the woman and her social network and to the support available to all. It is also linked to the situation and what else is happening within the lives of those participating. Caregivers need to be assessed for specific psychological, social, and spiritual distress. Healthcare professionals need to make a united effort to identify and implement effective interventions for supporting families and caregivers.

Assisting families and caregivers in finding the significance of the cancer in their own lives and to think about the consequences of the cancer will assist the woman, her family, and her caregivers to live with the cancer, finding sources of hope wherever possible. Nurses should ensure that caregivers are directed toward support services, such as social workers, psychologists, support groups, and bereavement counseling. Family conferences to facilitate difficult decision making or to address conflicts within families can also lend support. While not all concerns can be eliminated, support and awareness of the impact of cancer and its treatment on all persons is vital to improving the quality of life for the woman with cancer and her family.

References

1. Lammers SE, Schaefer KM, Ladd EC, Echenberg R. Caring for women living with ovarian cancer: recommendations for advanced practice nurses. *J Obstet Gynecol Neonatal Nurs.* 2000;29(6):567–574.

2. McCarron EG. Supporting the families of cancer patients. *Nursing95.* 1995;June:48–51.

3. McCorkle R, Pasacreta J. Enhancing caregiver outcomes in palliative care. *Cancer Control.* 2001;8(1):36–45.

4. Lev EL, McCorkle R. Loss, grief, and bereavement in family members of cancer patients. *Semin Oncol Nurs.* 1998;14(2):145–151.

5. Zacharias DR, Gilg CA, Foxall MJ. Quality of life and coping in patients with gynecologic cancer and their spouses. *Oncol Nurs Forum.* 1994;21(10):1699–1706.

6. Lowdermilk D, Germino B. Helping women and their families cope with the impact of gynecologic cancer. *J Obstet Gynecol Neonatal Nurs.* 2000;29(6):653–660.

7. Yates P. Family coping: issues and challenges for cancer nursing. *Cancer Nurs.* 1999;22(1):63–71.

8. Speice J, Harkness J, Laneri H, et al. Involving family members in cancer care: focus group considerations of patients and oncological providers. *Psychooncology.* 2000;9:101–112.

9. Grbich C. The emotions and coping strategies of caregivers of family members with a terminal cancer. *J Palliat Care.* 2001;17(1):30–36.

10. Flanagan J, Holmes S. Social perceptions of cancer and their impacts: implications for nursing practice arising from the literature. *J Adv Nurs.* 2000;32(3):740–749.

11. Oberst MT, Gass KA, Ward SE. Caregiving demands and appraisal of stress among family caregivers. *Cancer Nurs.* 1989;12:209–215.

12. Primomo J, Yates BC, Woods NF. Social support for women during chronic illness: the relationship among sources and types of adjustment. *Res Nurs Health.* 1990;13:153–161.

13. Steginga SK, Dunn J. Women's experiences following treatment for gynecologic cancer. *Oncol Nurs Forum.* 1997;24(8):1403–1408.

14. Nikoletti S, Kristjanson LJ, Tataryn D, McPhee I, Burt L. Information needs and coping styles of primary family caregivers of women following breast cancer surgery. *Oncol Nurs Forum.* 2003;30(6):987–996.

15. Chambers M, Ryan AA, Connors SL. Exploring the emotional support needs and coping strategies of family carers. *J Psychiat Mental Health Nurs.* 2001;8:99–106.

16. Kristjanson LJ, Ashcroft T. The family's cancer journey: a literature review. *Cancer Nurs.* 1994;17(1):1–17.

17. Northouse P, Northouse L. Communication and cancer: issues confronting patients, health professionals, and family members. *J Psychosoc Oncol.* 1987;5(3):17–46.

18. Lalos A. The impact of diagnosis on cervical and endometrial cancer patients and their spouses. *Eur J Gynaec Oncol.* 1997;18(6):513–519.

19. Rose KE. A qualitative analysis of the information needs of informal cares of terminally ill cancer patients. *J Clin Nurs.* 1999;8(1):81–88.

20. Wright, Dyck S. Expressed concerns of adult cancer patients family members. *Cancer Nurs.* 1984;7(5):371–374.

21. Burnet K, Robinson L. Psychosocial impact of recurrent cancer. *Eur J Oncol Nurs.* 2000;4(1):29–38.

22. Jansen C, Halliburton P, Dibble, Dodd M. Family problems during cancer chemotherapy. *Oncol Nurs Forum.* 1993;20(4):689–696.

23. Ferrell BR, Grant M, Chan J, Ferrell BA. The impact of cancer pain education on family caregivers of elderly patients. *Oncol Nurs Forum.* 1995;22:1211–1218.

24. Schaefer KM, Ladd EC, Lammers SE, Echenberg RJ. In your skin you are different: women living with ovarian cancer during childbearing years. *Qual Health Res.* 1999;9(2):227–242.

25. Hardwick C, Lawson N. The information and learning needs of the caregiving family of the adult patient with cancer. *Eur J Cancer Care.* 1995;4:118–121.

26. Zhang AY, Siminoff LA. The role of the family in treatment decision making by patients with cancer. *Oncol Nurs Forum.* 2003;30(6):1022–1028.

27. Lobchuk MM, Degner LF. Symptom experiences: perceptual accuracy between advanced-stage cancer patients and family caregivers in home care setting. *J Clin Oncol.* 2002;20:3495–3507.

28. Cameron J, Franche R, Cheung AM, Stewart DE. Lifestyle interference and emotional distress in family caregivers of advanced cancer patients. *Cancer.* 2002;94:521–527.

29. Dodd MJ, Dibble SL, Thomas ML. Predictors of concern and coping strategies of cancer chemotherapy outpatients. *Appl Nurs Res.* 1993;6:2–7.

30. Fitch MI, Bunston T, Elliot M. When mom's sick: changes in a mother's role and in the family after her diagnosis of cancer. *Cancer Nurs.* 1999;22(1):58–63.

31. Northouse LL. The impact of cancer in women on the family. *Cancer Pract.* 1995;3(3):134–142.

32. Oberst MT, James RH. Going home: patient and spouse adjustment following breast surgery. *Top Clin Nurs.* 1985;7:46–59.

33. Northouse LL, Peters-Golden H. Cancer and the family: strategies to assist spouses. *Semin Oncol Nurs.* 1993;9:74–82.

34. Compas BE, Worsham N, Epping-Jordan JE, et al. When mom or dad has cancer: markers of psychological distress in cancer patients, spouses, and children. *Health Psychol.* 1994;13(6):507–515.

35. Christ GH, Siegel K, Sperber D. Impact of parental terminal cancer on adolescents. *Am J Orthopsychiat.* 1994;64(4):604–613.

36. Hinds C. The needs of families who care for patients with cancer at home: are we meeting their needs? *J Adv Nurs.* 1985;10:575–581.

37. Darrow SL, Speyer J, Marcus AC, Maat JT, Krome D. Coping with cancer: the impact of the cancer information services on patients and significant others. *J Health Comm.* 1998;3(suppl):86–96.

Chapter 16

Living with Recurrent Cancer

Sheryl Redlin Frazier, RN, BSN, OCN®

Carol Larson, RN, MSN

Over the last decade, the notion of living with cancer and the role of cancer survivorship has become a reality for many. This change is the welcomed result of a technologically advancing scientific community of researchers, many of them nurses and physicians, dedicated to cancer treatment and discovery. Although cancer recurrence is devastating, in many instances, it no longer presents an immediate sentence of death. In fact, the concept of viewing cancer as a chronic disease is now a reality. However, this growing group of survivors presents complex disease and symptom management challenges. Gynecologic malignancies are no less enigmatic.

Ovarian Cancer

There is little doubt that ovarian cancer still poses the greatest concern for recurrent disease management of all the gynecologic malignancies. The 2008 American Cancer Society (ACS) statistics estimate that 21,650 women will be diagnosed with ovarian cancer, with an estimated death rate of 15,520 women.[1] Even though there has been a modest, although statistically significant, decline in the incidence—3.0%

from 2001 to 2005[2]—only approximately 75% of women survive at least 1 year after diagnosis and less than half (45%) are alive 5 years after diagnosis.[1] If ovarian cancer is diagnosed in an early stage, the survival rate is 92%; however, there has been virtually no improvement in early detection, and the majority of women are still diagnosed with advanced stage III or IV disease.[1] Unlike ovarian cancer, cervical and endometrial cancers are much more likely to be detected early and consequently have an overall survival advantage. Conversely, in the setting of recurrence, ovarian cancer survivors have a long-term survival advantage over women living with recurrent endometrial or cervical cancer.

Endometrial Cancer

As the most commonly occurring gynecologic malignancy, endometrial cancer incidence has increased significantly over the last few decades ranking, in 2008, as the fourth most common cancer in women, with an overall lifetime risk of 1 in 41.[3] The 5-year survival rate for localized disease is 95.5%; the survival rate is 67.5% and 23.6% for regional and distant spread, respectively.[4] Local recurrence is more likely to occur within the vagina at the cuff or in the vaginal wall, with an excellent chance for cure using pelvic radiotherapy, particularly in radiation-naïve patients.[5] Distant metastases or recurrence within a previously radiated field, however, pose a much more difficult problem because chemotherapy, though endometrial cancer is chemosensitive, has proven to be only marginally beneficial for long-term survival.[6,7] Chemotherapeutic benefits offer limited long-term survival, with overall response rates ranging from 21% to 36%.[7] Hormonal therapy is helpful by minimizing the impact of treatment on quality of life, but it doesn't usually confer more than a 25% response rate (ranges from 9% to 56.2%), with a short time to progression.[8] If the disease is confined to the pelvis, a pelvic exenteration may be considered. The success rates for exenterative procedures are usually around 20%.[7]

Cervical Cancer

The 5-year survival rates for cervix cancer are also dependent upon the stage of the disease at diagnosis, but nearly 30%–50% of women with advanced cancer will have persistent or recurrent disease following first-line therapy.[9] As many as 75% of recurrences happen within the first 2 years following therapy.[10] Symptoms of recurrent disease include pain, weight loss, vaginal bleeding, cachexia, and lower extremity edema (see **Table 16-1**). Recurrent cervical cancer has a very poor prognosis; it is usually insensitive to chemotherapy. Many regimens have been explored, and cisplatin was once thought to be the most effective agent, with an overall response rate of 19%. However, recent trials have shown response rates of 27% and 39% when cisplatin is used in combination with other agents, such as paclitaxel or topotecan, respectively.[11] Radiation can be successfully used in patients who have not received radiation as prior therapy and in whom the recurrent disease is confined to a well-defined area.[9] Radiation is also helpful to palliate symptoms, such as pain, or to control local problems like vaginal bleeding. Surgery in the form of pelvic exenteration is another possibility if the disease is confined to the pelvis. Few women with recurrent cervical cancer are candidates for an exenterative procedure. The

---

Table 16-1 PRESENTING SYMPTOMS OF PATIENTS WITH RECURRENT OR PERSISTENT CERVIX CANCER.

Weight loss
Leg edema
Pelvic, thigh, or buttock pain
Vaginal discharge
Progressive ureteral obstruction
Supraclavicular lymphadenopathy
Persistent cough/hemoptysis

Source: Adapted with permission from DiSaia PJ, Creasman WT. *Clinical Gynecology*. 5th ed. St Louis, MO: Mosby Year Book, Inc; 1997:86.

challenges of the exenteration are many; even of those patients who are selected and undergo the procedure, many are found to have unresectable disease and the completion procedure is modified or abandoned.[9] For those women who successfully complete the procedure, whether it is a total, anterior, or posterior exenteration, the challenges are sometimes overwhelming. Women should receive extensive counseling prior to the procedure and should be selected not only on the appropriateness of the treatment but also on the individual's psychological and social steadfastness.

Cancers of the Vulva and Vagina

Recurrent cancer of the vagina has a similar prognosis as cancer of the cervix, with the treatment options for recurrent disease much the same. Surgery for recurrent disease would involve a vaginectomy, perhaps with vaginal reconstruction. Radiation and chemotherapy are used in cases where surgical removal is not possible. Vulvar cancer recurs in approximately 30% of patients following primary therapy.[12] In a review of cases, most recurrences are local, and treatment is based upon size, location, depth of invasion, and whether there is lymph node involvement.[12] Women who are diagnosed with vaginal and vulvar cancers have issues of body image changes that can be very difficult to cope with, and nurses must be aware of this impact.[13] Because of treatment sequelae, women will have difficulty with intimacy related to surgical disfigurement, changes in anatomy that prevent normalization of prediagnosis sexual activity and intercourse, fear and anxiety related to pain that is real or anticipatory, and

for some women, resumption of sexual activity will never take place.[13] Nurses must advocate for privacy during the clinical course, be aware of sexuality and intimacy needs, and be in tune to help solve or mediate any circumstances that arise in the management of recurrent disease in these women.

Clinical Nursing Implications — Confounding Factors of Recurrent Disease

Recurrent gynecologic cancers span a spectrum of disease- and treatment-related sequelae. The problems of recurrent disease affect all aspects of the life of each woman dealing with recurrence, and the overall impact is immeasurable. Certain confounding factors that must be considered are age, ethnicity, comorbidities, nutrition, resources, and social support.

The Older Woman

The increased incidence of gynecologic cancers in the elderly woman is undisputed. Cervical cancer has a peak incidence in women under 45 years of age, but the death rate is nearly doubled in women over 65 years of age.[9] Endometrial cancer occurs most often in postmenopausal women between the ages of 55 and 64 years.[4] Cancers of the vulva and vagina are more likely to occur in women age 70 years and older.[14,15] Ovarian cancer occurs most frequently in the seventh decade, and women aged 65 years and older are twice as likely to die within 5 years of diagnosis as their younger counterparts.[2] The propensities for cancer development are due, in part, to the biology of cancer and aging.

In the recurrent disease phase, selection of treatment modalities must be modified to consider age, renal function, and functional and cognitive status, as well as nutritional and social status.[16] Treatments for recurrent disease are not contraindicated in the elderly patient; nevertheless, comorbid conditions must be considered in treatment planning.[16] In radiotherapy, impaired circulation may result in tissue hypoxia, thereby decreasing tumor sensitivity and decreasing response potential, but also increasing the risk of damage to normal tissue. Damage to normal tissue can result in fistulae formation, lymphedema, or other organ failure.[17] Chemotherapy in the elderly must be individualized, accounting for glomerular filtration rates, bone marrow reserve, gastrointestinal function, albumin and nutritional status, and functional status. Slowed absorption, metabolism, and excretion all have potentially harmful effects when combined with chemotherapy.[17] Many of the new biotherapies (targeted therapies) affect body systems and interact with medications in ways not previously encountered; therefore, a careful review of comorbidities and medications, prescribed and over the counter, must be accounted for prior to beginning treatment. The oncology nurse, as a part of the healthcare team, must assess and assert her knowledge of the patient when recurrent disease treatment of an elderly woman is being implemented.

Impact of Ethnicity

The incidence and mortality of gynecologic malignancies is higher in women with ethnic differences. In African-American women, cervical cancer has a poorer outcome, and for Asian-Pacific Islanders, endometrial cancer has a poorer outcome.[18] Whether the differences of incidence and mortality for ethnic women

when compared to white women are relative to access to quality health care, tumor biology, or other comorbid conditions is not well defined. The fact remains that these women are at a disadvantage when diagnosed and should be given careful consideration when undergoing treatment for recurrence. Historically, participation in clinical trials by nonwhite women has been poor; therefore, participation in clinical trials should be encouraged because the answers to some of the questions regarding differences in response rates, time to progression, and disease-free intervals may be answered more quickly.[19]

Nutrition and Complementary Therapies

Nutritional compromise of some sort is present in most women with disease recurrence. Good nutrition is essential to avoiding some of the morbidity of recurrent disease and treatment. Poor nutrition or habits result in poor wound healing and compromised response to treatment; poor gastrointestinal function, symptoms of constipation, diarrhea, malabsorption, nausea, and vomiting, whether caused by disease or treatment, all contribute to anorexia and weight loss. There are numerous resources to combat poor nutritional intake, and the oncology nurse must take the opportunity to educate the woman and her support system on the ways to best meet her needs.

The threat of recurrent disease and death is a strong motivator for some women to seek complementary and alternative medicine (CAM) as a source for treatment and cure. Unfortunately, replacing food intake with supplements in various forms or extreme diets, such as macrobiotics and rigorous fasting diets, are more often harmful than helpful. There is a multitude of resources, both good and bad, that outlines and defines therapies that women with recurrent disease may utilize. The *American Cancer Society's Guide to Complementary and Alternative Cancer Methods* is a valuable and comprehensive text on complementary and alternative therapies.

The Social Challenges

Women are typically the center of the family social universe, around which all the activities of the family revolve. For the woman with recurrent cancer, the challenges become more profound. Physiological changes, such as loss of femininity, sexual dysfunction, ostomies, fistulae, and odor all have devastating psychologic impact.[20] The ability to remain part of the workforce is challenged or eliminated altogether, and the loss of income and insurance has a dreadful effect on the woman, her family, and her support system. The elderly woman may have a frail or deceased caregiver and have no support to rely upon. Identifying ways to cope with recurrent disease are interventions the oncology nurse can implement. The woman and her family should be encouraged to maintain normalcy as much as possible, think positively, maintain a sense of humor, consider professional counseling with a psycho-oncologist or clergy member, and maintain a focus on the present.[21]

Cancer Symptom Management

Over the past decade, because of the movement of the bulk of care to the outpatient area, oncology nurses have had to become more astute at symptom management via telephone triage and outpatient visits. Using knowledge and communication skills, the oncology nurse is able to monitor and assess symptoms related to treatment and disease. The nurse uses this symptom information to define the frequency,

duration, and severity of the symptoms.[22] Utilization and management of this information is an art and a science that is particularly well suited for nursing. The following are the most commonly occurring symptoms and problems associated with recurrent disease, as well as suggestions for management of those problems.

The Problems of Recurrent Disease

Gynecologic malignancies present particular challenges to the cancer survivor and to healthcare providers. Effusions in the form of pleural effusions and ascites are more common to recurrent ovarian cancer and are very difficult to manage if treatment is unsuccessful. Similarly, fistulae formation, whether in a recurrent disease setting or not, is emotionally and physically devastating. The problems presented here are an overview of the most commonly encountered problems seen in gynecologic malignancies.

Pleural Effusions

Malignant pleural effusion is an abnormal accumulation of fluid in the intrapleural space that results in debilitating symptoms, including dyspnea, pleuritic chest pain, cough, and fatigue.[23] Approximately 25%–30% of women in advanced stages of ovarian cancer will develop pleural effusions as a sign of recurrent or refractory disease. On physical examination, the provider will find markedly decreased breath sounds, most frequently in the lung base.[24] In addition to physical symptoms, a chest X-ray or CT scan can confirm the diagnosis. Ideally, chemotherapy is the best means of treatment, but if this fails or if the results are not quick enough, a more invasive means of treatment will need to be employed. Treatment of pleural effusions is usually done for palliation, mean survival is 6 months, and it is important to explain to the patient that the fluid can accumulate rapidly.[23] Treatment options can include: thoracentesis, a tube placed into an intercostal space for a single episode of drainage of fluid; a catheter, which can indwell indefinitely with a one-way valve that can be drained intermittently as needed for fluid reaccumulation; or thoracostomy with chest tube insertion, introduction of a sclerosing agent, and pleurodesis.[23] Thoracentesis, without pleurodesis, is a temporary solution for removal of fluid because most malignant pleural effusions will reaccumulate; consequently, chemotherapy treatment must be started right away.[23] The thoracentesis procedure is relatively simple and can be done on an outpatient basis. A local anesthetic is injected in the costal space prior to the thoracentesis. After analgesia is achieved, a thoracentesis needle is inserted, and the cavity is drained. The needle is then withdrawn, pressure is applied, and a sterile dressing is placed. The amount of fluid evacuated will be guided by the patient's symptoms (cough and chest discomfort). It is important that the woman understands that malignant pleural effusions reaccumulate in 4 to 5 days without initiation of systemic therapy.[24] This can be very frustrating, and emotional support needs to be provided. The goal of repetitious therapeutic thoracenteses is to provide transient relief of symptoms and avoid hospitalization for patients with limited survival expectancy and poor performance status.[25] Given that the thoracentesis without chemotherapy or pleurodesis is not an effective long-term solution, the insertion of a chest tube may be utilized for better long-term management. The placement of large- and small-bore tubes can be performed at the bedside. Various drainage systems are used, but the concept of a closed, usually wet suction system connected to a collection device is the most common setup.[23] Mild to moderate chest pain can be associated with the insertion of the intercostal tube. Small-bore tubes should be considered initially for the drainage of malignant effusions because of the potential advantages, including reduced patient discomfort, ease of placement, and comparable pleurodesis success rates.[25]

The goal of pleurodesis is to obliterate the pleural space through fibrosing (scarring) of the tissues, thus preventing reaccumulation of fluid. The most common side effects of pleurodesis are pleuritic chest pain and fever. Pleurodesis is an uncomfortable procedure, and many who undergo this procedure experience anxiety.[25] Opioids, emotional support, and patient education need to be provided so that the patient can remain calm during the procedure. Agents that are used for sclerosing include bleomycin, tetracycline, doxycycline, and sterile talc. Of the many agents used for sclerosing, talc has proven to be the most effective.[25] Serious complications can arise with the use of talc, including adult respiratory distress syndrome (ARDS) or acute pneumonitis leading to acute respiratory failure.[25] Candidates for pleurodesis should be assessed carefully, and the chosen method of treatment should be individualized.

Ascites

Ascites, the accumulation of abdominal fluid, is thought to occur when tumor implants block or impede normal peritoneal lymph flow and when peritoneal surfaces, in response to the irritation of tumor, produce an increased amount of fluid.[26] The most common manifestation of ascites includes abdominal distention, loss of appetite, shortness of breath, fatigue, nausea, pain, decreased bowel motility, constipation, potential bowel obstruction, and decreased bladder capacity.[27] In the healthcare setting, it is abdominal distention that is seen as the most common and obvious manifestation of ascites. Several means of assessment can be performed, including measurement of the abdominal girth, percussion of the abdomen, detection of a fluid wave, and a review of the patient's symptoms. When percussion is performed, free fluid in the abdomen can be detected. A minimum of 500 ml of fluid must be present for the fluid to be palpated. There are two means to assess for the presence of fluid, including shifting dullness and a fluid wave.[28] To detect shifting dullness, the woman needs to recline on her back so the healthcare provider can percuss her flank area. If fluid is present, a tympanic sound will be heard over the midabdomen, and dullness will be heard in the flank area. To further confirm the diagnosis, the patient can lie on her side and the procedure can be repeated. If there is ascitic fluid present, the fluid will shift to the dependent flank. Confirmation is achieved when dullness is heard close to the umbilicus and a tympanic sound is heard in the upper flank area.[28] When diagnosing ascitic fluid by a fluid wave, the presence of two clinicians is needed. One clinician needs to place the ulnar side of her hand on the midline of the patient's abdomen and apply a firm amount of pressure. The second clinician will then place her hand along the patient's flank area. Ascitic fluid is present if a wave is felt along the palpating hand.[28] Diagnosis can also be achieved through the use of an ultrasound or CT scan, and a radiologically guided needle aspiration can provide a definitive diagnosis.[29]

The therapeutic paracentesis is widely employed for symptomatic malignant ascites.[27] This procedure is minimally invasive and can be combined with abdominal ultrasound surveillance to better localize the fluid collection.[27] Repeated paracenteses are often required because the fluid can reaccumulate rapidly, but each paracentesis places the patient at risk for injury to the intra-abdominal organs, infection, and discomfort.[30] Nutrition, pain control, and emotional support need to be addressed with women who are experiencing ascites. The healthcare provider needs to ensure that further electrolyte abnormalities, hypoalbuminemia, and hypovolemia do not occur. Ascitic fluid contains large amounts of proteins, and many women who experience this problem already suffer from malnutrition. By repeating the procedure, the patient is put at further risk for developing electrolyte imbalances, increased stress, and pain associated with the procedure.[31]

In some instances, women may request a diuretic for management, but malignant ascites respond poorly to fluid restriction, decreased salt intake, and diuretic therapy.[27] The use of diuretics places the woman at further risk for developing fluid and electrolyte derangement.

A peritoneovenous shunt (PVS) can be used for the relief of recurrent ascites. Success rates vary with shunting, depending on the nature of the ascites and the pathology of the primary tumor. It is reported that ovarian cancer patients with malignant ascites do extremely well with the use of the shunt to achieve palliation.[30] There are concerns with the use of a PVS, though, including the risk of occlusion, bleeding, infection, venous obstruction, and death, in addition to limited effectiveness.[30] Women should be carefully selected for this procedure, and it may not be appropriate for all patients.

Intraperitoneal chemotherapy and sclerosing agents have also been used to help treat malignant ascites.[29]

Emotionally, the problem of recurrent ascites, as with pleural effusions, is devastating. It is indicative of failure to respond to treatment, as well as being disfiguring, and contributes to body image depression. These women experience great frustration because of the rapid reaccumulation of ascitic fluid, and response to further treatment is often unlikely. Frustration can easily lead to depression; therefore, the nurse must listen sympathetically while providing comfort and support.

Intestinal Obstruction

In the recurrent disease setting, intraperitoneal spread of disease will lead to eventual intestinal obstruction.[32] The causes of the obstruction may range from benign postoperative adhesions to a focal malignant or benign deposit, or, as in relapse, a diffuse carcinomatosis.[33] Usually, at the time that an obstruction develops, women are functional, not in significant pain, and not suffering from major organ system failure. These women are often admitted to an inpatient hospital setting for treatment, which may include intravenous fluid and placement of a nasogastric drainage tube. For many women, obstructions will resolve with bowel rest and intravenous fluids. However, in some cases, in spite of resting the bowel, the obstruction is unrelieved. The physician will discuss options for management with the woman and her family. Women who develop an intestinal obstruction tend to have a poor prognosis and usually do not survive more than a year from the onset of the obstruction.[34] The symptoms that are almost always present are intestinal colic, continuous abdominal pain, and nausea and vomiting.[34] Current medications should be reviewed and the abdomen should be examined for distention, resonant percussion, visible peristalsis, tenderness, and bowel sounds. An abdominal X-ray is performed to determine whether the obstruction is due to fecal impaction or ileus or mechanical obstruction.[34]

When an intestinal obstruction is confirmed and appears to be related to progression of disease, many physicians consider the disease incurable and focus treatment in terms of palliative care. Dr. Rubin stated, "Put very simply, can the obstruction be relieved and how long will the patient live?"[35] The obstruction can be categorized as acute or chronic. For an acute event, surgery, such as a loop colostomy, can be performed to relieve the obstruction. A chronic obstruction, one that is not amenable to surgical intervention, is managed in a less invasive fashion. Some factors that are considered include the amount of disease present, the organs involved, previous treatment regimens, and the chances of further response. There are certain prognostic factors that must be taken into consideration, such as nutritional status, performance status, concurrent illness and comorbidities, ascites, tumor burden, age, prior radiotherapy, and the tolerability of postoperative chemotherapy, psychological health, and social support.[34] After these factors are considered, the method of treatment is determined. Surgery to relieve the obstruction is followed by the initiation of treatment. In less fortunate cases, the obstruction is evidence that disease has significantly progressed, leaving the patient with few or no options. At this time, treatment options focus on comfort and include the use of a nasogastric tube or some other gastric or duodenal decompressive intervention, antiemetics, antispasmodics, and sometimes pain medications and steroids. In the event of an obstruction that is persistent and unrelieved, the placement of a percutaneous endoscopic gastrostomy (PEG) tube can be placed for drainage of gastrointestinal contents.[36]

The problem of intestinal obstruction is both mechanical and absorptive. Women who have recurrent cancer and in whom the obstruction cannot be bypassed will have life-threatening malnutrition. Instituting total parenteral nutrition (TPN) or enteral feedings is controversial when short-term survival is predicted.[37] However, it is important not to underestimate the value of quality of life and the potential of therapeutic intervention. Many women and their support systems will inquire about the utility of supportive nutritional therapy, and the oncology nurse, in concert with the healthcare team, must be prepared to answer this question.

Lymphedma

Chronic lymphedema of the lower extremities is a frequently encountered morbidity seen in gynecologic malignancies. Lymphedema occurs when the lymphovascular system is interrupted or impaired, either by radiation, surgical interruption of the lymphovascular system, or for extrinsic reasons such as tumor compression. Lymphedema can be unilateral or bilateral. The consequence of the body's inability to maintain tissue homeostasis can lead to distortion of the size, shape, and function of the extremity(ies), as well as exerting a profound impact on quality of life.[38] The symptoms of lymphedema are swelling; sensations such as pain, fullness, heaviness, and tightness; and onset of cellulitis.[38] When women who are at risk complain of the onset of symptoms associated with lymphedema, an office visit assessment should be obtained to evaluate the lymphedema and initiate patient education.

Educating the woman about the impact of lymphedema is essential to avoiding the morbidities of the disease. Some of the interventions that have been modestly successful in managing lymphedema of the lower extremities include compression stockings, sequential compression devices, and manual lymphatic drainage.[39] It is important to note that although diuretics are often considered, they are rarely effective.[38] Protection of the involved limb(s) from harm and infection is essential. Women need to be taught careful foot and skin surveillance, cautious care of toenails and shaving, and alterations in shoes and clothing to accommodate the potential harm that can be encountered with chronic lymphedema. Finally, the emotional impact of lymphedema can be devastating. The conflict women feel between cancer survivorship and treatment sequelae is profound and should never be overlooked.[38]

Fistulas

In gynecologic cancers, fistulas are physiological phenomena that are frequently encountered. A fistula is a tract that communicates between one organ and another or an organ to the surface or to a hollow cavity. Some of the most commonly encountered are vesicovaginal (bladder to vagina), ureterovaginal (ureter to vagina), colovaginal and enterovaginal (large or small bowel to vagina), and enterocutaneous (small bowel to skin) fistulae. Some fistulas that are purposefully and surgically created are called mucous fistulas. These are created to preempt the formation of a fistulous tract that the human body would create in an effort to drain the mucous generated by the bowel to the surface. When the bowel is bypassed surgically, in some cases the surgeon will create a mucous fistula. The drainage from this type of fistula is often small and easily captured on a 2-inch gauze pad. Other fistulas are less amenable to such management.

Fistula formation is more often seen in radiated fields and most often in radiated fields that have recurrent disease or have had some sort of surgical intervention. Often there are prodromal symptoms that precede the eruption, such as pain in one particular area that is associated with fever, an above-normal white blood cell count, and malaise. Management of fistulas is often very difficult and greatly affects a woman's body image. The content of the output is body waste and is accompanied by offensive odors, skin breakdown, and large amounts of drainage.[40] The oncology nurse and wound ostomy continence nurse (WOCN) frequently team together to manage the fistula with wound care products, drainage collection systems, and odor management products. The creativity of this team should never be underestimated. In some circumstances, fistulas can be surgically managed, but when that is not possible, the oncology nurse and healthcare team must make every effort to assist the patient in the management of the problem.

Pain

For patients with cancer, pain can be the most common and distressing symptom. For all types of gynecologic cancer, the symptom of pain can exist whenever the cancer has recurred. It is an ongoing goal of the oncology nurse to manage a person's pain through regular assessment, intervention planning, and the administration of pharmacologic and nonpharmacologic treatments.[41] Although pharmacotherapy is the foundation of pain management, with the use of opioids as a mainstay, understanding the various aspects of pain and suffering are necessary in helping to relieve the pain.[41] There are multiple pain problems in people who are living with cancer that frequently go untreated.[42] Cancer pain can be caused by tumor progression, surgeries, toxicities of treatment, infection, or muscle aches when the patient has limited physical activity.[43] Quality of life is greatly impacted when people are experiencing pain. Pain can affect physical, psychological, social, and spiritual well-being.[42] Spiritual pain manifests itself as meaninglessness and worthlessness of living, emptiness, loneliness, or anxiety.[44] Many patients experience fear of the unknown and fear of death. It is important for the oncology nurse to listen empathically, provide a safe environment, and affirm the need and right to self-expression.[45]

Physical pain can be nociceptive and/or neuropathic.[46] Regardless of the etiology of pain, it is essential that nurses assess, advocate, and institute measures for alleviating and relieving pain.[47] The World Health Organization (WHO) recommends a three-step approach to pain management, which allows increases of analgesia as the pain increases.[41] Step 1 is treatment of mild pain and recommends the use of a nonopioid analgesia. Step 2 is for moderate pain and recommends the use of a weak opioid, such as codeine or oxycodone, along with a nonopioid. Step 3 is for severe pain, and the ladder recommends the use of a strong opioid, such as morphine or hydromorphone, combined with a nonopioid.[42] In all three steps, it is critical to identify the level of pain so that effective and appropriate analgesia can be prescribed.

Social pain is the pain of isolation and/or separation from society, friends, and family or pain from financial burdens. This type of pain manifests in feelings of loneliness, isolation, and rejection.[48] As with any issue, listening and providing appropriate resources can be beneficial to the woman and her family.

Lastly, spiritual pain describes the search for meaning, hope, acceptance, and dignity as disease progresses.[49] Providing spiritual support may be difficult for some nurses, and it is important to not let personal spiritual beliefs influence or bias care and support. Offering to pray with the patient or providing companionship during prayer may develop a rapport, which will build further trust in the relationship.

Pain control can be difficult to fully achieve in all circumstances, but a person has the right to relief of pain and suffering. Education regarding pain relief is critical for the oncology nurse because lack of knowledge and awareness is usually the reason for poor management of pain. Women who experience recurrence will ultimately have pain at some point in time, and it should be the primary goal of the patient's healthcare providers to make her as comfortable as possible for the duration of her disease.

Conclusion

For women who are experiencing the pain, emotional or physical, of recurrent disease, the oncology nurse must amplify advocacy and support. Giving consideration to the confounding factors of age, disease, prior therapies, site(s) and problems of recurrence, and presenting symptoms, the nurse supports and nurtures the woman through the difficult course of recurrent disease management and palliative care. The recurrent disease setting is often a long and richly lived period of time, and the art of nursing excellence is seen in the way in which nurses assist these women to live as well as possible with the problems of recurrent disease.

References

1. American Cancer Society. What are the key statistics about ovarian cancer? www.americancancersociety.org. Published 2008. Accessed June 24, 2008.
2. National Cancer Institute. (2008). Surveillance epidemiology and end results (SEER) for ovarian cancer. http://seer.cancer.gov/statfacts/html/ovary.html?statfacts_page=ovary.html&x=4&y=17. Published 2008. Accessed July 7, 2008.
3. American Cancer Society. What are the key statistics about endometrial cancer? www.americancancersociety.org. Published 2008. Accessed July 6, 2008.
4. National Cancer Institute. Surveillance epidemiology and end results (SEER) cancer stat fact sheets—cancer of the corpus and uterus, NOS. http://seer.cancer.gov/statfacts/html/corp.html. Published 2008. Accessed July 7, 2008.
5. Petignat P, Jolicoeur M, Alobaid A, et al. Salvage treatment with high-dose-rate brachytherapy for isolated vaginal endometrial cancer recurrence. *Gynecol Oncol.* 2006;101:445–449.
6. Bakkum-Gamez JN, Gonzales-Bosquet J, Laack NN, Mariani A, Dowdy SC. Current issues in the management of endometrial cancer. Mayo Clinic Proceedings. 2008;83(1):97–112.
7. Greer BE, Koh WJ, Abu-Rustum N, et al. Uterine neoplasms. NCCN practice guidelines in oncology,™ (Version 1.2008). 2008 National Comprehensive Cancer Network, Inc. http://www.nccn.org. June 6, 2008.
8. Pectasides D, Pectasides E, Economopoulos T. Systemic therapy in metastatic or recurrent endometrial cancer. *Cancer Treat Rev.* 2007;33(2):177–190.
9. Chi D, Lanciano R, Kuldelka A. Cervical cancer. In: Chi D, Lancianoa R, Kuldelka A, eds. *Cancer Management: A Multidisciplinary Approach.* Manhassett, NY: CMP; 2004:419–447.
10. Friedlander M, Grogan M. Treatment of recurrent and metastatic cervical cancer. *Oncologist.* 2002;7(4):342–347.
11. Tewari KS, Monk BJ. Gynecologic oncology group trials of chemotherapy for metastatic and recurrent cervical cancer. *Cur Oncol Rep.* 2005;7(6):419–434.

12. Fonseca-Moutinho JA. Recurrent vulvar cancer: an update on vulvovaginal disorders. *Clin Obstet Gynecol.* 2005;48(4):879–883.

13. Janda M, Obermair A, Cella D, Crandon AJ, Trimmel M. Vulvar cancer patients' quality of life: a qualitative assessment. *Int J Gynecol Cancer.* 2004;14:875–881.

14. Vapiwala N, Shinohara ET. Who gets vaginal cancer? In: *Vaginal Cancer: The Basics.* http://www.oncolink.org/types/ article.cfm?c=6&s=20&ss=798&id=9501. Published February 23, 2008. Accessed July 6, 2008.

15. Whitcomb B. Gynecologic malignancies. *Surg Clin North Am.* 2008;88(2):301–317.

16. Burdette-Radoux S, Muss H. Adjuvant chemotherapy in the elderly: whom to treat, what regimen? *Oncologist.* 2006;11(3):234–242.

17. Stone H, Coleman N, Anscher M, McBride W. Effects of radiation on normal tissue: consequences and mechanisms. *Lancet Oncol.* 2003;4(9):529–536.

18. Kost ER, Hall KL, Hines JF, et al. Asian-Pacific Islander race independently predicts poor outcome in patients with endometrial cancer. *Gynecol Oncol.* 2003;89(2):218–226.

19. Jemal A, Murray T, Samuels A, Ghafoor A, Ward E, Thun MJ. Cancer statistics, 2003. *CA Cancer J Clin.* 2003;53(1):5–26.

20. Lauver D, Connolly-Nelson K, Vang P. Stressors and coping strategies among female cancer survivors after treatment. *Cancer Nurs.* 2007;30(2):101–111.

21. Hodgkinson K, Butow P, Hunt G, Wyse R, Hobbs K, Wain G. Life after cancer: couples' and partners' psychological adjustment and supportive care needs. *Support Care Cancer.* 2007;15:405–415.

22. Rosenfeld A. *The Truth About Chronic Pain: Patients and Professionals on How to Face It, Understand It, Overcome It.* New York, NY: Basic Books; 2003.

23. Khaleeq G, Musani A. Emerging paradigms in the management of malignant pleural effusions. *Respir Med.* 2008;102:939–948.

24. Porcel J, Light R. Diagnostic approach to pleural effusion in adult. *Am Fam Physician.* 2006;April:1211.

25. Antunes G, Neville E, Duffy J, Ali N. BTS guidelines for the management of malignant pleural effusions. *Thorax.* 2003;58(Suppl II):ii29–ii38.

26. Larrison E. Palliative care in end stage ovarian cancer. *J Gynecol Oncol Nurs.* 2003;13(1):10–14.

27. Rosenberg R. Palliation of malignant ascites. *Gastroenterol Clin North Am.* 2006;35:189–199.

28. Rushing J. Assessing for ascites. *Nursing.* 2005;35(2):68.

29. Becker G. Medical and palliative management of malignant ascites. *Cancer Treat Res.* 2007;134:459–467.

30. Seike M, Maetani I, Sakai Y. Treatment of malignant ascites in patients with advanced cancer: peritoneovenous shunt versus paracentesis. *J Gastroenterol Hepatol.* 2007;22(12):2161–2166.

31. Brooks R, Herzog T. Long-term semi-permanent catheter use for palliation of malignant ascites. *Gynecol Oncol.* 2006;101:360–362.

32. Sartori E, Chiudinelli F, Pasinetti B, Zanagnolo V. Palliative care in advanced ovarian cancer patients with bowel obstruction. *Gynecol Oncol.* 2005;99:S215–S216.

33. Mangili G, Aletti G, Frigerio L, et al. Palliative care for intestinal obstruction in recurrent ovarian cancer: a multivariate analysis. *Int J Gynecol Cancer.* 2005;15:830–835.

34. Helyer L, Easson A. Surgical approaches to malignant bowel obstruction. *J Support Oncol.* 2008;6(3):105–113.

35. Rubin SC. Intestinal obstruction in advanced ovarian cancer: what does the patient want? *Gynecol Oncol.* 1999;75(3):311–312.

36. Pothuri B, Montemarano M, Gerardi M, et al. Percutaneous endoscopic gastrostomy tube placement in patients with malignant bowel obstruction due to ovarian carcinoma. *Gynecol Oncol.* 2005;96:330–334.

37. Brard L, Weitzen S, Strubel-Lagan S, et al. The effect of total parenteral nutrition on the survival of terminally ill ovarian cancer patients. *Gynecol Oncol.* 2006;103:176–180.

38. Ryan M, Stainton MC, Jaconelli C, Watts S, MacKenzie P, Mansberg T. The experience of lower limb lymphedema for women after treatment for gynecologic cancer. *Oncol Nurs Forum.* 2003;30(3):417–423.

39. American Cancer Society. *Lymphedema: Understanding and Managing Lymphedema after Cancer Treatment.* Atlanta, GA: American Cancer Society; 2006:63–101.

40. Burke C. Rectovaginal fistulas. *Clin J Oncol Nurs.* 2005;9(3):295–297.

41. Panke J. Difficulties in managing pain at the end of life. *J Hospice Palliative Nurs.* 2003;5(2):83–90.

42. Slatkin N. Cancer-related pain and its pharmacologic management in the patient with bone metastasis. *Support Oncol.* 2006;4(2)(Suppl I):15–21.

43. Wells N, Murphy B, Wujcik D, Johnson R. Pain-related distress and interference with daily life of ambulatory patients with cancer with pain. *Oncol Nurs Forum.* 2003;30(6):977–986.

44. Tamura K, Kikui K, Watanabe M. Caring for the spiritual pain of patients with advanced cancer: a phenomenological approach to the lived experience. *Palliat Support Care.* 2006;4(2):189–196.

45. Tsai J, Wu C, Chiu T. Symptom patterns of advanced cancer patients in a palliative care unit. *Palliat Med.* 2006;20:617–622.

46. Swarm R, Anghelescu DL, Benedetti C, et al. (2008). Adult cancer pain. NCCN Clinical Practice Guidelines in Oncology,™ (Version 1.2008). 2008 National Comprehensive Cancer Network, Inc. http://www.nccn.org/professionals/ physician_gls/ PDF/pain.pdf. Accessed July 6, 2008.

47. Gordon DB, Dahl JL, Miaskowski C, et al. American pain society recommendations for improving the quality of acute and cancer pain management. *Arch Intern Med.* 2005;165(14):1574–1580.

48. Eisenberger N. Identifying the neural correlates underlying social pain: implication for developmental processes. *Hum Dev.* 2006;49(5):273–293.

49. Mako C, Galek K, Poppito S. Spiritual pain among patients with advanced cancer in palliative care. *J Palliat Med.* 2006;9(5):1106–1113.

Chapter 17

Cultural Aspects in Women's Cancers

Lois Anaya
Winkelman, MS,
RN, AOCN®

Marylou S. Anton,
MSN, RN, OCN®

Introduction

As immigration into the United States and the population of ethnic Americans increases, we are finding our society more culturally diverse than ever. Identification of different ethnic groups and how cultural components influence a patient's experience in the healthcare system is only the beginning. Improvements in early detection, prevention, cancer treatment, quality of life, and survival rates in minorities can only be achieved by increasing our knowledge of cultural, social, and economic differences, as well as identifying cultural health behaviors and beliefs. To increase cultural competence, it is also necessary to examine one's own culture and the feelings/opinions one has regarding members of other cultures.[1] This knowledge can then be applied to patient care that is culturally sensitive. Healthcare providers, especially nurses, will need to include cultural components in the nursing care, education of, and support of the patient and family.

Nowhere is the challenge greater than in the field of oncology, specifically in gynecologic malignancies, where the cancers and the treatment influence physical, psychological, sexual, and spiritual aspects of the individual and the family. The nature of cancer therapies encompasses all treatment modalities— surgery, radiation, chemotherapy, and hormonal therapy—either separately or in combination. The experience of cancer and its treatment affects the patient's body image, self-image, role in the family, communication, sexuality, and spirituality. For patients of a different culture, whose concepts, definitions, and experience of these same components may be different than the healthcare provider's, the challenge is even greater.

Conceptual Framework

There are many definitions of culture. The terms culture and ethnicity are oftentimes used interchangeably. A person is born into an ethnic group and shares common cultural characteristics that include heritage, language, race, food preferences, religious faith, values, traditions, folklore, and physical appearance traits.[2] Culture describes a sense of identification with a particular ethnic group. For the purposes of this chapter, the definition of culture will refer to the many learned, shared, and transmitted values, beliefs, norms, and life ways of a particular ethnic group that guide thinking, decisions, and actions in patterned ways.[2]

Culture plays an important role in forming and influencing the human experience.[3] Culture socializes us to know what is acceptable to others. Culture is a potent force in shaping beliefs, moderating behaviors, and giving meaning to experiences.[4] Beliefs and customs influence health behaviors, which in turn affect health outcomes.[5] Patients bring cultural identity, language, and customs into the healthcare arena that influence their response to illness.[6]

Caring for an individual from a different culture requires awareness of the concepts of assimilation, acculturation, and ethnocentrism. *Assimilation* occurs when people take on the values, beliefs, and behaviors of the major culture and abandon their own traditions.[7] *Acculturation* occurs when people accept their own culture and other cultures, adapting to both.[7] The concept of *ethnocentrism* is defined as a view that a particular culture's way of doing things is the right and natural way. Ethnocentrism involves judgment against a culture different than one's own.[7]

Cultural relativity is an attempt to view or interpret the behavior of a culturally different individual within the context of those of the healthcare providers. It is an acknowledgement that behavior that is appropriate in one culture may not be acceptable in another. This does not require the nurse to accept the beliefs and values of the other culture, but the nurse must recognize that behavior is based on a different value system.[8]

Culturally competent care describes care that is provided with awareness and appreciation of cultural differences between the healthcare provider and patient. Care is individualized and respects the patient's cultural background and beliefs.[9] The development of cultural competence requires that the nurse self-evaluate his or her own cultural influences and overcome any tendencies toward ethnocentrism.[10] Competent holistic nursing results from incorporation of this awareness into the care we give patients.[11]

Literature Review

Data from National Cancer Institute (NCI) and research studies attempt to describe causation between certain ethnic groups and the higher incidence of certain cancers, based on genetic predisposition, environmental exposures, lifestyles, health beliefs, and behaviors. Higher mortality rates are associated with decreased access to care, less education about the early signs of cancers, philosophy of "fatalism," and economic reasons such as poverty, as well as barriers to care that include transportation issues, lack of medical insurance, language barriers, and use of folk medicine instead of established "Western" medical technology.

Topics of women's health include sexuality, fertility, body image, changes in body function, obstetric issues, mental health, and menopause. Issues of sexuality and fertility arise more in the gynecologic oncology literature because of the direct effect of cancer on the female reproductive system. Specific descriptions of gynecologic oncology patients and the impact of culture are also available, although due to a decreased incidence of gynecologic cancers overall, the number of available articles is limited. Minorities' underutilization of early detection and preventive measures, such as Pap tests and mammography, resulting in advanced cancer, is frequently investigated. Advanced disease at diagnosis contributes to higher mortality rates despite lower cancer incidence rates among ethnic groups.

It is difficult to generalize information because of the many subcultures within an ethnic group. For example, although African Americans make up the largest minority group in the United States, different subcultures exist depending on geographic location. Hispanics encompass Puerto Ricans, Mexicans, Cubans, and South Americans. Asians include Chinese, Japanese, Vietnamese, Thai, Filipino, and other sects within each. Native Americans have only recently been identified as a separate ethnic group with many tribes, each with different philosophies and geographic locations. Research studies also have methodology limitations, such as the inability to accurately translate questionnaire tools into another language, contributing to a lack of cross-cultural validity, reliability, and generalizability.[12]

A major effort has been made to understand how culture impacts patient/family experience in the healthcare setting. Several references have identified language barriers, lack of interpreters, lack of healthcare providers who are the same ethnic heritage as the patient, and lack of teaching tools for instruction in the patient's native language as major weaknesses in the system. This identification gave rise to the concept of transcultural nursing and the development of standards of care for ethnic patients.

Transcultural nursing is not necessarily a new concept. In 1880, Florence Nightingale saw the need for cultural care.[13] Transcultural nursing as a concept can easily be understood as a strategy of caring for people who, due to their cultural needs, require consideration of their culture, specific values, beliefs, and practices.[14] The purpose of transcultural care is to direct caregivers in understanding the values

and beliefs of a different culture and to respond to such cultural differences and similarities in a sensitive and knowing way.[14]

Discussion

Culture influences how women respond to the fact and meaning of cancer, how side effects will be understood and experienced, and how emotions will be expressed.[12]

Cultural Values and Beliefs: Areas of Influence

The following values and beliefs have different meanings for each individual culture. Nurses should assess the patient and her cultural influence for each of these concepts.

- Body image
- Meaning of death
- Drug metabolism
- Gender roles
- Social support
- Concept of dependency

- Concept of disability and impairment
- Use of traditional medicine
- Visiting patterns
- Pain response
- Communication patterns
- Dietary differences

Textbooks, nursing journals and professional organizations, and Web sites are dedicated to cultural components and cultural assessment tools for nurses. Transcultural nursing is holistic in nature, embracing a comprehensive range of cultural factors, as well as spirituality, economics, politics, and kinship in diverse contexts. Several transcultural nursing theorists exist. Leninger[14] was the first to develop a transcultural assessment tool. Leninger's "sunrise model" (2006) depicts dimensions of cultures and social structures. Six dimensions are identified in this model:

1. Cultural values, beliefs, and practices
2. Religion, philosophies, or spiritual beliefs
3. Economic factors
4. Technology views
5. Kinship and social ties
6. Political and legal factors

In 2002, Narayanasamy[15] described components of transcultural nursing in the *ACCESS* model. The *ACCESS* model includes *A*ssessment, *C*ommunication, *C*ultural negotiation and compromise, *E*stablishing respect and support, *S*ensitivity, and *S*afety.

In 2000, Andrews and Boyle[7] provided these components in their transcultural assessment tool:

- Cultural affiliation
- Cultural sanctions and restrictions
- Health-related beliefs and practices
- Socioeconomic considerations
- Organizations available to provide support
- Cultural aspects of disease incidence
- Developmental considerations

- Values orientation
- Communication
- Nutrition
- Educational background
- Religious affiliation
- Bicultural variations

Giger and Davidhizar's transcultural assessment tool[16] in 2004 identified six essential cultural phenomena that include communication, concept of space, social organization, concept of time, environmental control, and biological variation.

The goal of a cultural assessment tool is to improve the care of the ethnic patient. In addition, an assessment can provide the healthcare provider an avenue to identify his/her own cultural prejudices and deficits in cultural knowledge, and an opportunity to identify ways of incorporating cultural concepts into care delivery. Nursing care should encompass sensitivity and individual considerations of each culture and its specific values, beliefs, and practices. Any of the assessment tools mentioned would be excellent to use in the holistic care of the gynecologic oncology patient.

Incidence of Women's Cancers in the Four Major Ethnic Groups

Although there are many ethnic groups to consider, the following four major groups will be explored in more detail, as these groups are encountered more frequently: African-Americans, Asian/Pacific Islanders, Hispanics, and Native Americans/Alaska Natives.

African Americans

About 152,900 new cancer cases were expected to be diagnosed in 2007, with an estimated 62,780 cancer deaths.[17] African Americans are more likely to develop and die from cancer than any other racial or ethnic group. The death rate for cancer among African American females is about 17% higher than among white females.[18] Cancers among African Americans are more frequently diagnosed after the cancer has metastasized and spread to regional or distant sites.[17]

Breast cancer is the second most common cause of cancer death among African American women, surpassed only by lung cancer. The most common gender-related cancer among African

American women is breast cancer (27%).[17] Although breast cancer incidence is lower among African Americans (27%), mortality rates among African American women are approximately 19% higher than among white women.[18] Despite increases in the survival rate for breast cancer in recent decades for the African Americans, these women are still less likely than white women to survive 5 years after diagnosis.[17]

Factors that may explain differences in survival rates include biological and genetic differences in tumors, the presence of risk factors, barriers to healthcare access (lack of insurance), health behaviors, and later stage of disease at diagnosis. Participation in annual mammography screening and treatment of disease at its earliest stages offers the best opportunity for decreasing mortality and improving survival. Several studies have documented treatment differences between African Americans and white women.[17] In a review of past cancer treatment and survival studies by Shavers and Brown,[19] a person's race and ethnicity influenced his or her access to and use of medical services. Three studies found racial variations in the treatment of cervical cancer, resulting in survival disparities as well.[20] Similar findings in the treatment of breast cancer among African Americans and whites were cited in 12 studies reviewed by Shaver and Brown,[19] with the findings from six studies being statistically significant.[21]

Asian/Pacific Islanders

Asian American refers to persons whose familial roots originate from many countries, ethnic groups, and cultures of the Asian continent, including (but not limited to): Asian Indian, Bangladeshi, Bhutanese, Burmese, Cambodian, Chinese, Filipino, Hmong, Indonesian, Japanese, Korean, Laotian, Malayan, Mien, Nepalese, Pakistani, Sikh, Sri Lankan, Thai, and Vietnamese.[22] According to US census data, the Asian American population consists of these percentages of ethnicities: 23.8% Chinese, 20.4% Filipino, 12.3% Japanese, 11.8% Asian Indian, 11.6% Korean, and 8.9% Vietnamese.[22] Seventy percent of US Asians are immigrants who entered the United States during one of three distinct immigration waves: before 1975, between 1975 and 1979, and 1980 or later.[23] Most Asian Americans who have arrived since 1965 still live in the 10 largest metropolitan areas.

These Asian-born individuals emigrated from countries with the overall lowest breast cancer rates in the world.[24–26] Despite this fact, since 1980 cancer has been the number one killer of Asian American women.[27] They are the first American population to experience cancer as the leading cause of death.[22]

Breast cancer is the leading cancer among Chinese, Filipino, Hawaiian, Japanese, and Korean women. Among Asian American or Pacific Islander women, breast cancer incidence (78.1 per 100,000) and mortality rates (11.0 per 100,000) are lower than Caucasian and African American women.[28] Incidence and mortality rates vary from group to group. However, aggregate data may mask the fact that for particular subgroups, such as immigrants, native Hawaiians, the economically disadvantaged, and the elderly, breast cancer incidence and mortality risk may be higher. For Asian Americans who immigrated to the United States at least a decade ago, risk of breast cancer is 80% higher than that of new immigrants. For those born in the United States, the breast cancer risk is similar to that of Caucasian women.[29] Young Asian women have lower participation in breast self-examination (BSE) and Pap tests.[30] Some studies indicate that approximately 79% of Asian-born Asian American women with breast cancer have a greater proportion of tumors larger than 1 cm at diagnosis.[22,31] A major problem in Chinese women is that approximately 22% often use herbal remedies when diagnosed with breast cancer.[32]

The most commonly occurring cancer in Vietnamese females in the United States is cervical cancer.[33] Cervical cancer incidence rates are five times higher among Vietnamese American women than white women.[34] It is the number one incident cancer in Vietnamese women, whereas breast cancer is the number one incident cancer for all racial and ethnic groups.[34]

Cervical cancer is also a significant health problem in Korean American women.[23] A significant number of Korean Americans have never heard of the Pap smear test.[35] Forty-eight percent of Filipino and 41% of Korean women receive Pap smear tests within the recommended time.[36] Southeast Asian women have higher invasive cervical cancer incidence rates and lower Pap testing frequencies than most other ethnic groups in the United States.[37] According to some studies, a large number of Vietnamese women cannot correctly explain what a Pap test is used for.[19]

Hispanics

The five most frequently diagnosed cancers among Hispanic women are breast, colon and rectum, lung and bronchus, cervix uteri, and corpus uteri.[34] The five most common types of cancer deaths among Hispanic women are breast, lung and bronchus, colon and rectum, pancreas, and ovary.[34] Uninsured Hispanics are two to three times more likely to have

cancer diagnosed at a later stage, making it less treatable.[38]

Hispanic/Latina women show lower breast cancer screening rates than non-Hispanic/Latina white women and tend to seek and attain healthcare services less frequently than other ethnic groups.[39] The breast cancer incidence rate in Hispanic women is about 40% lower than that of non-Hispanic white women. This may partly result from protective reproductive patterns (lower age at first birth and larger number of children) and less hormone replacement therapy.[40] Studies consistently show that low income, low educational attainment, lack of health insurance, inability to speak English, lack of awareness of breast cancer risks and screening methods, acculturation level, and lack of physician referral play important roles in the lower rates of screening utilization by Hispanic/Latina women.[29,40] Hispanic women tend to seek and attain healthcare services less than other ethnic groups.[39–41]

Among Mexican Americans and Puerto Rican women, cervical cancer incidence is two to three times higher than in non-Hispanic white women.[41] Hispanics experienced the highest invasive cervical cancer incidence rates (16.2 per 100,000) of any group, other than Vietnamese, and twice the incidence of non-Hispanic women (7.9 per 100,000).[41,42] This risk differential has not appreciably improved over the last decades. Cervical cancer mortality is also markedly higher among Latinas.[43]

Factors related to higher mortality of cervical cancer among Latinas are most certainly due to the underutilization of Pap smear screening in this population. As an illustration, a large multiethnic Hispanic population study conducted by Ramirez et al.[43] shows significant variations in Pap smear screening across Hispanic groups in the United States (from 53% among Mexican American women age 40 years and older in Laredo, Texas to almost 80% among younger Mexican American women in San Diego, California). Comparing this study's results to the Healthy People 2010 target of 85% of all women, only Central American women in San Francisco, Mexican American women in California, and Cuban women in Miami, Florida, are approaching these goals.[43,44]

Native Americans/Alaskan Natives

Native Americans/Alaskan Natives consist of over 560 federally recognized tribes and over 100 state-recognized tribes, of which each has its own unique culture. There is great diversity within American Indian and Alaska Native political, social, cultural, and spiritual communities. Likewise, American Indians and Alaska Natives continue to be among the poorest populations in the United States.[45–47] Because cancer is primarily a disease that affects older people, the younger median age of the Native American population partially explains why cancer appears to be less common among selected Native communities. There are 217 native languages spoken today, and most, if not all, indigenous languages do not include a word for "cancer."[48]

The types of cancer experienced within Native communities vary significantly by geographic region with some unusual patterns (e.g., colon and lung cancer among Alaska Natives; lung, cervical, breast, and prostate cancer among Northern Plains tribes; stomach and gallbladder cancer among Southwestern tribes).[49–51] Cervical cancer occurs primarily among older Native American women.[31]

Wilson et al.'s study on the quality of breast cancer care for women living in New Mexico found significant disparities in time to first cancer-directed surgery for Native American women for every interval examined, compared to non-Hispanic white women. Controlling for age, stage, grade, and census-tract poverty level, Native American women were four times more likely to receive their first cancer-directed surgery more than 6 months (186 days) after diagnosis.[52]

Meaning of Cancer/Illness

Each culture has its own definition of health and illness. The diagnosis of cancer instills fear of pain and death in all people. A gynecologic malignancy compounds that fear with shame and embarrassment. Because of language barriers and lack of educational resources and availability to healthcare services, many cultural groups maintain beliefs about cancer that are not grounded in scientific fact. Religious beliefs and myths that involve the supernatural influence how patients will react to the diagnosis and treatment of their cancer.

As culture shapes the explanation and meaning one has for a disease, it also determines how one believes that disease is to be treated and cared for psychosocially. Kleinman[53] observed that while healthcare providers typically focused on the disease itself, the patient, family, and folk practitioners addressed the disease as an experience in its social and spiritual context. Patients therefore seek healing and holistic care in addition to cure. They seek personally and socially meaningful explanations of disease.

Rituals for healing the spirit or the proposed cause of the illness are common in certain cultures. Patients may try these first before seeking medical attention or may combine them with standard treatment. Most cultures trust their own recommended "folk" remedies or herbal therapies. Consequently, it is important that healthcare providers know what patients may be subscribing to. Healthcare providers should support the patient's beliefs, even if they do not agree or understand, as long as there is no harm to the patient. Attempts to increase knowledge of these herbal remedies or rituals, and even including the "healer" in the treatment plan, would be helpful to gaining patient trust.[12]

Questions that the nurse should ask the patient include:

- What does a cancer diagnosis mean to you?
- What do you think caused this cancer?
- What do you fear about cancer and the treatment?
- How do you think cancer spreads?
- Do you think cancer is a punishment or curse?
- Are you taking any special herbs, medicines, or foods for your cancer?
- Is there a special healer who can be involved in your care?

Assessing what the patient believes will help guide the goals of patient education and help dispel myths. Nurses who are interested in decreasing the burden of cancer must know the threat posed by cancer and its meaning to the patient. Nurses are in a primary position to initiate this process.

Health Beliefs and Practices—Ethnicity and Cancer

The ethnicity of each individual group plays a large role in how cultures respond to a cancer diagnosis, providing a guideline for practice. There can be subgroups within the four major ethic groups, dependent on the geographic location of the subgroup along with their cultural beliefs and practices.[2]

African Americans

African Americans have a tendency to categorize events as either desirable or undesirable. Illness is categorized as undesirable, along with bad luck, unemployment, and poverty. There is a strong relationship between faith and healing. To some, cancer is believed to be an unnatural illness caused by sinful behavior or is supernatural and untreatable by Western medicine. Illness may be perceived as a result of discord and conflict in one or more aspects of a person's life. This discord or conflict usually falls into the areas of divine punishment, impaired social relationships, and environmental hazards. Some may present with somatic, psychological, and spiritual complaints because they cannot distinguish between physical and mental illness and spiritual problems. God sends blessings and is the only one who can heal the sick. Some African Americans respond to pain stoically because they may view pain as God's will.

African Americans are more fatalistic about cancer, tending to be less knowledgeable about cancer than whites.[2] They are less likely to see a doctor when they have signs or symptoms and are less aware of the benefits of preventive medicine and screenings for specific cancers. Because of this, many tend to be diagnosed with cancer at a later stage and therefore have a poorer prognosis, leading to higher mortality rates.

Many African Americans prefer to remain ignorant of their cancer diagnosis and are less likely to consent to chemotherapy, surgery, or radiation therapy because they are less optimistic about chances for survival. Research done on patient utilization of early detection practices among African Americans found that 64% believed cancer to be a death sentence, and 65% believed that the treatment was worse than the disease.[54] Eighty percent believed that cancer spread by surgery, and 20% indicated they would rather not know that they had cancer. For many of these reasons, nurses may find patients to be unwilling, uncooperative, or noncompliant in their care and treatment.[55]

African American attitudes about the United States healthcare system may be explained partially by history. After slavery, African Americans often received poor health care and inferior treatment in hospitals and clinics that served to enforce their negative view of Western medicine. Because of the history of past medical and research atrocities committed against African Americans, healthcare providers are still often viewed with suspicion and mistrust. Poor and less educated African Americans who receive care in public clinics and hospitals feel particularly vulnerable to medical misconduct and experimentation. They may voice complaints about feeling disrespected or "talked down to" by healthcare providers of different ethnicities.[56] African Americans may choose not to seek care if they perceive that their values will not be respected. To help these patients and families, the nurse may need to convey an added measure of caring and understanding.

Asian/Pacific Islanders

The group known as Asian/Pacific Islanders (API) is the fastest growing ethnic minority in the United States. The group is composed of people from 28 Asian countries and 25 Pacific Island cultures. This is a very culturally diverse group because there are many subgroups, with additional variations. Many APIs have good incomes, but approximately one out of eight live in poverty. Many APIs have college degrees or postgraduate educations, with contrasting significant numbers who are functionally illiterate.[57]

Many APIs practice traditional health beliefs and practices that are carried out to varying degrees within each subgroup. Because of the influence of the Chinese culture, there are similarities among groups. A shared commonality among all subgroups is the most common belief that health is a state of harmony in body, mind, and spirit with nature and the universe.[58] Hawaiians, although not of Chinese decent, have the same belief that harmony with nature is an important health belief.

In Chinese, Japanese, and Korean culture, there must be a balance between the yin and the yang. In these life forces, yin (cold) is characterized as female, dark, negative energy, and yang (hot) is male, light, positive energy. The APIs also believe that there must be a balance between hot and cold to have good health. Illness, therefore, is a result of an imbalance between the two forces of hot and cold. The treatment aim is to reestablish a balance between the two forces. For example, cancer is a yin or cold illness and is treated with foods, herbs, and healing ceremonies that possess hot qualities. The cultures from the Philippines, India, and Southeast Asia also have similar beliefs that there must be a hot and cold balance for health.

The belief that suffering is part of life is widespread among APIs and may be the reason why there is postponement in seeking medical treatment. For the Filipino culture, the fatalistic belief of *bahala na,* or "it is in God's hands," leads them to view pain and illness as a punishment. In the Japanese culture, *shoganai*, meaning misfortune, is viewed as "it can't be helped" and also reflects a fatalistic approach to illness. Chinese Americans also believe that they lack control over nature.[59]

The fear exhibited by many APIs over venipunctures is related to the belief that blood is a life force that cannot be replaced, or if taken it can disrupt the balance in the body and cause weakness or even death. Many reluctantly receive blood transfusions because of a belief that the donor's spirit will enter their body through the transfusion. For the Chinese and Vietnamese, the removal of organs or body parts is a very difficult decision because they believe that the human body must be intact at the time of death to avoid potential consequences in the afterlife. Vietnamese believe that surgery is a last resort and associate it with death, therefore avoiding it whenever possible. Surgery is viewed as a releasing of the body's spirits through the incision, causing an imbalance.[60]

Hispanics

Hispanics are identified by their culture values and language, not by geography. "Hispanic" is a term that has been used by the US government to classify people who have ties to Spain in their heritage. "Latino" is a term to describe all Latin Americans and those immigrants from Spanish-speaking countries where the integration of Spanish and African people occurred. It is usually an individual preference to be called Hispanic or Latino. Some people have strong preferences, while others do not. "Chicano" is also a term used when discussing Hispanics, and it refers to all Americans of Mexican descent.[2]

For Hispanics, health is believed to be the result of good luck or a reward from God for good behavior. Religion has a very strong influence on Hispanic beliefs in health and illness. Terminal illnesses are a result of some indiscretion against God. There is a fatalistic view that a person is at the mercy of the environment and has little control over what happens. Because Hispanics believe they are not personally responsible for present or future successes or failures in regard to their health, personal efforts toward improving health or preventing disease are limited. Traditionally, neither prevention nor health promotion are valued.[61]

The Hispanic culture has several categories of disease. The Chinese concept of yin and yang is similar to the hot and cold imbalance held by Hispanics. To ensure good health, Hispanics believe that an individual must ingest both hot and cold foods. Changes in the balance of hot and cold can be caused by internal factors, such as change in body temperature, and external factors, like the foods eaten. For example, a stomach ulcer is a hot illness caused by eating too much hot food. It is believed that excesses of heat developing from within the body and extended outward cause cancer.[2]

Hispanics have a strong belief that cancer is God's will, and they believe that it goes against principle to treat cancer aggressively. Family members, especially the elderly, are often not informed that they have cancer. It is believed that it can be deadly if told and would elicit great fear. Cancer is viewed as contagious and hard to prevent because many things cause it. Many Hispanics believe chemotherapy does not work, that radiation causes cancer, and that cancer remains in the body even after surgery. Some even believe the side effects of some treatments will be passed on to family members. This is seen often in radiation therapy where the family members believe they can/will become radioactive.[62]

The belief that there is no need to see a doctor unless a person is very ill is very common amongst Hispanics. Hospitals are a place where people go to die. Medical attention is not sought unless there are symptoms that develop and the family cannot care for an individual. Many Hispanics believe they should only receive health care that they can afford; therefore, if they cannot pay, they may not seek medical care.

Hispanics believe that they are at the mercy of their environment and have little control over what happens to them. People of Hispanic origin often think that they should not ask questions of those caring for them because they have a great fear of authority. The health-care team members, especially the doctor, are viewed as the authority, and Hispanics believe that compliance and subservience are required to prevent angering them. Doctors, who have more education than they do, should be treated respectfully.[2] Maintaining a good relationship with their doctors is important. Because Hispanics believe that physical touch promotes healing, if the provider of care does not touch them during a visit, they have derived no benefits from the visit.[61]

Native Americans/Alaskan Natives

Native Americans include natives of the continental United States, Aleuts, and Alaskan Eskimos. This very large group consists of many tribes and over 400 federally recognized nations, each of which has its own traditions and cultural heritage. There are approximately 2.1 million descendants of native North American residents that make up the smallest of the defined US minority groups. There are 33 states with Indian reservations. The largest Native American tribes are Navajo, Cherokee, Sioux, Chippewa, and Choctaw, with the largest groups living in Oklahoma, Arizona, California, New Mexico, and Alabama.[63]

For the Native American, religion is something that surrounds an individual at all times and has a profound influence on the entire being.[64] Wellness is harmony in body, mind, and spirit, as well as resilience, the ability to survive under exceedingly difficult circumstances. It is the patient's response or attitude toward circumstances that creates harmony.[2]

Native Americans believe that humans have an intimate relationship with nature and the earth is felt to be a living being with a will and desire to be well. The earth, like humans, has periods of wellness and illness. Native Americans are also expected to treat both the physical body and the earth with respect. If someone causes harm to the earth, he or she consequently causes harm to himself or herself. Humans should respect their bodies and nature by seeking and participating in proper treatment.[2]

Witchcraft and evil or negative energies are believed to be the cause of illness. It can be premeditated, so Native Americans feel they must be careful how they think or talk because bad thoughts can cause illness. The cause of disease, injury, damage to property, or continued misfortune is felt to be traceable to breaking a taboo or contacting a ghost or witch. Consequently, the treatment for illness must be focused on external factors in addition to the illness or injury itself. Supernatural powers or forces are believed to be the cause of illness or disease. Treatment must focus on the origin of the bodily aliment.[2] Sickness is viewed as a discord with the laws of nature and is most often caused by sorcery or witchcraft, taboo violation, disease or object intrusion, spirit intrusion, being possessed by spirits, or loss of soul.[2] Attributing illness to viruses, malfunctioning of a body part, or poor nutritional intake is not acceptable to a Native American.

Many Native Americans use traditional medicine and Western medicine, often simultaneously. One doctor helps the individual to heal by restoring harmony, while the other treats the physical disease. To treat the mind and spirit of a person, the healer must understand the reason why the disease occurred and help resolve the conflict that is occurring in the mind, body, and spirit. In most cases, the two systems of care are complimentary and should be supported.[65]

Preventive measures are practiced in an effort to ward off the effects of witchcraft, to reestablish harmony, and/or to prevent evil spirit possession. Sometimes a medicine person will instruct the Native American to wear a garment (buckskin) or a headpiece (talisman) that has preventive or curative powers. The nurse must be careful not to remove any items without permission because the patient may believe that if it is removed, there could be serious consequences.[65]

Surgery can be a problem for some Native American tribes because they are not receptive to invasive bodily procedures. The patient may be reluctant to have the recommended procedure. Having family members or relatives donate blood is also difficult because many feel that if the recipient dies, the donor will also die. Native Americans should always be asked if they want a body part back after surgery because some tribes believe the body must be intact for burial and that body parts can be used as a conduit for spirits to enter the body and cause harm.[65] Native Americans are not always comfortable with Western healthcare providers because of a history of inconsistent care and disrespectful

treatment. Long waits in a clinic, being separated from family, unfamiliar routines of hospital care, and the often demanding and demeaning attitudes of nurses and physicians cause many Native Americans to either respond with silence or leave, never to return again.[58] When treatment is sought, medication is generally expected. If none is given, the Native American will be disappointed because their expectations were not met.[65] To work successfully with the Native American patient, helpful interventions should include: conveying acceptance without judgment of physical appearance, beliefs, or practices; recognition of unique cultural beliefs and behaviors; and making staff and services available when the need arises rather than by scheduling an appointment. Native Americans will become discouraged and not use the health system if an unwillingness to accept traditional healing beliefs and practices are perceived.

Incorporating Cultural Components with Gynecologic Oncology Issues

Because of the nature of female reproductive cancers and treatments, several delicate issues arise when caring for the gynecologic oncology patient. These issues are even more sensitive when caring for a patient of a different cultural heritage. The impact of cancer and its treatments—surgery, radiation, chemotherapy, and hormonal treatments on sexuality, fertility, self-image, role changes, meaning of illness, experience of side effects, communication styles, barriers to care, and spirituality issues regarding death and grieving rituals—will be different for each culture. Gynecologic oncology nurses need to identify how each ethnic group responds and reacts to each of these issues and incorporate the concepts of transcultural nursing into their care, education, and support of the patient and her family.

Barriers to Care

Ethnic minorities continue to have increased cancer mortality rates when compared to white Americans. Despite medical advances, several socioeconomic factors are identified as major causes for this disparity.[66] Inadequate education, unemployment, and underemployment play a key role in perpetuating the "legacy of poverty" and an inability to obtain health insurance. Living conditions of the poor are usually overcrowded, substandard housing arrangements with possible exposure to noxious agents and physical stresses, which also impact their access to care. The stress of trying to survive daily challenges and threats to self and family makes health promotion and maintenance a low priority for most ethnically diverse women.[67]

Decreased access to medical care by ethnic minorities has also been attributed to decreased availability of resources in their communities, inability to afford health care, transportation and child care issues, and lack of time or ability to lose time from work. Fear of death, the medical community, and being mistreated add to this dilemma. Despite public education efforts, the underutilization of early detection and cancer screening, such as the Pap smear and mammogram, by ethnic minorities reveals a weakness in the system and contributes to increased numbers of patients who present with advanced disease, resulting in higher death rates. The inability of the medical community to "cure" patients may, in turn, perpetuate the

attitude of "fatalism" among certain cultures, whose philosophy is that this is their fate or "God's will." As in the case of treating gynecologic malignancies, a patient may require continuous treatments, such as chemotherapy or radiation. These barriers to care compound difficulties with complying with therapy.

A nursing assessment should include questions regarding the patient's social situation, economic factors, and family or community support systems that the patient may have available to them. Assisting patients with referrals to social services, government programs, and community resources will lessen the burdens of the patient.

Body Image/Self-Concept

Culture's definition of femininity and beauty is based on certain physical attributes. In gynecologic malignancies, the treatments of surgery, radiation, chemotherapy, and even hormonal therapies cause changes in the physical appearance of the patient. Surgical scars, radiation therapy tattoos, weight loss or gain, and hair loss all affect a patient's body image. A patient may no longer feel attractive. Members of her culture or of the opposite sex may even exacerbate these feelings by treating her differently now that she has cancer.

Changes in energy levels, pain, and neurological toxicities can affect a patient's ability to perform usual roles, impacting her self-concept. If she is unable to function in her usual capacity, she may feel diminished as a woman and mother. It is important to note if and how family members support her.

Issues to consider include:

- What role do women have in her culture?
- How does the culture define femininity?

- How does an illness such as cancer affect that role?
- How does the patient feel about her ability to perform her usual roles?
- What physical symptoms interfere with her ability to perform her usual duties?
- What physical changes from the cancer and the treatment have occurred?
- What support does the patient have available to her?

Recognizing the cultural implications of the physical and emotional changes the patient may be experiencing while providing emotional support are important nursing interventions, particularly in the gynecologic oncology setting.

Sexuality/Fertility

Each culture assigns varying levels of importance to sexuality and fertility. Because of the involvement of the female reproductive system with gynecologic cancers, sexuality and fertility are of major concern for the patient, her family, and her healthcare team. In cancer therapy, where saving lives is the primary goal, healthcare providers may view these issues as secondary priorities.

The gynecologic exam alone brings up issues of who is considered to be acceptable to examine a female patient, who should be present for the exam, and how communication should occur during the exam.[2] Some cultures require same-sex healthcare providers to perform the pelvic exam; others may require that a same-sex family member be present. Concerns related to modesty, shame, and embarrassment for having her "private" area exposed is a major source of discomfort to the patient.

If surgery is required, as with most gynecologic cancers, the removal of the reproductive organs and how it affects sexual identity and function of the patient will have a different meaning for each culture. Even if surgery is not required, as in the case of treatment with radiation or chemotherapy, loss of fertility is still an issue for a woman of childbearing age. If a culture's definition of a woman includes her ability to reproduce, loss of fertility may affect her meaning for living and status in her community. Even for a woman who is not of childbearing age, her sexual identity as a woman may be shaken. Changes in feelings of sexual identity and sexual attractiveness will affect how she relates to others.

Cancer and its treatment can also influence the patient's desire for and enjoyment of sexual activity. Surgery can cause pain, possible shortening of the vagina, and removal of the cervix. During radiation therapy, toxicities to the genital area, such as vaginal dryness, vaginal discharge, bleeding, and insertion of radiation implants, can all influence the sexual desire and function of most women. Side effects of chemotherapy or hormonal therapies, such as weight loss or gain, hair loss, fatigue, nausea, and vomiting can also influence a woman's sexuality. Stress of the cancer diagnosis and treatments can result in depression, anxiety, and emotional distress. Relationships with significant others and other members of her community may be negatively affected by all of these changes in her sexuality and fertility.

Questions to keep in mind when caring for an individual of a different culture include:

- How does the treatment influence the sexual desire, function, and identity of the patient?
- What does the loss of fertility mean to this patient and her culture?

- What role changes are affected by infertility?
- Are there changes in the patient's status due to her sexuality/fertility changes?
- How are relationships affected?
- Does the patient have a supportive network to draw upon?
- Are there resources available for the patient to assist with these issues?
- Is there a member of the patient's cultural group who can assist the healthcare team to further understand the patient's concerns?

The nurse can advocate for the patient by clarifying what is acceptable to her and communicating that to other healthcare providers. Nursing interventions that can provide relief from toxicities caused by treatment will help alleviate physical symptoms, resulting frequently in an improvement in the patient's sense of sexual well-being. If necessary, making appropriate referral for counseling can assist patients in coping with sexuality and fertility issues. Providing emotional support during pelvic exams and throughout the treatment continuum is critical.

Communication

Culture shapes how people respond to disease. It influences how the patient interprets symptoms and labels, understands, and communicates with others about them.[68] Each culture has established acceptable norms regarding verbal and nonverbal communication. Nonverbal communication includes body posture, eye contact, and touch. Verbal communication used by healthcare providers should always be respectful, informative, and sensitive to the patient's needs. Being knowledgeable about the cultural influences a patient brings to the healthcare environment is the first step in ensuring that the exchange between the patient and the healthcare team is one that is a sensitive two-way exchange. It is imperative that healthcare providers be aware of what is appropriate for each culture and respect boundaries whenever possible.

To combat language barriers, involving an interpreter may be necessary. Although it is acceptable to use a family member or friend for interpretation, it is recommended that a third party who is familiar with medical terminology be utilized so that bias and personal input can be avoided. Because the patient's heritage may view the institution of family as more important than the individual, it is still necessary to understand that a designated family member who is viewed as decision maker for all major medical decisions be available for critical discussions.

Because of the high value of family held by many cultures, a patient will receive most of her physical and psychological support from members of her family. It is important to make time for the families to visit and assist the patient. Establishing visiting hours and allowing family to be actively involved in the patient's care shows a spirit of cooperation and the unified goal of wanting what is best for the patient.

Written information to reinforce patient teaching should be in the patient's native tongue. There are many resources available for this purpose (see the resources list at the end of this chapter). Well-informed patients are frequently more empowered and tend to be active participants in their care. Nurses should encourage sharing of concerns and questions with all who are involved in their care.

How a patient expresses and requests relief from side effects, symptoms of cancer, and its treatment may vary depending on her cultural background. Some cultures expect to have pain and suffering in life, not expecting or requesting relief from the discomforts they might experience. Some patients may suffer in silence, while others may express their symptoms loudly, depending on their culture.

Questions to ask during the initial and ongoing therapy include:

- What discomforts are you experiencing?
- Are the prescribed medicines helpful to you?
- Who in your family should be included in important discussions?
- Is the written information helpful to you?

Nurses contribute to and often create the open and caring climate that allows patients to feel safe in communicating their needs. By allowing patients to express themselves, free of judgment from the staff, and asking questions in an honest and respectful manner, nurses can communicate their desire to know and care for the patient better. A caring approach can be understood in any language.

Developing relationships and an open communication with significant family members and healers will also help the nurse improve his or her understanding of the cultural influences and belief system of the patient.

Spirituality

Spirituality influences an individual's response to cancer. Most cultural groups have a formal religious affiliation they turn to in times of crisis. Having a spiritual connection and belief system that provides strength and purpose to life can be a major asset for patients.

By becoming familiar with these components, the healthcare team can utilize this resource to assist the patient in coping with her illness and possible death.

Questions frequently arise about the meaning of life and death, one's purpose in life, and beliefs about life after death. Individuals are forced to look at their mortality and its impact on their family. With cancer comes pain and suffering at many levels, emotional as well as physical. The meaning of suffering is different for each culture. For many cultures, suffering is expected with illness; thus patients may not request relief from their suffering or pain. They may view suffering as an opportunity to atone for sins, leading to spiritual enlightenment; others may feel it is a punishment for sins and find great emotional distress in their experience. Becoming knowledgeable about what view the patient holds will assist the nurse in planning appropriate interventions for relief of suffering. A discussion with the patient regarding alternatives to suffering and focusing on the potential improvement in quality of life for spending precious time with her family may be the outcome focus needed.

Unfortunately for many gynecologic malignancies, it is not uncommon for patients to succumb to their disease. Spiritual beliefs and cultural background greatly influence how an individual views what death is, prepares for death, and mourns losses resulting from death.[68] Rather than attempt to control death, many cultures accept the dying process as natural and view its manipulation as inappropriate. For Hispanics and African Americans, God's will determines whether there will be a cure or death. Ersek et al.[69] described cultural practices and attitudes related to end-of-life care and the use of advance directives, concluding that nonwhite patients are less likely to know about and have an advance directive. Even when approached about advance directives, nonwhites may refuse or relegate the decision to the family. Many minorities are less likely to agree to discontinue life support and believe that full disclosure to the patient is not desired.[69]

Including a religious leader from the patient's spiritual community can provide an alternative approach to religious observances that is compatible with Western healthcare practices.[68] Every culture has rituals surrounding the dying process and the care of the dying patient. Honoring beliefs and respecting wishes is an important part of closure for everyone, including healthcare providers.

It is unrealistic for nurses to expect to be experts on comparative religions or cultures. What is important is that the nurse sensitively and respectfully assesses spirituality and provides spiritually nurturing care.

Some questions to consider are as follows:

- What is the patient's belief system and religious affiliation?
- What does suffering mean to the patient?
- What are the rituals that provide spiritual comfort?
- What end-of-life issues need to be addressed?
- Is the patient informed of her prognosis?
- Does the patient have or believe in an advance directive?
- Is there a religious leader who should be involved in meeting the patient's spiritual needs?

To be supportive of culturally diverse patients' spiritual beliefs and practices, the nurse must assume an attitude of receptivity and acceptance. Nurses should respond to patients in a way that allows them to integrate their spiritual expressions and requests into their care.[12] Respectful attention to spiritual beliefs and practices can assist the patient with a gynecologic cancer to create meaning and find comfort.

Future of Transcultural Nursing in Gynecologic Oncology

Becoming culturally competent can be difficult for even the most conscientious nurse. Even though transcultural nursing has existed since the 1960s, growth in the healthcare field has been slowed by national trends and patterns, including lack of minority healthcare professionals, the dominance of the Western medicine model, limited cultural knowledge and racism, stressors in the managed care work environment, and limited cultural-specific curricula and teacher preparation in higher education.[70] As the population becomes more culturally diverse, nurses will need to think and act in ways that are culturally sensitive. Similar expectations permeate the corporate and educational institutions and other organizations within our society that must now serve an increasingly diverse clientele.

Nurse Education

Developing cultural competence focuses on enhancing self-awareness, gaining knowledge about ethnic groups, strengthening intercultural communication and assessment skills, and identifying and managing cultural conflicts. There are several ways to increase cultural competence. First, become aware of your own professional values instilled through your nursing education and your personal values about your culture and other cultures.[1] Examine your own cultural biases. To avoid ethnocentrism, one must understand how our perspectives impact our responses to patients' needs. This does not mean abandoning one's own values, beliefs, and cultural practices, but respecting those of others.[70]

Improving Patient Care

Cultural competence can be incorporated into all stages of the cancer continuum: prevention/early detection, diagnosis, treatment, follow-up, and end-of-life care. Nurses should adopt a cultural assessment model to ensure the systematic collection of relevant cultural data for developing care plans.[70] Utilizing a cultural assessment tool will increase the nurse's knowledge about how culture influences the cancer experience of the patient and her family. A cultural assessment tool will improve nursing care at all stages: assessment, nursing care, education, and emotional support of the patient. Armed with the knowledge learned from such a tool, patient education, both written and oral, will improve. Including additional resources from the patient's family, community, and spiritual affiliation will improve social, psychological, and spiritual support to the patient. Several resources have already been presented.

Access to Care

To reduce the gap between ethnic minorities' and white Americans' access to medical care, several programs have been developed. Data has been evaluated in an effort to determine best practices for improving the numbers of ethnic groups that are served. Identification of what factors are necessary in developing early detection, cancer prevention, and access to medical treatments are imperative. Recognizing the limitations that minorities experience and their health beliefs may help improve their participation in these programs. If cancer can be detected early and treatment is available, survival rates will improve. Prevention programs that focus on lifestyle, genetic predisposition, and diet may also further improve cancer incidence statistics for these groups.

Clinical Cancer Trials

Involving minorities in clinical trials and evaluating that research will add to the knowledge about culture-specific cancer causes, treatment response, toxicities, quality of life, survival, and health behaviors unique to each culture. Historically, minorities have been underrepresented in clinical trials. The two barriers identified are distrust of outsiders doing research in their communities and lack of culturally sensitive and specific education materials.[2] Other barriers correspond with the barriers to care previously listed. Afraid of being taken advantage of and not understanding the value of research, minorities decline participation.

In an effort to recruit more minorities in National Cancer Institute (NCI)-sponsored clinical trials, NCI developed the minority-based community clinical oncology program (CCOP). Since its inception in 1990, the fundamental factor that facilitated progress of this program has been the healthcare provider's respect for and increased understanding of the unique cultures that they serve.[71] Involvement in cancer prevention trials is still a problem. One reason may be that minorities are disproportionately economically disadvantaged. With immediate survival needs taking priority over participating in cancer prevention trials, the benefits to the individual are meaningless.[71,72]

To overcome these barriers, McCabe[73] identified factors that might facilitate participation:

- Adequate information and education about risks, benefits, cost, and time commitment
- Peer group norms that are supportive of the goals of the trial
- Endorsement of trial goals by the church, the cultural or social group leaders, or the employers
- A perceived benefit to the individual for participating
- Minimal actual cost in terms of time lost from work, transportation, and child care

Several challenges exist in conducting ethnic research: selection of samples, appropriate instruments, and research methodologies and translation of research instruments. Strategies to overcome these potential problems include accurately identifying the group being studied; developing instruments that are culturally sensitive, and pilot testing research instruments with the appropriate group to exhibit reliability.[74]

As the US population becomes more culturally diverse, there is an obvious need for more cancer research involving ethnic minorities. Expertise is needed to incorporate cultural considerations where cancer research studies are developed and conducted. Continued government support and funding to researchers, as well as educational grants that support opportunities for minorities to enter the healthcare field, will enhance "human" resources available to assist with future clinical research.

Conclusion

The US Census Bureau predicts growth rates of ethnic minority groups will redefine the population composition of our country. In an effort to decrease disparity between medical advances and lower-than-normal survival rates, health care and health status of these groups has become a national priority. To provide culturally competent care for women with gynecologic cancers, nurses should be familiar with the practices and customs important to the ethnic populations in the area of the country where they practice. Cultural beliefs and customs that reflect traditional culture may not be practiced universally by all members of the cultural group. Variables such as a subculture within the primary group, degree of acculturation, assimilation, education, income level, and amount of contact with older generations can influence the extent to which the person practices these customs.[11] Sensitivity to not only individual differences but also to cultural and ethnic traditions is an ethical imperative for nurses.

Resources

Books

St. Hill P, Lipson JG, Meleis AI. *Caring for Women Cross Culturally.* Philadelphia, PA: FA Davis; 2003.

University of Washington Medical Center. *Culture Clues.* Seattle, WA: Staff Development Workgroup, Patient and Family Education Committee; 1999. http://depts.washington.edu/pfes/cultureclues.html.

Web sites

The National Woman's Health Information Center: A project of the U.S. Department of Health and Human Services, Office on Women's Health: http://www.4woman.org

Intercultural Cancer Council: http://iccnetwork.org/cancerfacts/

American Cancer Society translation materials. Languages include: Spanish, Chinese, French, Haitian, Creole, Hindu, Korean, and Russian: http://www.cancer.org/docroot/PRO/content/PRO_3_Easy_Reading_Health_information.asp

American Cancer Society. Cancer Facts and Figures Annual statistics: http://www.cancer.org/docroot/stt/stt_0.asp

National Comprehensive Cancer Network: www.nccn.org

Translation of English to Spanish Web site: http://babelfish.altavista.com/translate.dyn

Oncology Nursing Society. (2000). Multicultural Tool Kit: http://www.ons.org/clinical/Special/toolkit.shtml

Nursing Journals

Journal of Transcultural Nursing
605 Worchester Rd.
Towson, MD 21286-7834
Editor's office: 877-843-0508
www.tcns.org

Minority Nurse
Contact: Pam Chwedyk
Sr. Editor, Editorial Manager
Minority Nurse magazine
211 W. Wacker Dr., Suite 900
Chicago, IL 60606
Phone: 312-525-3095
www.minoritynurse.com

Journal of Multicultural Nursing and Health
Chautauqua Institution
P.O. Box 889
Chautauqua, NY 14722
Phone: 716-357-2479
Fax: 716-357-2479

Suggested Readings on Cultural Assessment Tools

D'Aranza C. *Pocket Guide to Cultural Health Assessment.* 4th ed. St. Louis, MO: Mosby; 2008.

Giger JN, Davidhizar RE. *Transcultural Nursing: Assessment and Intervention.* 5th ed. St Louis, MO: Mosby; 2008.

Luckman J, Munoz C. *Transcultural Communication in Nursing.* 2nd ed. South Africa: Delmar; 2005.

Spector R. *Cultural Diversity in Health and Illness.* Upper Saddle River, NJ: Pearson Prentice Hall; 2004.

References

1. Gerrish K, Papadopoulos I. Transcultural competence: the challenge for nurse education. *Br J Nurs.* 1999;8(1):453–457.

2. Itano JK. Cultural diversity among individuals with cancer. In: Yarbro CH, Frogge MH, Goodman M, eds. *Cancer Principles and Practice.* 6th ed. Sudbury, MA: Jones and Bartlett Publishers; 2005:69–94.

3. Cowles KV. Cultural perspectives of grief: an expanded concept analysis. *J Adv Nurs.* 1996;23:287–294.

4. US Department of Health and Human Services. Report of the secretary's task force on black & minority health, vol 1, executive summary. Bethesda, MD: National Institutes of Health; 1985.

5. The National Cancer Institute Cancer Screening Consortium for Underserved Women. Breast and cervical cancer screening among underserved women. Baseline survey results from six studies. *Arch Fam Med.* 1995;4(7):617–624.

6. Gordon C. The effect of cancer pain on quality of life in different ethnic groups: a literature review. *Nurs Practition Forum.* 1997;8(10):10–13.

7. Andrews MM, Boyle JS, eds. *Transcultural Concepts in Nursing Care.* Philadelphia, PA: Lippincott Williams & Wilkins; 2000:38–41.

8. Lowdermilk DL, Perry SE. *Maternity Nursing.* 7th ed. St. Louis, MO: Mosby; 2006:32.

9. Leninger M, McFarland MR. *Transcultural Nursing—Concepts, Theories, Research and Practice.* 3rd ed. New York, NY: McGraw-Hill; 2002:117–143.

10. Flores G. Culture and the patient-physician relationship: achieving cultural competency in healthcare. *J Pediatr.* 2000;13:14–23.

11. Bowers P. Cultural perspectives in childbearing. Nursing Spectrum Career Fitness online. http://www.nurse.com/ce/CE26360.

12. Kagawa-Singer M. Socioeconomic and cultural difference on cancer care of women. *Semin Oncol Nurs.* 1995;11:109–119.

13. Muss HB, Junter CP, Wesley M, et al. Treatment plans for black and white women with stage II node-positive breast cancer. The National Cancer Institute black/white cancer survival study experience. *Cancer.* 1992;70:2469–2477.

14. Leninger M. The theory of culture care diversity and universality. In: Leninger MM, McFarland MR, eds. *Culture Care Diversity and Universality: A Worldwide*

Nursing Theory. 2nd ed. Sudbury, MA: Jones and Bartlett Publishers; 2006.

15. Narayanasamy A. The ACCESS model: a transcultural nursing practice framework. *Br J Nurs.* 2002;11: 645–650.

16. Giger JN, Davidhizar RE. Introduction to transcultural nursing. In: Giger JN, Davidhizar RE, eds. *Transcultural Nursing: Assessment and Intervention.* 4th ed. St. Louis, MO: Mosby; 2004:3–19.

17. American Cancer Society. *Cancer Facts and Figures for African Americans 2007–2008.* Atlanta, GA: American Cancer Society; 2007.

18. American Cancer Society. *Cancer Facts and Figures 2008.* Atlanta, GA: American Cancer Society; 2008.

19. Shavers VL, Brown ML. Racial and ethnic disparities in the receipt of cancer treatment. *J Natl Cancer Inst.* 2002;94(5):334–357.

20. Howell EA, Chen YT, Concato J. Differences in cervical cancer mortality among black and white women. *Obstet Gynecol.* 1999;94:509–515.

21. Boyer-Chammard A, Taylor TH, Anton-Culver H. Survival differences in breast cancer among racial/ethnic groups: a population-based study. *Cancer Detect Prev.* 1999;23:463–473.

22. Asian American Network for Cancer Awareness, Research and Training. http://www.aancart.org/apicem/index.htm. Published 2003.

23. Department of Commerce. Bureau of the Census. *We the American Asians.* Washington, DC: US Government Printing Office; 1993.

24. Shinagaw LH. The impact of immigration on the demography of Asian Pacific Americans. In: Hing B, Lee R, eds. *Reframing the Immigration Debate.* Los Angeles, CA: LEAP Asian Pacific American Public Policy Institute and UCLA Asian American Studies Center; 1996.

25. Houn F. Breast cancer in Asian Americans. Presented at: First Annual Conference of the National Asian Women's Health Organization; November 17, 1995; San Francisco, CA.

26. Ziegler RG, Hoover RN, Pike MC, et al. Migration patterns and breast cancer risk in Asian American women. *J Natl Cancer Inst.* 1993;85(22):1819–1827.

27. National Center for Health Statistics. *Health, United States, 1998 with Socioeconomic Status and Health Chartbook.* Hyattsville, MD: National Center for Health Statistics; 1998.

28. American Cancer Society. *Breast Cancer Facts and Figures 2007–2008.* Atlanta, GA: American Cancer Society; 2007.

29. Susan G. Komen Foundation. ABC's of Breast Cancer Guide. http://cms.komen.org/komen/AboutBreastCancer/TheABCsofBreastCancerGuide/index.htm.

30. Tang TS, Solomon LJ, Yeh CJ, Worden JK. The role of cultural variables in breast self-examination and cervical cancer screening behavior in young Asian women living in the United States. *J Behav Med.* 1999;22(5):419–436.

31. Hedeen AN, White E, Taylor V. Ethnicity and birthplace in relation to tumor size and stage in Asian American women with breast cancer. *Am J Public Health.* 1999;89(8):1248–1252.

32. Lee MM, Lin SS, Wrensch MR, Adler SR, Eisenberg, D. Alternative therapies used by women with breast cancer in four ethnic populations. *J Natl Cancer Inst.* 2000;92(1):42–47.

33. Schulmeister L, Lifsey DS. Cervical cancer screening knowledge, behaviors, and beliefs of Vietnamese women. *Oncol Nurs Forum.* 1999;26(5):879–887.

34. Ries LAG, Harkins D, Krapcho M, et al., eds. SEER cancer statistics review, 1975–2003, National Cancer Institute. Bethesda, MD. http://seer.cancer.gov/publications/survival/surv_race_ethnicity.pdf. Published 2006.

35. Kim K, Yu ES, Chen EH, Kim J, Kaufman M, Purkiss J. Cervical cancer screening knowledge and practices among Korean American women. *Cancer Nurs.* 1999;22(4):297–302.

36. Maxwell AE, Bastani R, Warda. US Demographic predictors of cancer screening among Filipino and Korean immigrants in the United States. *Am J Prev Med.* 2000;18(1):62–68.

37. Taylor VM, Schwartz SM, Jackson JC, et al. Cervical cancer screening among Cambodian-American women. *Cancer Epidemiol Biomarkers Prev.* 1999;8(6):541–546.

38. American Cancer Society. *Cancer Facts and Figures for Hispanics 2006–2008.* Atlanta, GA: American Cancer Society; 2006.

39. Ramirez AG, Talavera GA, Villarreal R, et al. Breast cancer screening in regional Hispanic populations. *Health Educ Res.* 2000;15(5):559–568.

40. American Cancer Society. *Cancer Facts and Figures for Hispanics 2006–2008.* Atlanta, GA: American Cancer Society; 2006.

41. Ramirez AG, Suarez L. The impact of cancer in Latino population. In: Aguirre-Molina M, Molina C, Zambrana R, eds. *Health Issues in the Latin Community.* San Francisco, CA: Jossey-Bass; 2001:211–244.

42. Ries LAG, Eisner MP, Kossary CL, Hankey BF, Miller BA, Edwards BK, eds. SEER cancer statistics review, 1973–1997. Bethesda, MD: National Cancer Institute; 2000.

43. Ramirez AG, Suarez L, McAlister A, et al. Cervical cancer screening in regional Hispanic populations. *Am J Health Behavio.* 2000;24(3):181–192.

44. Parker SL, Davis KJ, Wingo PA, Ries LAG, Heath CW. Cancer statistics by race and ethnicity. *CA Cancer J Clin.* 1998;48(1):1–48.

45. US Department of Commerce. Bureau of the Census. *We the First Americans.* Washington, DC: US Government Printing Office; 1993:Pub. No. 350-631.

46. Dixon M, Roubideaux Y, eds. *Promises To Keep.* Washington, DC: American Public Health Association; 2001.

47. Ramirez AG, McAlister A, Gallion K, Villarreal R. Targeting Hispanic populations: future research and prevention strategies. *Environ Health Perspec.* 1995;103(8)(suppl):287–290.

48. Burhansstipanov L, Hollow W. Native American cultural aspects of nursing oncology care. *Semin Oncol Nurs.* 2001;17(3):206–219.

49. Cobb N, Paisano RE. Patterns of cancer mortality among Native Americans. *Cancer.* 1998;83(11):2377–2383.

50. Burhansstipanov L, Hampton JW, Wiggins C. Issues in cancer data and surveillance for American Indian and Alaska Native populations. *J Regist Manage.* 1999;26(4):153–157.

51. Burhansstipanov L, Olsen S. Cancer prevention and early detection in American Indian and Alaska Native populations. In: Frank-Stromberg M, Olsen SJ, eds. *Cancer Prevention Diverse Populations: Cultural Implications for the Multidisciplinary Team.* St. Louis, MO: Mosby; 2001.

52. Wilson RT, Adams-Cameron M, Amir-Fazli A, et al. Racial/ethnic differences in breast cancer treatment patterns among American Indian, Hispanic and non-Hispanic white women using SEER-Medicare linked data: New Mexico and Arizona, 1987–1996. 2001:8–22.

53. Kleinman AR. Concepts and a model for the comparison of medical systems as a cultural system. *Soc Sc Med.* 1978;12:85–93.

54. Bloom JR, Hayes WA, Saunders F, et al. Physician and patient-induced utilization of early cancer detection practices among black Americans. *Adv Cancer Control Innov Res.* 1989;293:270–296.

55. Kosary CL, Ries LAG, Miller BA, et al. (1989). SEER cancer statistics review, 1973–1992. National Cancer Institute, NIH. Publication No. 95-2789. Bethesda, MD.

56. St Hill P. African-Americans. In: St Hill P, Lipson JG, Meleis AI, eds. *Caring for Women Cross Culturally.* Philadelphia, PA: FA Davis Company; 2003: 11–27.

57. Frank-Stromberg M. Changing demographics in the United States: implications for health professionals. *Cancer.* 1991;67:1772–1778.

58. Spector RE. Health and illness in American Indian and Alaska Native populations. In: Spector RE, ed. *Cultural Diversity in Health and Illness.* 6th ed. Upper Saddle River, NJ: Pearson Prentice Hall; 2004: 185–201.

59. Chin P. Chinese. In: St Hill P, Lipson JG, Meleis AI, eds. *Caring for Women Cross Culturally.* Philadelphia, PA: FA Davis Company; 2003:92–108.

60. Stauffer RY. Vietamese-Americans. In: Giger JN, Davidhizar RE, eds. *Transcultural Nursing: Assessment and Intervention.* 4th ed. St. Louis, MO: Mosby; 2004:455–491.

61. Kemp C. Mexicans and Mexican-Americans: health beliefs and practices. http://www3.baylor.edu/~Charles_Kemp/hispanic_health.htm. Published 2003.

62. Cohen RJ, Rohasly JA. Cancer prevention and screening among Hispanic populations. In: Frank-Stromberg M, Olsen SJ, eds. *Cancer Prevention in Minority Populations: Cultural Implications for Heath Care Professionals.* St. Louis, MO: Mosby Year Book; 1993:203–238.

63. US Census Bureau. National population estimates: May 2000. http://www.census.gov/main/www/cen2000.html.

64. Hanley CE. Navajos. In: Giger JN, Davidhizar RE, eds. *Transcultural Nursing: Assessment and Intervention.* St. Louis, MO: Mosby; 2004:255–278.

65. Primeaux M, Henderson G. American Indian patient care. In: Henderson G, Primeaux M, eds. *Transcultural HealthCare.* Menlo Park, CA: Addison-Wesley; 1981:239–254.

66. Kolb B, Wallace AM, Hill D, Royce M. Disparities in cancer care among racial and ethnic minorities. *Oncology.* 2006;20(10):1256–1261.

67. Loehe PJ Sr, Gregar HA, Weinberger M, et al. Knowledge and beliefs about cancer in a socioeconomically disadvantaged population. *Cancer.* 1991;68:1665–1671.

68. Taylor EJ. Spirituality, culture, and cancer care. *Semin Oncol Nurs*. 2001;17:197–205.

69. Ersek M, Kagawa-Singer M, Barnes D, et al. Multicultural considerations in the use of advance directives. *Oncol Nurs Forum*. 1998;25:1683–1690.

70. Kersey-Matusiak G. An action plan for cultural competence. Nursing Spectrum Career Forum online. http://www.nurse.com/ce/CE255. Published 2003.

71. Brawley CW. Minority accrual and clinical trials. *Oncol Issues*. 1995:22–24.

72. Millon-Underwood S, Sander E, Davis M. Determinants of participation in state-of-the-art cancer prevention, early detection/screening and treatment trials among African-Americans. *Cancer Nurs*. 1993;18:25–33.

73. McCabe MS, Varricchio CG, Padberg RM. Efforts to recruit the economically disadvantaged to national clinical trials. *Semin Oncol Nurs*. 1994;10:123–129.

74. Munet-Vilaro F. Methodological issues in the implementation of a Latino population. Proceedings of the third national conference on cancer nursing research. Atlanta, GA: American Cancer Society; 1994: 39–43.

Index

A

AASECT (American Association of Sexuality Educators, Counselors and Therapists), 210

Abdominal/pelvic CT scan, 90–91

Abnormal Pap Smears: What Every Woman Needs to Know (Rushing & Joste), 130

ACCESS model for transcultural nursing, 314

Access to care, cultural aspects, 328

Acculturation, defined, 312

Acetylcholine, 255

ACIP. *See* Advisory Committee on Immunization Practices

ACOG. *See* American College of Obstetrics and Gynecology

ACS. *See* American Cancer Society

Adenocarcinomas, 138

Adjuvant therapy. *See also* Chemotherapy; Platinum-based chemotherapy

breast cancer and, 50, 51–52

cognitive dysfunction and, 248–255

endometrial cancer and, 72

gynecologic sarcomas and, 177, 178

invasive cervical cancer and, 145

juvenile granulosa cell tumors and, 111

nonepithelial ovarian malignancies and, 104, 105

ovarian sex cord stromal tumors and, 107–108, 110

Sertoli-Leydig and, 113

Adoption and adoption resources, 222–223

Adult granulosa cell tumors (AGCTs). *See* Granulosa cell tumors

Adult respiratory distress syndrome (ARDS), 302

Advisory Committee on Immunization Practices (ACIP), 21, 22

AFP (alphafetoprotein), 105, 106

African American women

cervical cancer and, 300

endometrial cancer and, 24, 59–60

epithelial ovarian cancer and, 86

gynecologic sarcomas and, 174

health beliefs and practices of, 318–319

incidence rates for, 314–315

mortality rate, 315

nonepithelial ovarian malignancies and, 100

osteoporosis and, 235

vasomotor symptoms and, 229

AGCTs (Adult granulosa cell tumors). *See* Granulosa cell tumors

Age at diagnosis of gynecologic cancer, 285–286

Age of onset

adult granulosa cell tumors, 108

breast cancer, 5

endometrial cancer, 23, 25, 59, 74, 78

epithelial ovarian cancer, 85–86

gynecologic sarcomas, 174

juvenile granulosa cell tumors, 111

menopause, 227

ovarian cancer, 9, 11

ovarian germ cell tumors, 100, 105

Sertoli cell, 112

Sertoli-Leydig, 112

sex cord stromal tumors, 107, 108, 114

thecoma, 111

vaginal cancer, 28, 155–156

vulvar cancer, 30, 155, 156

AIDS. *See* HIV

Alaskan Natives/Native Americans

health beliefs and practices of, 321–322

incidence rates for, 317

Alcohol intake, 4, 229

Alkylating agents, 221

Almog, B., 129

ALND (Axillary lymph node dissection), 48–49, 50

Alpha fetoprotein (AFP), 105, 106

Alternative medicine, 300–301. *See also* Herbal therapies

Alternative sexual practices, 211–212

Alternative therapies for menopause symptoms, 238–240

ALTS (ASCUS/LSIL Triage Study), 20

Alzheimer's disease, 233

American Association of Sexuality Educators, Counselors and Therapists (AASECT), 210

American Cancer Society (ACS)

assistance to cancer patients, 150

breast cancer screening, 5, 6, 46

cervical cancer screening, 18, 19, 127, 130, 136–137

cervical cancer statistics, 133

endometrial cancer, 26, 59, 63

ovarian cancer statistics, 297

smoking, 57

vaginal cancer screening, 158

vulvar and vaginal cancer statistics, 155